Major Partners
supporting the European Vascular Course

AngioDynamics®

AtriCure®

Boehringer Ingelheim

COOK® MEDICAL

Cordis® a Johnson & Johnson company

COVIDIEN positive results for life™

Edwards

esaote

GORE Creative Technologies Worldwide

LR

MAQUET

medi

Medtronic

PHILIPS

VASCUTEK TERUMO

EVC 2010 is supported by:

Maastricht UMC+
azM academisch ziekenhuis Maastricht | Maastricht University
AZM en UM werken samen onder de naam UMC+

provincie limburg

Best Practice in Vascular Procedures

Best Practice in Vascular Procedures

Edited by

Michael Jacobs, MD

University Hospital, Maastricht, The Netherlands

University Hospital, Aachen, Germany

EDIZIONI MINERVA MEDICA

TURIN 2010

ISBN 13: 978-88-7711-667-3

LIST OF CONTRIBUTORS

Wissam AL-JUNDI
Sheffield Vascular Institute
Northern General Hospital
Sheffield, South Yorkshire, UK

Jonathan BEARD
Sheffield Vascular Institute
Northern General Hospital
Sheffield, South Yorkshire, UK

Jean-Pierre BECQUEMIN
Department of Vascular Surgery
Henri Mondor Hospital University
Paris, France

Luca BERTOGLIO
Department of Vascular Surgery
IRCCS H. San Raffaele
Milan, Italy

Andrew W. BRADBURY
Department of Vascular Surgery
University of Birmingham NHS Foundation Trust
Birmingham, UK

Deborah BRAMBILLA
Division of Vascular and Endovascular Surgery
University of Perugia
S. Maria della Misericordia Hospital
Perugia, Italy

Piergiorgio CAO
Unit of Vascular Surgery
S. Maria della Misericordia Hospital
Perugia, Italy

Fabio CALLIARI
Department of Vascular Surgery
IRCCS H. San Raffaele
Milan, Italy

Laurent CHICHE
Department of Vascular Surgery
Pitié-Salpêtrière University Hospital
Paris, France

Roberto CHIESA
Department of Vascular Surgery
IRCCS H. San Raffaele
Milan, Italy

Efrem CIVILINI
Department of Vascular Surgery
IRCCS H. San Raffaele
Milan, Italy

Frédéric COCHENNEC
Department of Vascular Surgery
Henri Mondor Hospital University
Paris, France

Giovanni COPPI
Department of Vascular Surgery
IRCCS H. San Raffaele
Milan, Italy

Eike Sebatian DEBUS
Department of Vascular Medicine
Vascular Surgery–Endovascular Interventions–Angiology
University Heart Center Hamburg-Eppendorf
Hamburg, Germany

Paola De RANGO
Division of Vascular and Endovascular Surgery
University of Perugia, Maria della Misericordia Hospital
Perugia, Italy

Nuno DIAS
Vascular Center Malmö-Lund
Malmö Univeristy Hospital
Malmö, Sweden

Holger DIENER
Department of Vascular Medicine
Vascular Surgery–Endovascular Interventions–Angiology
University Heart Center Hamburg-Eppendorf
Hamburg, Germany

Konstantinos P. DONAS
Department of Vascular Surgery,
Center of Vascular and Endovascular Surgery
St. Franziskus Hospital and Münster University Hospital
Münster, Germany

Gianluca FAGGIOLI
Vascular Surgery
University of Bologna
Bologna, Italy

Gustav FRAEDRICH
Department of Vascular Surgery
Medical University
Innsbruck, Austria

Francesca FRATESI
Vascular Surgery
University of Bologna
Bologna, Italy

Antonio FREYRIE
Vascular Surgery
University of Bologna
Bologna, Italy

Mauro GARGIULO
Vascular Surgery
University of Bologna
Bologna, Italy

Federica GIOVANETTI
Vascular Surgery
University of Bologna
Bologna, Italy

Caroline GOULFIER
Department of Vascular Surgery
Pitié-Salpêtrière University Hospital
Paris, France

Stéphan HAULON
Biomaterials Research Group
Biophysical Laboratory, Faculty of Medicine
University of Lille II
Service of Vascular Surgery, Cardiology Hospital
CHU de Lille, University of Lille II
Lille, France

Rob HINCHLIFFE
St Georges Vascular Institute
St Georges Healthcare NHS Trust
London, UK

Peter HOLT
St Georges Vascular Institute
St Georges Healthcare NHS Trust
London, UK

Maya HUIJBERTS
Department of Internal Medicine,
University Hospital Maastricht
Maastricht, The Netherlands

Giacomo ISERNIA
Division of Vascular and Endovascular Surgery
University of Perugia, Ospedale Maria della Misericordia
Perugia, Italy

Michael JACOBS
European Vascular Center Aachen-Maastricht
Department of Vascular Surgery
Maastricht University Medical Center
Maastricht, The Netherlands

Stephan KISCHE
Department of Cardiology
Medical Clinic I
Rostock AöR University Hospital, Center for Internal Medicine (ZIM)
Rostock, Germany

Thomas KOEPPEL
European Vascular Center Aachen-Maastricht
Vascular Surgery Clinic
Aachen University Hospital
Aachen, Germany

Axel LARENA-AVELLANEDA
Department of Vascular Medicine
Vascular Surgery–Endovascular Interventions–Angiology
University Heart Center Hamburg-Eppendorf
Hamburg, Germany

Ian LOFTUS
St Georges Vascular Institute
St Georges Healthcare NHS Trust
London, UK

Davide LOGALDO
Department of Vascular Surgery
IRCCS H. San Raffaele
Milan, Italy

Nicolas LOUIS
Department of Vascular Surgery
Henri Mondor Hospital University
Paris, France

Filippo MAIOLI
Vascular Surgery
University of Bologna
Bologna, Italy

Martin MALINA
Vascular Center Malmö-Lund
Malmö Univeristy Hospital
Malmö, Sweden

Enrico Maria MARONE
Department of Vascular Surgery
IRCCS H. San Raffaele
Milan, Italy

Germano MELISSANO
Department of Vascular Surgery
IRCCS H. San Raffaele
Milan, Italy

Natascia MUCCINI
Vascular Surgery
University of Bologna
Bologna, Italy

Ross NAYLOR
Department of Vascular Surgery
Clinical Sciences Building
Leicester, UK

Christoph NIENABER
Department of Cardiology
Medical Clinic I
Rostock AöR University Hospital, Center for Internal Medicine (ZIM)
Rostock, Germany

Noel O'BRIEN
Biomaterials Research Group
Biophysical Laboratory, Faculty of Medicine
University de Lille II
Service of Vascular Surgery
Cardiology Hospital
CHU de Lille, University of Lille II
Lille, France

Gianbattista PARLANI
Division of Vascular and Endovascular Surgery
University of Perugia, Maria della Misericordia Hospital
Perugia, Italy

Barbara RANTNER
Department of Vascular Surgery
Medical University
Innsbruck, Austria

Tim RESCH
Vascular Center Malmö-Lund
Malmö Univeristy Hospital
Malmö, Sweden

Geert-Willem SCHURINK
European Vascular Center Aachen-Maastricht
Department of Vascular Surgery
Maastricht University Medical Center
Maastricht, The Netherlands

Björn SONESSON
Vascular Center Malmö-Lund
Malmö Univeristy Hospital
Malmö, Sweden

Andrea STELLA
Vascular Surgery
University of Bologna
Bologna, Italy

Matt THOMSPON
St George's Vascular Institute,
St George's Hospital
London, UK

Giovanni Battista TORSELLO
Department of Vascular Surgery
Center of Vascular and Endovascular Surgery
St. Franziskus Hospital and Münster University Hospital
Münster, Germany

Giovanni Federico TORSELLO
Department of Vascular Surgery
Center of Vascular and Endovascular Surgery
St. Franziskus Hospital and Münster University Hospital
Münster, Germany

Yamume TSHOMBA
Department of Vascular Surgery
IRCCS H. San Raffaele
Milan, Italy

Rao VALLABHANENI
Regional Vascular Unit
Royal Liverpool University Hospital
Liverpool, UK

Frank VERMASSEN
Ghent University Hospital
Gent, België

Fabio VERZINI
Division of Vascular and Endovascular Surgery
University of Perugia, Ospedale Maria della Misericordia
Perugia, Italy

Martin WINKLER
Department of Vascular Medicine
Vascular Surgery–Endovascular Interventions–Angiology
University Heart Center Hamburg-Eppendorf
Hamburg, Germany

FOREWORD

The main mission of the European Vascular Course (EVC) is to offer an educational program in which theoretical, practical and technical issues of vascular interventions are addressed. In addition, EVC focuses on optimal clinical outcome and integration of scientifically proven evidence which altogether determine best practice for our patients. Therefore the 2010 topic of the European Vascular Course is Best Practice in Vascular Procedures *and the 20 selected subjects cover the wide spectrum of our daily vascular activities.*

The first part of the book describes the surgical and endovascular techniques of carotid artery revascularization, followed by evidence-based strategies for symptomatic and asymptomatic carotid artery disease. The second part concentrates on lower limb arterial bypass surgery and endovascular revascularization in critical limb ischemia. Guidelines for open and endovascular treatment and the management of the diabetic foot complement the subject of critical limb ischemia. Following, treatment of thoracic aortic pathology is addressed: open and endovascular treatment of type A dissection, innovative treatment of arch aneurysms, surgical and endoluminal management of descending and thoraco-abdominal aortic aneurysms. Subsequently, open and endovascular surgery of infra- and suprarenal abdominal aortic aneurysms are described in detail, followed by endovascular strategies in acute and ruptured aneurysms. Based on existing scientific evidence, guidelines for abdominal aortic aneurysms are defined. The last part of this textbook consists of four subjects which play a major role in the future of our vascular activities: the ideal educational curriculum, centralization of vascular procedures, cost-effectiveness of interventions and finally the hybrid operating room as our new working environment.

I am most indebted to all authors who invested so much effort in preparing the chapters for this book. Dr Nabil Sedki and Mrs. Claudia Lenssen have significantly contributed to the editorial work. Having this high quality textbook edited, printed and ready to distribute at the start of EVC is also due to the fantastic cooperation with Mrs. Eugenia Battaglio and Mrs. Cecilia Ponsat from our publisher Minerva Medica.

The production and appearance of this book is only possible with the continuous support of our major partners from the medical industry to whom I would like to express my sincere gratitude.

Maastricht-Aachen, February 2010

Michael Jacobs

CONTENTS

List of Contributors VII

Foreword XI

1 How to Perform Carotid Artery Surgery
Giovanni Federico Torsello, Konstantinos P. Donas, Giovanni Battista Torsello 1

2 How to Perform Endovascular Carotid Revascularization
Fabio Verzini, Paola De Rango, Deborah Brambilla, Gianbattista Parlani, Giacomo Isernia, Piergiorgio Cao 9

3 Best Practice for Asymptomatic Carotid Disease
Laurent Chiche, Caroline Goulfier 21

4 Best Practice for Symptomatic Carotid Disease
Ross Naylor 37

5 Cruropedal Reconstructions in Peripheral Arterial Occlusive Disease
Eike Sebastian Debus, Holger Diener, Martin Winkler, Axel Larena-Avellaneda 51

6 How to Perform Endovascular Revascularizations
Mauro Gargiulo, Federica Giovanetti, Francesca Fratesi, Antonio Freyrie, Natascia Muccini, Gianluca Faggioli, Filippo Maioli, Andrea Stella 63

7 Bypass versus Angioplasty in Severe Ischemia of the Leg (BASIL) Trial
Andrew Bradbury 73

8 Diabetic Foot Disease
Maya Huijberts 85

9 Open and Endovascular Treatment of Type A Dissection
Christoph Nienaber, Stephan Kische 93

10 Innovative Treatment of Arch Aneurysms
Peter Holt, Rob Hinchliffe, Ian Loftus 99

11 Open and Endovascular Treatment of Descending Thoracic Aneurysms
Roberto Chiesa, Efrem Civilini, Yamume Tshomba, Enrico Maria Marone, Luca Bertoglio, Giovanni Coppi, Davide Logaldo, Fabio Calliari, Germano Melissano 109

12 Best Practice in Thoraco-Abdominal Aortic Aneurysm Repair
Stéphan Haulon, Geert-Willem Schurink, Noel O'Brien, Michael Jacobs 129

13 Open Repair of Infra- and Suprarenal Aortic Aneurysms
Barbara Rantner, Gustav Fraedrich 143

14 Endovascular Repair of Infra- and Suprarenal Aneurysms
Tim Resch, Björn Sonesson, Nuno Dias, Martin Malina 149

15 Endovascular Treatment of Ruptured Abdominal Aortic Aneurysms
Nicolas Louis, Frédéric Cochennec, Jean-Pierre Becquemin 159

16 Current Practice and Guidelines for AAA Treatment
Wissam Al-Jundi, Jonathan Beard 171

17 The Ideal Educational Curriculum of the Vascular Specialist
Thomas Koeppel, Michael Jacobs 181

18 Should Vascular Surgery Be Centralized?
Peter Holt, Matt Thompson 189

19 Cost-Effectiveness of Vascular Procedures
Frank Vermassen 199

20 Hybrid Operating Room: the New Working Environment
Rao Vallabhaneni 207

1

HOW TO PERFORM CAROTID ARTERY SURGERY

GIOVANNI FEDERICO TORSELLO, KONSTANTINOS P. DONAS,
GIOVANNI BATTISTA TORSELLO

Carotid atherosclerosis is one of the most common and devastating disorders dealt with in vascular surgery. Stroke ranks as the third leading cause of death in the United States, after ischemic heart disease and cancer. There are more than 700 000 incident strokes in the US each year, resulting in 160 000 deaths annually. Atherosclerosis within the carotid artery occurs most frequently within the common carotid bifurcation and proximal internal carotid artery (ICA). General risk factors for atherosclerosis such as hypertension, diabetes, old age, male gender, smoking and hypercholesterolemia apply also to carotid atherosclerosis. The pathogenesis of atherosclerosis is, roughly simplified, based on accumulation of lipoproteins within the intima, which may undergo oxidative modifications. These, in turn, may trigger a local inflammatory response, including mononuclear phagocytes to ingest lipids and thus becoming foam cells which form a fatty streak within the intima. As this evolves, smooth-muscle cells migrate from the media into the intima, creating the bulk of the advanced lesion, formed by extracellular matrix. As they advance, microscopic breaches in the endothelial integrity may occur in atherosclerotic plaques, which is one of the causes for atherothrombosis. The atherosclerotic plaque can therefore be either flow restricting, embolic or both. Among the numerous causes of ischemic stroke, thrombo-embolic stroke as a result of carotid atherosclerosis is one of the most frequent causes. The embolic source is mostly the rough surface of the plaque, whether it is ruptured or not. The aim of surgical revascularization is to remove the cause of cerebrovascular embolism and restore blood flow to the brain. In the present chapter we describe our strategy in the peri-operative management of patients with arteriosclerotic carotid disease.

Indications for carotid endarterectomy

Large, randomized clinical trials from the early 1990s have shown the superiority of carotid endarterectomy (CEA) and aspirin therapy in preventing stroke compared with aspirin alone for both symptomatic [1-5] and asymptomatic [6-8] carotid artery stenosis. On the basis of these trials, the most recent American Heart Association (AHA) guidelines recommend CEA for symptomatic patients with a stenosis of 50% to 99%, if the perioperative risk of stroke is less than 6% [9,10]. In asymptomatic patients, CEA is recommended for a stenosis of 60% to 99%, if the peri-operative risk of stroke or death is less than 3% [9,10].

Timing

The timing of CEA for symptomatic carotid disease is a key benchmark for secondary stroke prevention, because delays to surgery are associated with an increased risk of recurrent stroke. Potential reasons for delays include patients factors (delayed symptom recognition and presentation to medical attention), physician factors (delayed diagnosis and referrals), resource availability (rapid access to vascular imaging) and institutional factors relating to operating room availability and staffing. The recommendation to delay surgery for 4 to 6 weeks after acute stroke was suggested by the Joint Study of Extracranial Arterial Occlusion [3]. However, in the new era of computed tomography (CT) scanning and meticulous control of blood pressure during the immediate post-operative period, an effective patient stratification and adequate identification of the extent of pre-operative cerebral damage was achieved. Our experience correlates closely with several reports which reported no new neurologic peri- and post-operative deficits in patients with a small fixed stroke who underwent CEA within two weeks after stroke.

Pre-operative care

Before surgery, all patients undergo carotid Duplex sonography performed by the surgeon scheduled for the operation. In case of symptomatic lesions, cerebral CT scan is needed to detect the extension of the cerebral infarction and exclude other causes of neurological symptoms. CT-angiography with extra-cranial and intra-cranial views is generally preferred in order to exclude relevant stenosis of the origin of the common carotid artery (CCA) and also to estimate the morphology of the internal cranial artery in its entire length. All patients are examined by the neurologic staff of our institution in order to assess the pre-operative and post-operative neurological status. Antiplateled therapy is suspended at least 5 days before the operation and resumed at the first post-operative day. However, between March 2008 and March 2009, a prospective non-randomized study was conducted in our institution with two arms of patients with suspension or continuation of aspirin administration peri-operatively (unpublished data). The results of this study showed no differences between the two groups in terms of post-operative bleeding, so that aspirin is not discontinued anymore.

Anesthesia

Until today, there is no final consensus whether local/regional anesthesia or general anesthesia is safer. One potential advantage of local or regional anesthesia (LA) is the assessment of neurological function during carotid clamping, reducing the usage of shunts. Using less shunts, air and particulate embolism as well as artery injury and post-operative thrombosis are less likely to occur [11]. We shall refer to shunt-related complications later in this chapter. We prefer the use of general anesthesia (GA) because it is less stressful to both the surgeon and patient, especially in restless patients or patients developing a neurological deficit during the operation. Also, it is some author's opinion that general anesthesia, allowing controlled respiratory, cardiac and brain function facilitates brain tissue protection. Another argument brought forward by these authors is that more vasopressors are necessary under local anesthesia, thus resulting in higher myocardial infarction rates [12]. Gough [11] summarized all non-randomized and randomized findings, including the GALA Trial and a subsequent Cochrane Review. Analysis of the results showed no statistically significant difference between local and general anesthesia in terms of primary outcome events, such as stroke, death, fatal and non-fatal myocardial infarctions. Subgroup analysis showed no difference between LA and GA for patients older or younger than 75 years or for those considered to be high-risk patients. However, 10% of the patients with a contralateral carotid occlusion treated under general anesthesia experienced a primary outcome event. Significantly less patients of the same subgroup treated under local anesthesia experienced a primary outcome event (5%, p = 0.098) [11]. Lawrence et al. [13] also favor local anesthesia especially in patients with contralateral occlusion of the carotid. Local anesthesia also facilitates autoregulation of the blood pressure, which becomes important during carotid clamping. Under general anesthesia, anesthetists had to provoke rise of the systolic blood pressure pharmacologically in 43% of the cases (versus 17% in the LA group). In the end, both methods are proven to be safe. As stated above, patients with a contralateral occlusion might benefit more from LA, probably due to the facilitated autoregulation of blood pressure. However, taking into account that patient compliance might influence the accuracy of the surgery, which is in turn the key to success, method of anesthesia remains to be determined in each case individually.

TECHNIQUE

The surgical technique includes carotid eversion endarterectomy and endarterectomy with the use of synthetic material or vein patch. Only in selected patients vein graft interposition is used. After anesthesia induction and the placement of appropriate access and monitoring lines, the patient is positioned supine on the operating table with the head turned contralaterally to the operation site. The neck is moderately extended on the shoulders. The head of the table is flexed about 10-20 degrees to reduce venous pressure, which minimizes bleeding during dissection. Early experience with stroke after induction of the anesthesia in patients turned down from surgery showed that hypotension can be an important cause of cerebral infarction in patients with severe carotid disease. Especially in the phase between intubation and skin incision we observe a significant lowering of the blood pressure, which must be corrected. We prefer a longitudinal incision placed along the anterior border of the sternocleidomastoid muscle and centered over the carotid bifurcation. This incision can be extended proximally to the sternal notch for more proximal exposure of the CCA and distally to the mastoid process for extensive exposure of the ICA, when needed. The preparation is started at a cranial level of the ICA. The dissection plane is maintained along the anterior border of the sternocleidomastoid muscle, which permits anterior mobilization of the tail of the parotid gland rather than the bloody division of its substance, with risk of salivary fistula and injury of the buccal branch of the facial nerve. The jugular vein is visualized and mobilized until the common facial vein is identified. The common facial vein, which is a relatively constant landmark for the carotid bifurcation, is divided. Now the internal jugular vein can be mobilized laterally off the carotid bifurcation, providing excellent exposure. Particular care must be taken to check for anomalous course of vagus and hypoglossal nerve to avoid nerve injury. Another anomaly which often occurs on the right side of neck can be the occasional presence of a nonrecurrent laryngeal nerve that comes directly from the vagus on the way to innervate the vocal cord. This nerve can cross anteriorly to the carotid artery and may be mistaken for a part of the ansa hypoglossi, resulting in cord paralysis. The common, external and internal carotid arteries are then carefully dissected as far from cranially and caudally from the carotid bifurcation as possible. The carotid bulb is not dissected at this time to avoid peripheral embolism. After administration of 5 000 units of heparin intravenously and clamping of the ICA, the carotid bulb can be now sufficient mobilized and completely exposed. The dissection of the bulb and of the ICA is performed circumferentially in case of eversion endarterectomy and only in the ventral aspect in case of patching endarterectomy to avoid elongation of the vessel. The carotid bifurcation sheath is divided with scissors without irritating the glomus at the angle of the bifurcation. Proper preparation prior to clamping pays off when further arteriotomy is needed and therefore facilitates this procedure. In the open thrombo-endarterectomy approach, an arteriotomy is made on the lateral portion of the CCA and is extended toward the plaque and up the ICA with Pott's scissors. The arteriotomy is extended as far as necessary up the ICA to get beyond the plaque and to expose relatively normal artery. After the insertion of an internal shunt (Fig. 1) in the ICA first allowing backbleeding to evacuate air from the tube before inserting the common carotid end, a spatula is inserted beneath the plaque, developing the natural plane of separation between the plaque and the residual outer media and adventitia at the site of the external elastic lamella in case of patch endarterectomy. In case of eversion endarterectomy, the arteriotomy is made at the origin of the ICA circumferentially (Fig. 2). This approach normally requires a more extensive exposure of the ICA than the thrombo-endarterectomy approach. The intraluminal shunt

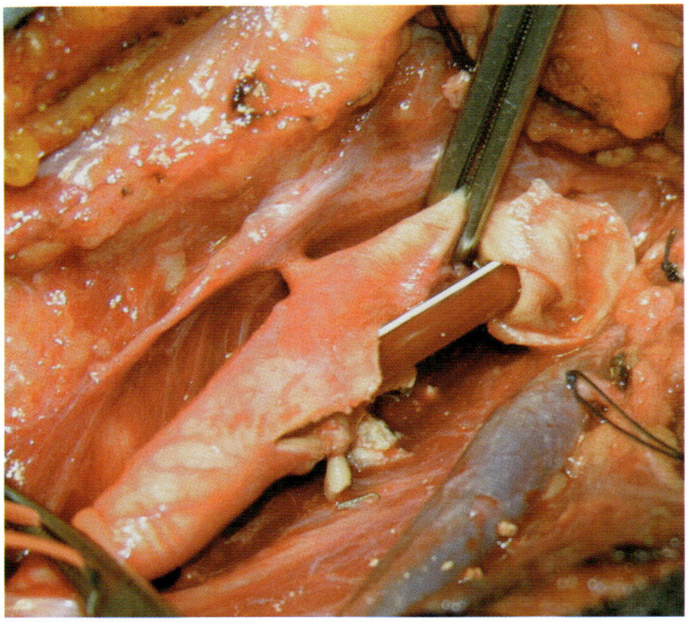

FIG. 1 An intraluminal shunt is placed into the carotid artery to maintain cerebral perfusion during endarterectomy.

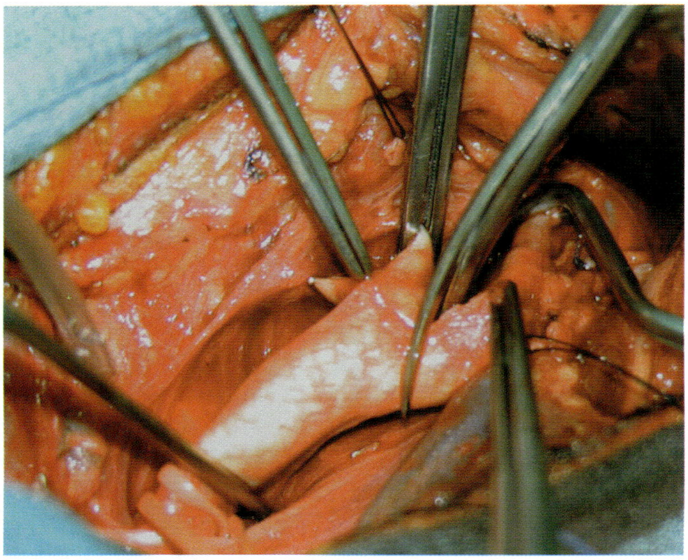

FIG. 2 Circumferential arteriotomy of the internal carotid artery.

is then placed in the same fashion as stated above. We keep the shunt in place proximally by using vessel loops like a tourniquet.

We seek to minimize shunt-related complications such as air and particulate embolism as well as artery injury and post-operative thrombosis caused by injury by using intraluminal shunts routinely. Moreover, the shunt acts as a hypomochlion that can aid in the closure of the internal carotid portion of the arteriotomy avoiding stenosis. Using intraluminal shunts routinely also facilitates the operation especially for surgeons in training and allows the surgeon to take the time he needs to work as accurately as possible. When taking the open thrombo-endarterectomy approach, the plaque often separates cleanly with traction alone. The muscularis of the media is removed along with the plaque to avoid residual thrombogenic material in the lumen and to reduce the risk of neointimal hyperplasia. The endarterectomy is ended at an appropriate point on the ICA where normal intimal and medial layers are present and adherent to the adventitia. In case of an unsmooth transition into the distal artery, the intimal step is leveled with a beaver knife. After removal of the plaque the luminal surface is cleared of residual circular medial fibers, removing them with a fine forceps and heparinized saline irrigation.

In the eversion endarterectomy approach, the transected vessel is peeled back over the plaque, allowing removal of the latter (Fig. 3). Sometimes, however, a tongue of atheromatous plaque extends beyond the location of the occluding clamp. Transitional opening of the clamp allows extracting of the residual plaque. The end point should be directly visualized. Avoiding unsmooth transition distally is equally important in this case, so intimal steps must be leveled. Therefore, the endarterectomized surface must be freed of all medial fibers and loose fragments. We usually do not apply tacking sutures. Clearing of the surface of residual circular medial fibers is also important in this approach. To avoid early thrombosis or restenosis, elongation of the carotid artery should be corrected by resection of the ICA after longitudinal arteriotomy or by longitudinal incision of the CCA and more proximal implantation after endarterectomy. However, before closing the arteriotomy in either of the two approaches, thrombo-endarterectomy of both external and the CCA is performed. The arteriotomy is closed in case of patch angioplasty by prosthetic material or vein. Myers et al. [14] concluded that saphenous vein patch did not deliver superior results to primary closure. AbuRahma et al. [15], however found, that patch closure with either saphenous vein, jugular vein or PTFE patches delivered better results in terms of cerebrovascular accidents (primary closure vs. patches, $p = 0.007$), reversible ischemic neurologic deficits (5.2% vs. 1.5%, $p = 0.04$) and early restenosis (primary closure vs. patches, $p = 0.008$). Although AbuRahma et al. [15] found no difference between PTFE and saphenous vein patches even if there was a higher incidence of ICA dilatation in the jugular vein group, causing the authors to recommend the other two patches. Other authors prefer autologous material because of the reduced risk of infection [12]. Vein patches, however, may rupture. Archie et al. [16] reported that small-diameter saphenous veins have a higher risk of rupture when used as a carotid patch. This corresponds with the findings of Riles et al. [17], who stopped using ankle vein in favor of groin saphenous vein patches.

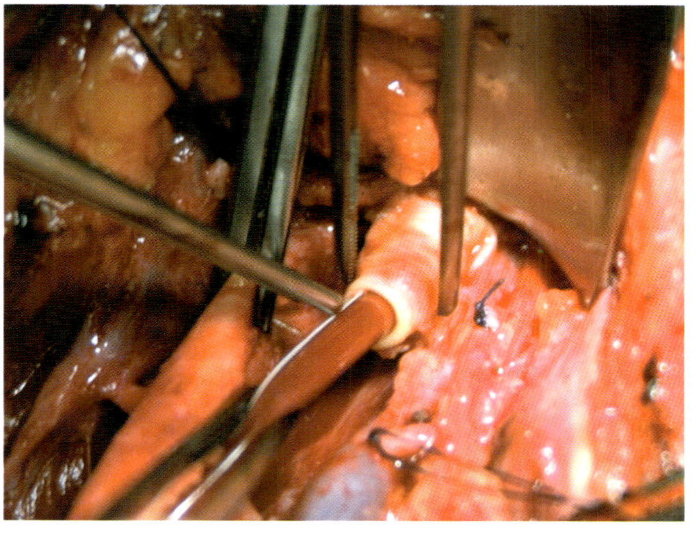

FIG. 3 Eversion of the internal carotid artery over the intraluminal shunt.

When taking the eversion approach, reanastomosis of the CCA and the ICA is circumferentially carried out with continuous 6/0 polypropylene sutures. By this technique, streamlined configuration and increase in diameter of the ICA are achieved without using any patch material. Comparing the two techniques Cao et al. [18] conducted a meta-analysis to determine whether eversion CEA was safer and more effective than the conventional thrombendatherectomy. Peri-operative stroke (1.7% versus 2%) and death (1.7% versus 2.4%) rates did not differ significantly. These findings correlate with the work of Peiper et al. [19]. In this study, a shorter clamping time, possibility of simultaneous shortening of an elongated ICA were found in the eversion CEA group. Peiper states that neither a PTFE patch nor autologous material — which demands a second skin incision — are needed in this approach, which would make the eversion CEA technically superior to the conventional CEA. Also according to other authors the choice of the technique should be based on the familiarity and the experience of the surgeon, preferring the eversion technique if the end point of the plaque can be easily reached. The shunt is removed before placement of the last few sutures. Air and debris are flushed out the bifurcation after release of the external clamp. The internal clamp is released last establishing blood flow first to the external and then to the ICA. We recommend the use of completion intra-operative quality control of the reconstruction by Doppler ultrasound or arteriography (Fig. 4). In a report, Lipski et al. [20]) showed that the incidence of residual disease and peri-operative neurologic complications was statistically significantly reduced in patients who had completion Duplex scanning compared to a control group who did not undergo completion imaging. We do not administer protamine after completion of the endarterectomy. Mauney et al. [21] found a significant difference (p = 0.045) in stroke rates when they compared patients who received protamine (stroke rate: 2.6%) with those who did not receive protamine (0%). After placement of the drainage, the platysma is closed with a running absorbable suture, and the skin is closed with an intracutaneous stitch.

Post-operative care

The first 12 hours are the most critical in the management of the patient after cerebral vascular reconstruction. Most important factors are observation of the patient's neurologic status, blood pressure control, and wound observation. The majority of patients can be sent to a regular room if they are neurologically and hemodynamically stable in the recovery room. The authors' practice is to resume anti-platelet drugs. We recommend aspirin 100 mg/daily. Post-operative carotid surveillance is performed with Duplex ultrasonography before discharge and in 6-month intervals during the first post-operative year and then once annually.

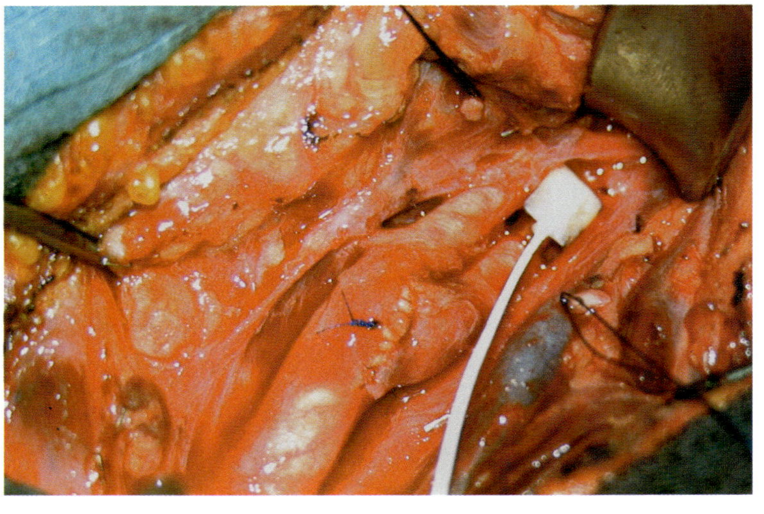

FIG. 4 Intra-operative Doppler ultrasound control as completion quality assessment.

Conclusion

The beneficial effects of CEA in selected symptomatic and asymptomatic patients with high-grade ICA stenosis have been well established in American and European trials [1-9]. There is no doubt that the value of CEA after a minor stroke, despite the increased surgical risk, is no longer open to question, however, issues about the timing of surgery and the risk of conversion of a non hemorhagic into a hemorrhagic infarct are still controversial. CEA can be more effective than best medical treatment preventing devastating stroke. The results are excellent if patient selection is adequate, operative technique is perfect and peri-operative management takes in to account the peculiarity of the carotid patient.

REFERENCES

1 Anonymous. Beneficial effect of carotid endarterectomy in symptomatic patients with high-grade carotid stenosis. North American Symptomatic Carotid Endarterectomy Trial Collaborators. *N Engl J Med* 1991; 325: 445-453.

2 Barnett HJ, Taylor DW, Eliasziw M et al. Benefit of carotid endarterectomy in patients with symptomatic moderate or severe stenosis. North American Symptomatic Carotid Endarterectomy Trial Collaborators. *N Engl J Med* 1998; 339: 1415-1425.

3 Anonymous. Randomised trial of endarterectomy for recently symptomatic carotid stenosis: final results of the MRC European Carotid Surgery Trial (ECST). *Lancet* 1998; 351: 1379-1387.

4 Anonymous. MRC European Carotid Surgery Trial: interim results for symptomatic patients with severe (70-99%) or with mild (0-29%) carotid stenosis. European Carotid Surgery Trialists´Collaborative Group. *Lancet* 1991; 337: 1235-43.

5 Mayberg MR, Wilson SE, Yatsu F et al. Carotid endarterectomy and prevention of cerebral ischemia in symptomatic carotid stenosis. Veterans Affairs Cooperative Studies Program 309 Trialist Group. *JAMA* 1991; 266: 3289-3294.

6 Hobson RW 2nd, Weiss DG, Fields WS et al. Efficacy of carotid endarterectomy for asymptomatic carotid stenosis. The Veterans Affairs Cooperative Study Group. *N Engl J Med* 1993; 328: 221-227.

7 Anonymous. Endarterectomy for asymptomatic carotid artery stenosis. Executive Committee for the Asymptomatic Carotid Atherosclerosis Study. *JAMA* 1995; 273: 1491-1502.

8 Halliday A, Mansfield A, Marro J et al. Prevention of disabling and fatal strokes by successful carotid endarterectomy in patients without recent neurological symptoms: randomized controlled trial. *Lancet* 2004; 363: 1491-1502.

9 Biller J, Feinberg WM, Castaldo JE et al. Guidelines for carotid endarterectomy: a statement for healthcare professionals from a Special Writing Group of the Stroke Council, American Heart Association. *Circulation* 1998; 97: 501-509.

10 Sacco RL, Adams R, Albers G et al. Guidelines for prevention of stroke in patients with ischemic stroke or transient ischemic attack: American Heart Association. *Circulation* 2006; 113: 409-449.

11 Gough MJ; GALA Trial Collaborators. The GALA Trial—A Summary of the Findings. *Eur J Vasc Endovasc Surg* 2008; 36: 505-506.

12 Sandmann W. Carotid Endarterectomy. In: Bell P, editor. *Vascular Surgery*. Philadelphia: Saunders; 1991. p. 111-21.

13 Lawrence PF, Alves JC, Jicha D et al. Incidence, timing, and causes of cerebral ischemia during carotid endarterectomy with regional anesthesia. *J Vasc Surg* 1998; 27: 329-337.

14 Myers SI, Valentine RJ, Chervu A et al. Saphenous vein patch versus primary closure for carotid endarterectomy: Long-term assessment of a randomized prospective study. *J Vasc Surg* 1994; 19: 15-22.

15 AbuRahma AF, Khan JH, Robinson PA et al. Prospective randomized trial of carotid endarterectomy with primary closure and patch angioplasty with saphenous vein, jugular vein and polytetraflruoroethylene: Perioperative (30-day) results. *J Vasc Surg* 1996; 24: 998-1007.

16 Archie JP, Green JJ. Saphenous vein rupture pressure, rupture stress, and carotid endarterectomy vein patch reconstruction. *Surgery* 1990; 107: 389-396.

17 Riles TS, Lamparello PJ, Giangola G et al. Rupture of the vein patch: A rare complication of carotid endarterectomy. *Surgery* 1990; 107: 10-12.

18 Cao P, De Rango P, Zannetti S. Eversion vs conventional carotid endarterectomy: a systematic review. *Eur J Vasc Endovasc Surg* 2002; 23: 195-201.

19 Peiper C, Nowack J, Ktenidis K et al. Eversion endarterectomy versus open thromboendarterectomy and patch plasty for the treatment of internal carotid artery stenosis. *Eur J Vasc Endovasc Surg* 1999; 18: 339-343.

20 Lipski DA, Bergamini TM, Garrison RN et al. Intraoperative duplex scanning reduces the incidence of residual stenosis after carotid endarterectomy. *J Surg Res* 1996; 60: 317-320.

21 Mauney MC, Buchanan SA, Lawrence WA et al. Stroke rate is markedly reduced after carotid endareterectomy by avoidance of protamine. *J Vasc Surg* 1995; 22: 264-270.

2

HOW TO PERFORM ENDOVASCULAR CAROTID REVASCULARIZATION

FABIO VERZINI, PAOLA DE RANGO, DEBORAH BRAMBILLA, GIANBATTISTA PARLANI, GIACOMO ISERNIA, PIERGIORGIO CAO

Treatment of carotid stenosis aims at prevention of ischemic neurologic events caused by cerebral embolization of atherosclerotic carotid plaque. Despite the proven efficacy of carotid endarterectomy (CEA) in the prevention of ischemic stroke, great interest has been generated in the last decades in carotid angioplasty and stenting (CAS) as an alternative to surgical therapy, due to its minimally invasive nature. Although CAS has clearly documented its feasibility and relatively safety, the appropriate clinical setting for its preferential use over CEA remains unclear. The potential for devastating neurologic complications significantly distinguishes endovascular treatment of the carotid artery from other vascular beds commonly treated by endovascular specialists. CAS requires careful patient selection, counseling and procedural planning.

Patient selection

CAS was initially targeted as a good alternative to CEA in loosely defined categories of high-risk patients. Gradually, it was also promoted as a valid substitute and a universal replacement for CEA in symptomatic and asymptomatic patients. However, current indications for CAS continue to be debated, being refined as more data of large studies are being accumulated. A number of additional factors have impacted the use and proposed indications for CAS including reimbursement coverage, industry pressure and subspecialty competition. Careful and objective patient selection is essential to guarantee the results. The indication to treatment of patients with carotid disease should consider different aspects:

1) neurological symptomatology;
2) degree of carotid stenosis;
3) medical co-morbidities;
4) vascular and local anatomical features; and
5) carotid plaque morphology.

In common practice, the basic indications for CAS do not differ from those of standard CEA. Patients eligible for CAS constitute three groups: asymptomatic patients with high-grade carotid stenosis (> 80%), symptomatic patients with at least 70% carotid stenosis and symptomatic patients with stenosis between 50% and 70% and ulcerated carotid plaque.

However, no randomized clinical trial (RCT) has proven the effectiveness of CAS in any specific subgroup, and the assumption that a patient can be treated with CAS when he has an indication to CEA has not been validated [1]. Furthermore, the role of symptoms in procedure selection remains unclear, since most of the good results of CAS have been achieved in populations with a large predominance of asymptomatic patients. Symptomatic patients seem to do worse with CAS, at least as evidenced by the recent international trials [2-4] even though a number of criticisms have been raised against the quality (early closure, inadequate sample size, inappropriate operators experience) of these trials to be assumed as the reference for providing guidelines for CAS treatment. Average-risk patients with symptoms should be preferentially treated with CEA, unless the patient is willing to enroll in a clinical trial. A number of randomized trials for low-risk CEA patients are currently underway, including the Carotid Revascularization Endarterectomy versus Stent Trial (CREST), the stent-protected angioplasty in asymptomatic carotid artery stenosis vs. endarterectomy (SPACE2) a three-arm randomized-controlled clinical trial, the Asymptomatic Carotid Surgery Trial (ACST2) and Carotid Stenting vs. Surgery of Severe Carotid Artery Disease and Stroke Prevention in Asymptomatic Patients (ACT-1) trials.

Paramount to the decision regarding which patients are eligible for CAS is indeed an understanding of exactly which patients are at "high risk" for CEA. The co-morbid conditions that would allow the designation as "high-risk" include a number of medical problems (i.e. congestive heart failure class III/IV, left ventricular ejection fraction < 30%, unstable angina), historical features and anatomic pathologies (i.e. recurrent stenosis, prior neck surgery, prior radiation treatment to the neck). While a number of surgical high-risk conditions are well recognized (and summarized in Table I), there is a number of patients groups that can be also included and others that can be excluded from this list and need to be identified. Recently more attention has been focused on identification of patients who are at greater risk for adverse outcomes during and after CAS, in an effort to refine indications. A number of anatomical unfavorable conditions can challenge the performance of CAS or CEA increasing the risks of the procedure (Ta-

Table I RISK FACTORS FOR CAROTID ENDARTERECTOMY (CEA)

Anatomic	*Clinical*
Radical neck surgery	Congestive heart failure class III/IV
Extensive neck radiation	Left ventricular ejection fraction < 30%
Tracheostomy	Multivessel coronary disease
Inaccessible anatomy (lesion or bifurcation)	Recent myocardial infarction
Infections	Severe chronic obstructive pulmonary diseases (FEV1 < 50% of predicted)
Spinal immobility	Renal failure on dialysis
Contralateral occlusion	Uncontrolled diabetes
Bilateral stenoses	Liver failure
Previous CEA with recurrent stenosis	Unstable angina
Contralateral vocal cord paralysis	

Table II Risk factors for carotid artery stenting

Anatomic	*Clinical*
Arch diseases and anomalies	Octogenarians
Severe tortuosity	Symptomatic patients
Echolucent lesion	Renal failure, chronic renal insufficiency
Tandem lesion	Preload dependent states, aortic valvular stenosis
Calcified/undilatable lesions	Previous-life threatening contrast reaction
Long lesion (> 15 mm)	
Very tight "string-sign" stenoses (99%)	
Lesions adjacent to carotid artery aneurysm	
Lesions containing fresh thrombus	

bles I and II). This is an area that is now beginning to be explored but requires further investigation to better define situations where CAS should not be attempted. Large clinical studies are needed to clarify these settings.

One clear clinical limitation of CAS has become evident in the last years, namely, the higher rate of adverse events in octogenarians. Investigators in the CREST lead-in phase reported 30-day stroke and death rate of 12% for octogenerians, compared to 3.23% among non-octogenarians [5]. This finding has been repeated with such alarming regularity in other studies that today CAS should be considered at least relatively contra-indicated in patients older than 80 years of age [6-8]. The increased risk with age might be at least partly related to depleted functional reserves (i.e. renal function, hemodynamic response) but also to hostile anatomic factors, such as adverse arch anatomy and vessel tortuosity that have been associated with increased risk of CAS and seem to be more prevalent in the elderly.

Many unfavorable anatomic characteristics, such as arch elongation, calcification and vessel tortuosity, can complicate performance of CAS even in younger patients and might delineate a group of patients who might not be appropriate candidates for CAS. Unfortunately there are also other anatomic elements remaining poorly defined and the data about clinical correlates is lacking.

Plaque characteristic has received attention as a high-risk anatomic feature for CAS, with some evidence that "soft" plaque with low echogenicity scores may be associated with significant neurologic adverse events [9]. This is another area where refinement of indications may be required, but many additional data are required to confirm these findings and facilitate patient selection. Plaque echolucency on ultrasound, or plaque hemorrhage, may be more common in recently symptomatic patients and can render CAS at higher risk of embolization more than CEA. Some other recently studied high-risk anatomic features associated with increased periprocedural adverse outcomes after CAS include the presence of long stenotic lesions (> 15 mm) and involvement of internal carotid ostium [10].

Procedural technique

Carotid stent procedures were performed early on in the development of catheter-based therapies: but only few centers persisted with experience in this area beyond the initial steps, at least until the mid-1990 when extensive experience began. The initial description of the technique of carotid stenting involved use of balloon expandable stents, initially approved in the biliary areas and coaxial systems placed over coronary guide wires through coronary guiding catheters. Since then, systems have been developed to perform the procedure with protection devices engineered for specific use during the carotid procedure, stents designed and approved for this purpose, and sheaths and delivery systems that have been optimized for use in the cervical carotid systems. It is impressive to note that the technological improvements have occurred during less than 10 years of time, and it is likely that we are still at a very early stage in the development process of these devices. Currently the procedure for performing CAS has been somewhat standardized, and involves: placement of an access guide or sheath into the common carotid artery below the area of stenosis, often followed by initiation of cerebral protection, eventual predilation of the lesion, stent placement and post-dilation of the stent.

Each of these sequential steps involves use of equipment that could be specifically designed for use in the carotid artery. It is through a better understanding of the interaction between the current devices available, patient anatomy and plaque morphology, and assessing the disadvantages of these technologies that outcomes of CAS can be improved.

Access technique

Access is typically through the common femoral artery, although cervical approach and access through the arm are also recognized. Full heparin anticoagulation is achieved prior to manipulations of catheters in the aortic arch and carotid vessels. Two techniques for advancing sheath into the common carotid artery have been utilized: access to the carotid arteries can be obtained with either a selective catheter followed by a straight sheath or directly with selective guiding catheter access. No clear advantages of one approach exist and different operator experiences and anatomical settings may drive the choice.

In the case of straight sheath, we usually use a 5 F selective catheter, the headhunter curve, for the right carotid and the Simmons 2 curve for the left. The angled catheter is positioned in the proximal common carotid artery and the initial cervical and intra-cranial angiograms are obtained in both antero-posterior and lateral projections. In case of straight anatomy, the same teflonated 0.035" guidewire with J tip used for arch access, is advanced into the distal common carotid, being careful not to cross the carotid lesion. Over this guidewire, the straight introducer sheath can be advanced with its tapered inner cannula exchanging the selective catheter. A pull and push maneuver can help in advancing the outer sheath over the dilator at the level of the angled common carotid origin.

Alternatively, with a telescopic technique, the sheath is premounted on the selective catheter and it is advanced over it once the guidewire and the selective catheter are in the correct place. As an evolution of this technique, the Guiding Sheath Systems (Shuttle Select, Cook Medical, Bloomington, In, USA) consist of a coil reinforced sheath with variable stiffness through its length and hydrophilic coating, combined with a 6.5 F braided curved selective catheter, tapered distally to 5 Fr, who matches proximally the inner lumen of the outer introducer to provide a smooth transition zone.

In case of tortuous anatomy, an exchange-length guidewire is advanced into the terminal branches of the external carotid artery (ECA) to gain secure fixation. An angled glide catheter (4 Fr or 5 Fr) is usually the initial catheter of choice and can be used in conjunction with 0.035-inch nitinol hydrophilic glidewire, that is then exchanged for a stiffer wire such as an Amplatz. The selective catheter is then removed and a long (70 to 90 cm) 6 Fr or 7 Fr shuttle sheath with its dilator is advanced over the Amplatz wire in the common carotid artery.

The advantage of gaining and maintaining a sheath access to the distal common carotid is due to the fact that once the 0.035-inch guide wire will be removed (and exchanged with a 0.014-inch wire for crossing the target lesion, cerebral protection and stent deployment), "support" for angioplasty and stent placement is provided solely by the sheath. If the sheath backs up into the aortic arch during the procedure, it is quite impossible to advance it again into the common carotid over a thin 0.014-inch guide wire. In excessively tortuous anatomies, a more secure fixation of the guiding sheath in place can be obtained with the use of a double guide wire: one with its tip parked into the ECA (buddy wire) and the other which crosses the lesion in the internal carotid artery.

Open cervical access to the common carotid has been suggested as a good option for some patients with difficult anatomy or situations where sheath transversal in the arch is not advisable, such as mobile atheroma.

Cerebral protection

Once the sheath is securely positioned in the common carotid artery, the optimal angle of the image intensifier is established to best visualize the carotid bifurcation and the entire carotid artery.

Currently, technology for protection system has been notably improved since the first use of distal occlusion balloon by Theron and a number of devices are available for clinical use. Soon after the initial use of distal balloon occlusion for the prevention of embolization it became evident that the use of filters for protection might provide a mechanism to allow continued perfusion of the vessel distally while potentially limiting distal embolization. Although no randomized trials attest the benefits of mechanical cerebral protection systems, the common practice level C recommendation suggests that carotid protection devices (CPD) are probably beneficial [11]. The first prospective RCT of CAS with or without a CPD was recently published and showed that new MRI lesions occurred in 72% of the CPD group and 44% in the no CPD group ($p = 0.09$), the stroke rate being equal between the two groups. The major limitation of this RCT was the exceptionally small number of cases included (36 CAS) due to the reluctance of patients to participate in a study without cerebral protection [12].

According to the basic design and conceptual mechanism of protection, a number of distal protection strategies (occlusive balloons or filters) and proximal protection strategies (flow interruption or flow reversal systems) are today available for cerebral protection. The main differences are related to the need for crossing (distal systems) or not (proximal systems) the target lesions before protection, and for requiring flow interruption (occlusion balloons and flow interruption/reversal) or allowing continued perfusion of cerebral arteries. Careful review and matching of the anatomic criteria and particular device specifications and pre-procedural imaging should help in device planning [13].

Distal protection strategies

Distal occlusive balloon

A distal protection strategy is based on the principle that neurological complications occur as a result of cerebral embolization of debris generated during angioplasty and stenting of the target vessel. The balloon is therefore placed distal to the target lesion and is inflated prior to angioplasty-stenting. Flow is typically redirected into the ECA or appears as a stagnant column. After the procedure is completed, this stagnant column of blood is aspirated to remove debris generated during the intervention prior to restoring cerebral flow. The distal occlusion system can offer some advantages (the lowest crossing profile, the ability to remove very small embolic particles and providing complete protection of the distal carotid artery) but shows evident disadvantages (as the need to cross the lesion first, inability to image by contrast injection following balloon inflation, incomplete removal of emboli at the balloon/artery interface and intolerance for clamping) and is less likely in use today. A newer catheter with an occlusive distal balloon, the TwinOne, has been recently introduced by Minvasys Company (Genevilliers, France). It holds the same concept of providing protection through distal internal carotid artery occlusion by a balloon, that is held in the same catheter of a dilation balloon used for post-stent angioplasty.

Filters

Unlike the distal balloons, filters are designed to trap larger embolic particles and debris released during the procedure without interruption of cerebral flow. The filter type of CPD is the most widely available and used device, with different filter devices commercially available. All these filters are mounted over an 0.014-inches wire platform and consist of a nitinol skeleton or hoop and a laser-cut polyurethane filter membrane (pore sizes range from 36 μm to 150 μm) or nitinol mesh. Filters are collapsed within a delivery sheath, which is then removed once the filter is positioned beyond the lesion and is again collapsed back within a recovery catheter at the end of the procedure for removal. Some differences in outcomes of various types of filter have been shown but results are conflicting and to date, no RCT has been performed [14-15].

Even if the profile is small, filters still have the potential for embolization during introduction and rarely it can be difficult to advance the devices across tortuous anatomy. Distal systems also require an adequate length for placement and minimal tortuosity and sufficient distance away from the lesion along the internal carotid artery. Finally, although all filters would trap large debris, the ability to filter small debris (< 50 μm) is limited.

Proximal protection strategies

Reversal of flow

This technique aims to reverse flow in the internal carotid artery and has some potential advantages compared to standard filter protection. The Gore Neuroprotection system (W L Gore, Flagstaff, Az. USA) consists of a balloon sheath, an external carotid balloon occlusion wire and an external filter connected with a line for femoral vein blood re-infusion. The balloon sheath is a dual-lumen catheter with a compliant balloon located at its most distal tip. The first lumen acts as the inflation lumen, while the second lumen allows for continual retrograde flow of blood with embolic particles and introduction of balloons and stents. The gradient between the internal carotid artery and the low-pressure femoral vein causes reversal of flow in the internal carotid artery. Disadvantages of the devices include the large introducer size (9 Fr), and the intolerance in about 3% to 9% of patients (especially in settings with contralateral carotid occlusion and impaired collateral cerebral circulation). However, even in these individuals, procedures can be completed under reversal protection with temporary deflation of the balloon sheath to allow adaptation with activation of collateral circulation [16].

Interruption of flow

The MOMA device (Invatec, Roncadelle, Italy) provides an "endovascular clamping" of vessels flow. This system consists of a common carotid balloon sheath and an external carotid balloon occlusion catheter integrated into the same sheath. No venous access is used and flow is simply halted in the carotid by inflation of the balloons on the system. Initial results with the device reflect a reasonable safety and efficacy [17].

Carotid angioplasty and stenting

Angiography is performed to verify proper positioning of the CPD and imaging of the carotid lesion before proceeding to ballooning and stenting. Because it is not uncommon for patients to have bradycardia and hypotension with carotid ballooning and stenting, hemodynamic assessment should be made continuously throughout the procedure. In order to limit the baroceptor response to carotid bulb manipulations, the patient is usually given a low dosage (0.4 to 1 mg) of intravenous atropine. Percutaneous transluminal angioplasty (pre-dilation) of the lesion is rarely performed in our experience with small (3 mm or 4 mm) angioplasty balloon, with "rapid-exchange" technology in case of very tight stenoses. Balloon length is usually chosen in the range of 1.5 to 2 cm in order not to dilate the healthy segment of the artery distal to the plaque.

A self-expanding stent is in every case of carotid angioplasty to prevent the risk of embolization. The CAVATAS randomized study recently reported the late results of carotid angioplasty, in which stent was used only as a bail-out procedure in only 26% of the patients undergoing endovascular treatment, compared to carotid endarterectomy. After 5 years, risk of restenosis (≥ 70% at Duplex examination) resulted 30.7% in the endovascular arm, significantly higher than 10.5% in the endarterectomy arm (HR 3·17, 95% CI 1·89-5·32). Interestingly, the incidence of restenosis was significantly lower after stenting compared to angioplasty alone, with a HR 0.43, CI 0.19-0.97; p = 0.04. In clinical terms, stenting was associated with a better prognosis, in fact the risk of ipsilateral nonperioperative stroke was lower after stenting than after angioplasty alone, but the number of events was small and the difference was not significant (0.66, 0.25-1.71) [18].

Stents have changed since the initiation of CAS procedure and currently there are different models approved (Table III). These modifications have included specific lengths and tapers for deployment in the carotid vessels, as well as miniaturization of the delivery systems , that have now been decreased to as small as 5 Fr.

Although it has been not universally noted, some authors hypothesized that stent design and application can influence outcomes [19]. The design of the stent alters stent flexibility, wall coverage, and scaffolding, all of which may impact outcomes in carotid stenting. Two main types of cell design in the metallic frame of the stent are now available: those with closed cell design, in which all the stent struts are interconnected, and those with open cell design in which not all the struts are interconnected, giving more flexibility to the stent structure. Most carotid lesions can be treated with either type. However, some lesions may be better suited for stenting with a specific cell design. Because open cell design is more conformable, this type of stent is often used when tortuous anatomy is encountered (Fig. 1). The closed cell design may lead to less plaque protrusion through the struts of the stent. Thus, a close cell stent is often used in ca-

Table III CHARACTERISTICS OF SOME OF THE CURRENTLY AVAILABLE CAROTID STENTING SYSTEMS

Manufacturer	*Stent*	*Cell Type*	*Tapered Configuration*
Abbott Vascular	Acculink	Open	Yes
Abbott Vascular	Xact	Closed	Yes
Bard	Vivexx	Open	Yes
Boston Scientific	Wallstent	Closed	No
Boston Scientific	Nexstent	Closed	No
Cordis	Precise Pro	Open	No
ev3	Protégé	Open	Yes
Invatec	Cristallo Ideale	Open/closed	Yes
Medtronic	Exponent	Open/closed	No
Optimed	Sinus	Open	Yes
W Cook	Zilver	Open	No

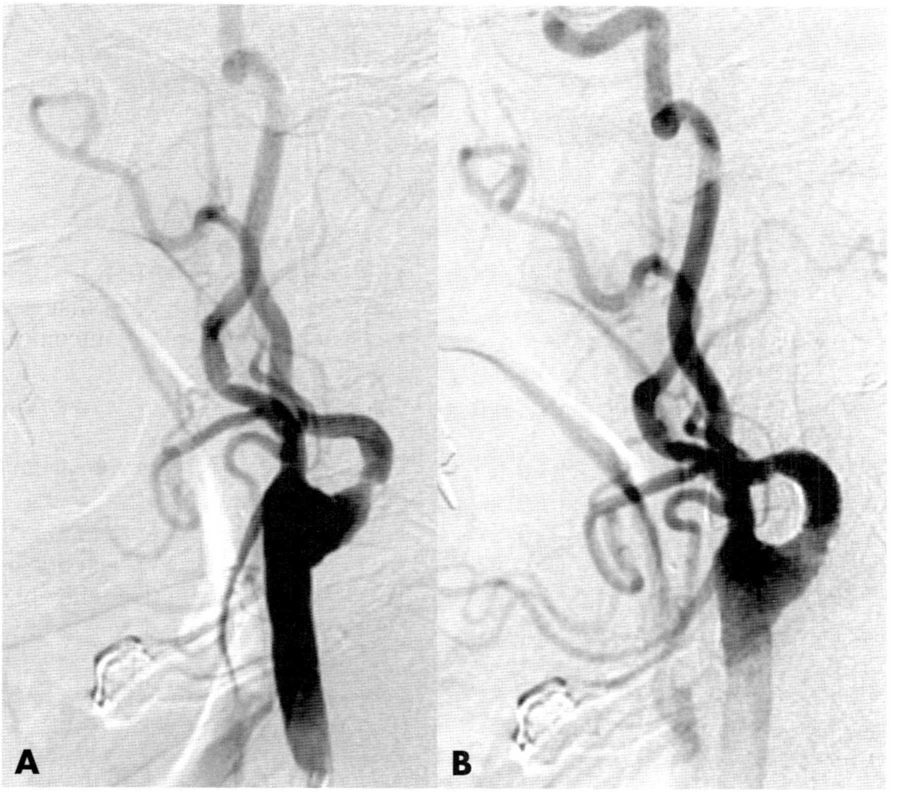

FIG. 1 A) Pre-operative angiogram showing a carotid severe stenosis in a tortuous internal carotid artery; B) Angiogram after stenting, an open cell design stent was used.

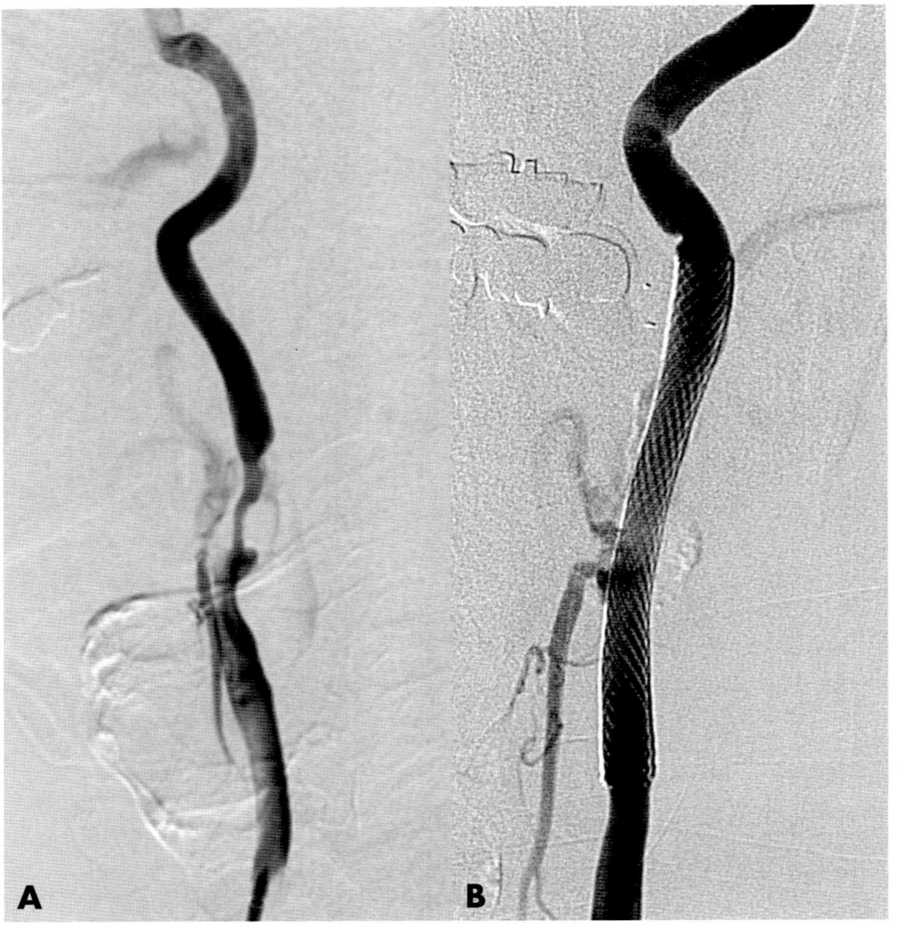

FIG. 2 A) pre-operative angiogram in a patient with severe stenosis, due to irregular plaque in a straight internal carotid artery; B) post-stenting angiogram, after deployment of a closed cell carotid stent

rotid stenoses that have a higher embolic potential as well as in straight anatomies (Fig. 2). Other important issues in the stent choice may be the radial force of the stent, which has to oppose the elastic recoil of the dilated plaque, and the free cell area of the stent, which might be important in reducing plaque protrusion and embolization.

Despite several changes in design and materials have been achieved in carotid stent, further improvements in technology are expected in the next years, since the interface between the diseased segment of the carotid artery and the device used to maintain patency of the vessel is the least understood aspect of endoluminal treatment of carotid stenosis. Interrogation of the lesion before treatment may suggest those lesions that will be at increased risk of embolic complications prior to treatment, thereby suggesting an alternative strategy in treating these patients. In these cases, stents would incorporate the ability to limit the trans-stent passage of plaque debris: either polymer coating, fabric coating or fine mesh coating of the stent would be helpful.

Once the stent is deployed, an angiogram is performed and the stent is post-dilated with expedient 5-mm to 6-mm balloon inflation to profile the stented segment; usually balloons no longer than 2 cm are used. It is wise to accept a mild residual carotid stenosis (< 30%) and avoid potential complications with repeated angioplasty or overdilation; the continuous force exerted by the self expanding stent will allow its full expansion with time. An angiogram is performed following stent deployment and before CPD removal to verify the patency of the internal carotid. The CPD is removed according to the device-specific instructions and completion angiogram images are obtained (anterior-posterior and lateral view). The sheath may be exchanged for a standard 6 Fr or 7 Fr short sheath and then this is removed with the assistance of a closure device.

INTRA-OPERATIVE COMPLICATIONS

Neurovascular rescue

Neurovascular complications may occur during CAS, some strictly related to the use of CPD. Management of these requires knowledge of vascular anatomy and collateral circulation, correct identification of the complication and its clinical implications. Many of the strategies used are not supported by literature, since rigorous, controlled data are lacking. If there is no flow through the internal carotid artery at the angiogram subsequent to stent deployment, one must consider a large burden of thrombus or atherosclerotic debris within a distal filter. Various techniques can be employed to clear the filter, such as aspirating with another catheter positioned in the filter basket. If a large embolus is identified within the filter, this is probably best managed by partially closing and removing the filter, if possible, or repeat usage of a lytic agent (e.g. rtPA) can be attempted. Associated spasm can be treated with nitroglycerine. Spasm at the site of filter deployment is common and in most cases is minor and does not require intervention.

Other causes of flow arrest are dissection and acute stent thrombosis. Flow limiting dissection is best managed with a further stent. An acute stent thrombosis is extremely rare, especially in patients adequately pretreated with aspirin/clopidogrel and heparin anticoagulated for the procedure and would probably best managed with a lytic agent with the protection system in place. Technical factors that may promote thrombosis include prolonged obstruction of a stenosed lumen with an occluding balloon or stent delivery catheter. If an in-stent filling defect is recognized, factors guiding management are the patient's neurologic response and severity of flow limitation. If the patient is neurologically stable, the problem can be addressed pharmacologically (IIb-IIIa inhibitors). Otherwise, balloon angioplasty or stent-in-stent can be employed, however, the risks of showering the intracranial circulation with multiple emboli are evident. A better option may be immediate open conversion to endarterectomy and stent removal in selected cases.

Intra-cranial embolism may become clinically apparent with acute hemispheric events or remain asymptomatic. Rarely, symptoms witnessed immediately on table are due to a large and visible embolus within the intracranial circulation: in these cases mechanical disruption, removal and lysis have all been successfully employed in rare cases and there is currently no suggestion to considered that one technique is better than the other. However, usually, no embolus is identified and the mechanism is probably diffuse distal micro-embolization. If this is confirmed with magnetic resonance and hemorrhage is excluded, the only option is to keep these patients anticoagulated to limit the extension of thrombus.

Intra-cranial hemorrhage has been the most dreaded complication of endovascular carotid approach especially with the use of the earliest large profile devices and stiff wires. However, today cerebral hemorrhage may still occur secondary to wire perforation of an intra-cranial vessel or to iatrogenic catheter/protection device trauma. Neurological/neurosurgical evaluation, reversal of anticoagulation and eventually abortion of an on-site procedure are mandatory.

Other complications

Hypotension and bradycardia immediately after CAS are common, but usually transient and rarely symptomatic. There is no consensus as to which patients provide vasopressor agents or prophylactic placement of a temporary pacemaker. Systematic use of low dosage of atropine has been suggested to prevent excessive response to carotid bulb manipulations [20]. Nevertheless, prophylactic administration of atropine has also been debated due to its potential side effects (e.g. tachycardia).

Major access-site complications occur around 3% of patients and include hemorrhage and arterial occlusion. Other complications (i.e. deterioration of renal function, contrast intolerance) are generic to all endovascular procedure.

Improving the outcome of carotid stenting

PROCEDURE STANDARDIZATION AND MONITORING

To improve outcome, CAS should follow a regular and defined protocol. The standardized approach for CAS also includes pre-procedural planning, patient monitoring and medical management.

Before the procedure

A pre-operative imaging study is preferable for the assessment and planning for carotid stent placement. A good quality contrast enhanced computed tomography or magnetic resonance angiography with arch, cervical and intra-cranial images may be used for evaluation of a patient's arch, carotid anatomy and CAS planning. This allows for proper selection not only of access catheters and sheaths but also cerebral protection devices and stents. Duplex ultrasound should be performed in an accredited vascular laboratory, ideally by the same lab that will be performing the procedure and the follow-up examinations

Medical therapy

Dual antiplatelet should be prescribed to all patients before the procedure and for at least 4 weeks following stent placement. Aspirin, 75 mg to 325 mg daily, and clopidogrel 75 mg daily are usually given for at least 5 days before the stenting procedure and then continued for at least 1 month after stent placement. If patients were not treated with clopidogrel before the procedure, 300 mg can be given in a single dose before the procedure. Ticlopidine is an alternative to those who are unable to take clopidogrel. All the procedures should be performed under full intravenous heparinization. Full heparin anticoagulation (typically 100 mg/kg) after arterial access is gained and prior to manipulation of catheters in the aortic arch and brachiocephalic vessels. It is likely that drugs intended to block the carotid baroceptors provide some protection against serious bradycardia and asystole during manipulation in the carotid bulb. Considering the beneficial effect of statins on patients undergoing CEA, it is reasonable to advocate their efficacy for patients undergoing CAS. However, no randomized prospective studies currently exist.

Procedure monitoring

A pre-operative neurological exam by a certified neurologist is essential in symptomatic patients, to understand neurological events eventually occurring in the peri-operative period. Neurologic assessment should be performed after sheath access and throughout the procedure: a noise-making device, is usually placed in the contralateral arm of the patient. It is squeezed throughout the procedure to assess the patient's monitor function and ability to follow verbal instructions. The patient's speech and cognitive abilities are followed throughout the procedure with a standard series of questions. Transcranial Doppler (TCD) can be used to monitor and record embolic and micro-embolic cerebral events. Hemodynamic changes related to stimulation (dilation, ballooning, stenting) of carotid baroceptors need to be assessed and treated by cardiac continuous monitoring.

After the procedure

The patient should be monitored after the procedure, usually until the following day, for hemodynamic and neurologic changes. A prolonged hospital stay is uncommonly due to hypotension and vasopressor requirement. Frequently, the pre-operative antihypertensive medications should be decreased before the discharge and the blood pressure closely monitored at home. Carotid Duplex ultrasound is usually performed before discharge, at one month of the CAS procedure, and every 6 months thereafter.

Quality control of the procedure: training, experience, facilities

Acquisition of appropriate competence and credentialing as well as the use of standardized protocols and materials significantly affect the outcome of CAS. Indeed, it has become evident that only if performed by an experienced and competent operator, CAS may offer a reasonable alternative to CEA [21].

Facilities

There are a number of "minimal requirements" that have been determined for "facilities" in performing CAS: adequate imaging, device inventory, experienced staff and infrastructure for a dedicated carotid stent program are mandatory. These include: high-resolution digital imaging, allowing for subtraction, magnification and road-mapping; advanced physiologic monitoring that should include real-time cardiac, blood pressure and cardiac rhythm management; emergent management and resuscitation system in place in the interventional room where the procedures would be performed; the presence of an anesthesiologist or another physician capable of maintaining adequate hemodynamic control is mandatory.

A database to collect information on all carotid stenting procedures and a carotid stent program should also be implemented for the monitoring quality process. The program should include a minimum case requirements for granting privileges and recording of complication rate.

Physician

When complex interventions are performed, one of the most important variables influencing outcomes might be the technical ability of the individual performing the procedure. A number of documents have been published to offer recommendations regarding the necessary training and the minimum physician competence levels prior to proceeding with performing the procedure independently. Despite there are no uniform official requirements on the experience and credentialing of the individual performing CAS, recommendations in Europe suggested at least 150 procedures of supra-aortic vessel engagement (during diagnostic as well as interventional procedures) within 2 years, of which at least 100 as the primary operator or at least 75 carotid stenting procedures, of which at least 50 as the primary operator [22]. Training regimen programs have been increasingly implemented by manufacturers and expert organizations to provide guidance for the credentialing process and to condense the learning phase while ensure performing CAS safely. Documentation of the eligibility to perform CAS must be also maintained and renewed every 2 years by providing additional confirmation (re-credentialing/re-certification).

Personal experience

In a now outdated matched case-control study comparing our CAS with CEA population, we found that stroke rate was significantly higher in CAS but the rate markedly decreased over the study period. To define the caseload necessary to perform CAS safely and the effect of the learning curve on CAS outcomes, we then reviewed all our CAS experience in 2006. We found that the caseload necessary to perform safe CAS, accepting a major stroke rate threshold as low as 2% per year, was reached only after the first 195 CAS (i.e., first 3 years 2001-2003), when the established yearly rate was achieved and remained stable at less than 2% for each of the following years.

In a more recent review of our experience on 1 170 CAS in a 7-year period, the overall 30-day stroke and death rate was 4.1% and the major stroke and death rate was 1.5%. When comparing the outcome of the first period of experience (2001-2003 years, Group I) wit the later one (2004-2008, Group II) it was evident that with increased clinical experience, the 30-day any stroke/death rate significantly decreased from 8.2% to 3.3% $p = 0.0045$, OR 2.61; 95% CI 1.4-4.8. There was a particular decrease in stroke rates occurring during the technical phase of placement of the sheath into the common carotid (from 2.0% to 0.1% for Groups 1 and 2, respectively, $p = 0.005$) and during the ballooning/stenting phase (from 5.1% to 1.3%, for Groups I and II, respectively, $p = 0.002$). Furthermore, the major stroke risk during the approaching phase was completely nullified in Group II (6 vs. 0). After filter retrieval, and within 30 days from intervention, the stroke rates were similar and lower than 2% in both groups [23].

The role of the learning curve in the decrease of all neurological complications during the study period as well as the different occurrence according to the different phases of the procedure is therefore evident. Both patient selection, avoiding unfavourable anatomy as diseased aortic arches, extremely tortuous epiaortic vessels, and a more careful manipulation of wires and catheters in approaching the target lesion have probably played a major role in results amelioration.

Conclusion

Recent trial results have not expanded indications for CAS and its use as the current evidence only supports its application in clinical trials or specific high-risk categories.

The approach to carotid disease is likely to evolve during the next several years as stenting technology and greater experience is acquired. Consequently, outcome of CAS will hopefully continue to improve. Once the influence of all anatomo-pathological factors, such arch anatomy and lesion characteristics, and clinical factors, such as age, symptoms, comorbidities, as well as genomics and proteomics will ultimately be well defined, a high-risk category for CAS as well as for CEA will likely emerge, to permit better selection of cases and improved outcomes.

Nevertheless, the benefit of either procedure in terms of stroke prevention, will still continue to strongly depend on technical perfection, institutional outcome and expertise level with both techniques.

REFERENCES

1 Ederle J, Featherstone RL, Brown MM. Randomised controlled trials comparing endarterectomy and endovascular treatment for carotid artery stenosis: a Cochrane Review. *Stroke* 2009; 40: 1373-1380.

2 Mas JL, Trinquart L, Leys D et al; EVA-3S investigators. Endarterectomy Versus Angioplasty in Patients with Symptomatic Severe Carotid Stenosis (EVA-3S) trial: results up to 4 years from a randomised, multicentre trial. *Lancet Neurol* 2008; 7: 885-892.

3 Eckstein HH, Ringleb P, Allenberg JR et al. Results of the Stent-Protected Angioplasty versus Carotid Endarterectomy (SPACE) study to treat symptomatic stenoses at 2 years: a multinational, prospective, randomised trial. *Lancet Neurol* 2008; 7: 893-902.

4 Anonymous. European Stroke Conference. ICSS: carotid endarterectomy superior to stenting, at least in the short term, *www.medscape.com/viewarticle/703471*; 2009

5 Hobson RW 2nd, Howard VJ, Roubin GS et al; CREST Investigators. Carotid artery stenting is associated with increased complications in octogenarians: 30-day stroke and death rates in the CREST lead-in phase. *J Vasc Surg* 2004; 40: 1106-1111.

6 Stanziale SF, Marone LK, Boules TN et al. Carotid artery stenting in octogenarians is associated with increased adverse outcomes. *J Vasc Surg* 2006; 43: 297-304.

7 Gray WA, Yadav JS, Verta P et al; CAPTURE Trial Collaborators. The CAPTURE registry: predictors of outcomes in carotid artery stenting with embolic protection for high surgical risk patients in the early post-approval setting. *Catheter Cardiovasc Interv* 2007; 70: 1025-1033.

8 Roubin GS, New G, Iyer SS et al. Immediate and late clinical outcomes of carotid artery stenting in patients with symptomatic and asymptomatic carotid artery stenosis: a 5-year prospective analysis. *Circulation* 2001; 103: 532-537.

9 Biasi GM, Froio A, Diethrich EB et al. Carotid plaque echolucency increases the risk of stroke in carotid stenting: the Imaging in Carotid Angioplasty and Risk of Stroke (ICAROS) study. *Circulation* 2004; 110: 756-762.

10 Sayeed S, Stanziale SF, Wholey MH et al. Angiographic lesion characteristics can predict adverse outcomes after carotid artery stenting. *J Vasc Surg* 2008; 47: 81-87.

11 Liapis CD, Bell PR, Mikhailidis D et al; ESVS Guidelines Collaborators. ESVS guidelines. Invasive treatment for carotid stenosis: indications, techniques. *Eur J Vasc Endovasc Surg* 2009; 37: 1-19.

12 Barbato JE, Dillavou E, Horowitz MB et al. A randomized trial of carotid artery stenting with and without cerebral protection. *J Vasc Surg* 2008; 47: 760-765.

13 Verzini F, Cieri E, De Rango P et al. Cerebral embolic protection during carotid artery stenting. In: Brancherau A, Jacobs M, editors (Eds). *Innovative Cardiovascular Procedures.* Turin: Edizioni Minerva Medica; 2009. pp. 157-166.

14 Hart JP, Peeters P, Verbist J et al. Do device characteristics impact outcome in carotid artery stenting? *J Vasc Surg* 2006; 44: 725-730.

15 Iyer V, de Donato G, Deloose K et al. The type of embolic protection does not influence the outcome in carotid artery stenting. *J Vasc Surg* 2007; 46: 251-256.

16 Rabe K, Sugita J, Gödel H, Sievert H. Flow-reversal device for cerebral protection during carotid artery stenting–acute and long-term results. *J Interv Cardiol* 2006; 19: 55-62.

17 Coppi G, Moratto R, Silingardi R et al. PRIAMUS–proximal flow blockage cerebral protectIon during carotid stenting: results from a multicenter Italian registry. *J Cardiovasc Surg (Torino)* 2005; 46: 219-227.

18 Bonati LH, Ederle J, McCabe DJH et al. Long-term risk of carotid restenosis in patients randomly assigned to endovascular treatment or endarterectomy in the Car*otid and Vertebral Artery* Transluminal Angioplasty Study (CAVATAS): long-term follow-up of a randomised trial. *Lancet Neurol* 2009; 8: 908-917.

19 Schillinger M, Gschwendtner M, Reimers B et al. Does carotid stent cell design matter? *Stroke* 2008; 39: 905-909.

20 Cieri E, De Rango P, Maccaroni MR et al. Is haemodynamic depression during carotid stenting a predictor of peri-procedural complications? *Eur J Vasc Endovasc Surg* 2008; 35: 399-404.

21 Verzini F, Cao P, De Rango P et al. Appropriateness of learning curve for carotid artery stenting: an analysis of periprocedural complications. *J Vasc Surg* 2006; 44: 1205-1212.

22 Cremonesi A, Setacci C, Bignamini A et al. Carotid artery stenting: first consensus document of the ICCS-SPREAD Joint Committee. *Stroke* 2006; 37: 2400-2409.

23 Verzini F, De Rango P, Parlani G et al. Carotid artery stenting: technical issues and role of operator's experience. *Perspect Vasc Surg Endovasc Ther* 2008; 20: 247-257.

3

BEST PRACTICE FOR ASYMPTOMATIC CAROTID DISEASE

LAURENT CHICHE, CAROLINE GOULFIER

Since nearly 20 years, remarkable efforts were undertaken to clarify the best treatment options and indications for patients with carotid artery disease. Several randomized controlled trials (RCTs), whose realization was ardently wished by the neurologists, made it possible to draw recommendations based on Grade I evidence for symptomatic and asymptomatic disease. Those relying on ACAS [1] and ACST [2] trials, respectively published in 1995 and 2004, relate to the treatment of asymptomatic disease. Not only for medical reasons but also for economic or even ethical reasons, these recommendations are nowadays the base of many controversies. The interest of any type of nonconservative treatment, either conventional open surgical treatment or endoluminal treatment, is even hardly questioned [3]. This chapter aims to focus on data and recent recommendations concerning the treatment of asymptomatic carotid disease, so that each physician being confronted can adopt on a case-by-case basis what he believes could be the most relevant therapeutic option.

Epidemiological background

Ischemic stroke represent a major health problem. It is the second leading cause of mortality in developed countries, after cardiopathies, and the leading cause of nontraumatic adult disability. The proportion of deaths caused by stroke is 10%-12% in western countries and 12% of these deaths occur in people less than 65 years of age [4]. During the first month following stroke, death rate varies from 20% to 25%. Survival rate at 5 years ranges from 39% to 60%. Prognosis appears even worse for hemorrhagic strokes as compared to ischemic strokes. A typical estimation, drawn from knowledge of stroke incidence and mortality, is that about 500 per 100 000 people live with the consequences of stroke. Because of the ageing population, the burden of stroke will increase greatly during the next 20 years, especially in developing countries. Because stroke mortality is probably decreasing faster than stroke incidence, the proportion of stroke survivors is likely to increase as well. Worldwide, strokes already consumes about 2%-4% of total health-care costs and in industrialized countries, it accounts for more than 4% of direct health-care costs. In the United States, stroke is currently estimated to cost the Health Services approximately $60 billion per year [3].

About 80% of all strokes are ischemic. Atherosclerosis accounts for up to one-third of all strokes. More precisely, atherosclerosis from supra-aortic vessels and especially from the common carotid bifurcation, is a major cause of recurrent ischemic stroke, accounting for almost 20% of all strokes [5]. Carotid occlusive disease amenable to revascularization accounts for 5%-12% of new strokes. The prevalence of > 50% carotid occlusive disease ranges from 5% to 10% in the global population aged > 65 years. It reaches 20% to 30% in patients with symptomatic coronary artery disease or lower limb occlusive disease. The annual incidence of cerebrovascular events, transient ischemic attacks and ischemic strokes, might differ due to methodological weaknesses in individual studies [6]. However, even in studies of the highest quality, it ranges from 240 for 100 000 people (standardized to the European population aged 45-84 years) in Dijon, France, to 600 to 100 000 people in Novosibirks, Russia [4]. This suggests important roles for both environmental and genetic factors.

Prevalence of stroke can be estimated by cross-sectional surveys, cohort studies, or by indirect calculations from incidence studies that have followed-up cases at uniform times after stroke onset. In their review of population-based studies of incidence, prevalence and case-fatality, published in 2003, Feigin et al. [6] identified from nine studies of stroke prevalence reported after 1990, a worldwide prevalence of stroke in all age-groups ranging from five to 10 per 1 000 population.

In the same study, Feigin et al. [6] showed that the age-specific incidence of stroke increased progressively with each decade of life. The average age of patients affected by stroke was 70 years in men and 75 years in women. More than half of all strokes occurred in people over 75 years of age. Age-standardized incidence of total stroke per 1 000 person-years for people aged 55 years or more was in the range 4.2-6.5 in 12 of 15 studies, although three studies reported higher values. For ischemic strokes, it ranged from 3.5 to 5.2 in 8 studies. The age-standardized prevalence rate of stroke in people aged ≥ 65 years ranged from 46 to 72 per 1 000 population. The variations in impact of classical risk factors of stroke by population, sex and age, were also analyzed in a recent study, within the framework of the MORGAM project [7]. Data were collected in 18 populations in 8 European countries with an average follow-up of 13.2 years. In 93 695 persons (5 1703 men) aged 19 to 77 years and free of major cardiovascular disease at baseline, total observation years were 1 234 252 and the number of stroke analyzed was 3 142, occurring in 1 851 men and in 1 291 women. For each year of age, the risk of stroke increased by 9% in men and by 10% in women. A 10-mmHg increase in systolic blood pressure involved a similar increase in men (28%) and women (25%). Across all Europe, smoking conferred a similar excess risk in women and in men. Higher high-density lipoprotein cholesterol levels decreased the risk of stroke more in women than in men. Risks appraissals identified the same risk factors for ischemic and hemorrhagic strokes. However, this study referred only to relative risks of stroke, which do not necessarily translate into risks of stroke in absolute terms. Determinants of variations in absolute risk for stroke between populations have to be addressed by forthcoming analysis within the MORGAM project.

When should we treat asymptomatic carotid disease? Lessons learned from the randomized trials

No single procedure has been the focus of more randomized trials testing standard medical treatment against surgical benefits of carotid endarterectomy (CEA). These trials underlied evidence-based guidelines and consensus statements providing recommendations for the use of CEA, either for symptomatic or for asymptomatic disease. However, despite the level I evidence supporting the role of CEA demonstrated by the two major randomized trials, ACAS [1] and ACST [2], considerable controversy remains regarding the management of patients with asymptomatic carotid disease.

The Asymptomatic Carotid Atherosclerosis Study (ACAS) [1] randomized 1 662 patients with 60%-99% carotid stenosis to either early CEA or differed treatment (best medical therapy until surgery was deemed necessary). Only surgeons having an excellent safety record were allowed to enroll the study. In all, ACAS rejected 40% of initial applicants, subsequently barring from further participation some surgeons who had adverse operative outcomes during the trial. The results were published in 1995 with a mean follow-up of 2.7 years, which represented 4 657 patient-years of observation. It was estimated that the aggregate 5-year risk of ipsilateral stroke and any peri-operative stroke or death was 5.1% for surgical patients and 11.0% for patients treated medically, leading to an aggregate risk reduction of 53%. Therefore, a Grade A recommendation to the use of CEA in selected asymptomatic patients with high-grade stenosis was given, provided that the rate of peri-operative stroke and death is 3% and life expectancy is at least 5 years.

Between 1993 and 2003, the Asymptomatic Carotid Surgery Trial (ACST) [2] randomized 3 120 patients with > 60% mainly asymptomatic (12% had symptoms at least 6 months previously) to immediate CEA plus medical treatment versus medical treatment alone or until the operation became necessary. An evidence of an operative risk ≤ 6% for their last 50 patients was required for the participating surgeons. However, none were excluded on the basis of the real operative risk during the trial. Carotid stenosis was assessed by Doppler ultrasonography, without any audit of the operator's performance. Selection of patients was based on the uncertainty principle, with very few exclusion criteria.

The Table details the design and main results of ACAS and ACST. It is important to notice that the two trials did not report similar end-points. Despite this fact and other differences in methods, the results of ACAS and ACST were quite similar. In both studies, the benefit of surgery in stroke prevention was modest and became apparent after one year in ACAS and two years in ACST. This benefit was only maintained when the peri-operative risks of stroke and death were below 3%. Actually, despite the inclusion of nearly 4 500 patients, the annual stroke and death rate after CEA was 1% versus 2% among patients who received medical treatment alone. In ACAS, the numbers of any strokes, any major strokes and ipsilateral strokes prevented per 1 000 CEA at 5 years were respectively 51, 27 and 29. In ACST, the numbers of any strokes and any major strokes prevented per 1 000 CEA at 5 years were respectively 54 and 26. In opposite to the symptomatic trials, neither ACAS nor ACST demonstrated any relationship between stenosis severity and late stroke risk. This counterintuitive observation was assumed to be attributable to a lack of statistical power in ACAS but cannot be dismissed with the additional data provided by ACST. Subgroup analysis in ACST, which had a larger sample size than ACAS, demonstrated that CEA significantly reduced the 5-year-risk of disabling or fatal stroke by 50%. Patients with a life expectancy of less than 5 years were unlikely to benefit from the modest risk reduction afforded by CEA. In fact, only ACST enrolled patients aged > 79 years showed that surgery did not benefit patients aged 75 years or older because of the excess mortality rate at follow-up in these patients. Males and females both gained significant benefit from surgery in ACST, although ACAS showed no significant benefit of prophylactic surgery in females. In ACST, the longer the follow-up, the greater was the benefit from CEA for women. It appeared that about three years were required to counterbalance the peri-operative risk in women, as compared to only 1.5 years in men. Finally, it is important to consider that in both trials, the enrolled patients constituted a highly selected group, not necessarily representative of patients routinely seen in clinical practice. Most of all, the medical arm of these studies was not uniformly defined and did not include what we can now consider as the best medical treatment, such as intensive control of blood pressure and lipid concentration. ACAS and ACST were published 5 to 14 years ago. There is now growing evidence that improvements in medical therapy have significantly reduced the risk of stroke, compared to that observed in both trials [8]. At least for this specific reason, prophylactic carotid artery revascularization for asymptomatic disease still remains a matter of debate. Another reason for this lack of consensus is the emergence of carotid artery stenting (CAS) over the preceding decade, which results remain under evaluation and should be compared to the current results of CEA.

CURRENT RESULTS OF CEA

Few surgical procedures have been scrutinized as thoroughly as CEA during the last two decades. Several techniques for CEA have evolved since the first case was performed in 1954. These techniques include the conventional endarterectomy, either followed by primary closure or by patch closure, and the eversion technique. In a recent review, AbuRahma [9] stated that based on the available data, meta-analysis and systematic review of prospective randomized trials with level I evidence, a grade A recommendation can be made that there

Table DETAILS OF THE TWO RANDOMIZED TRIALS, ACAS [1] AND ACST [2], COMPARING CAROTID ENDARTERECTOMY TO MEDICAL TREATMENT FOR ASYMPTOMATIC CAROTID DISEASE

	ACAS	*ACST*
Inclusion period	1987-1993	1993-2003
Countries	North America, 39 centres	Europe, 126 centres
N pts, sex-ratio	1 662, 66% male	3 120, 66% male
Carotid stenosis	≥ 60%, angiography or ultrasonography	≥ 60%, ultrasonography
Randomization	1/1, "surgery within 30 days" or "medical treatment" (aspirin, 325 mg)	1/1, "immediate surgery" or "delayed surgery or no surgery"
Follow-up duration	2.7 years	3.4 years
Mean age	67 years, inclusion from 40 to 79 years	68 years
Primary end point	Ipsilateral stroke + any stroke and perioperative death	Any stroke (ipsilateral, controlateral, vertebrobasilar) + death
30-day procedural risk of death and stroke	2.3%, (including a 1.2% rate of angiographic complications)	3.1%
Results (5-year risks)		
. *any stroke*	17.5% (BMT) vs. 12.4% (CEA), ARR = 5.1%	11.8% (BMT) vs. 6.4% (CEA), ARR = 5.4%
. *any major stroke*	9.1% (BMT) vs. 6.4% (CEA), ARR = 2.7%	6.1% (BMT) vs. 3.5% (CEA), ARR = 2.6%
. *Ipsilateral stroke*	11.0% (BMT) vs. 5.1% (CEA), ARR = 5.9%	5.1% (BMT) vs. 4.4% (CEA), ARR = 1.1%
. *Major ipsilateral stroke*	6.0% (BMT) vs. 3.4% (CEA), ARR = 2.6%	n/a

BMT: Best medical treatment; CEA: Carotid endarterectomy; ARR: Absolute risk reduction at 5 years

is no difference in stroke and death rates between conventional CEA with patch closure and eversion CEA. Eversion CEA yields a lower restenosis rate than CEA with primary closure. The incidence of significant restenosis with eversion CEA is quite similar to CEA with patch closure.

Actually, the current results of CEA, independently of the used surgical technique, can be estimated from single center publications, large registries and collective studies or from results of RCTs. In many studies, the specific results of CEA in the asymptomatic population were not detailed, thus complicating the extrapolation of short- and long-term risks of death and stroke.

Several recent single center studies have illustrated the excellent results of CEA. In a series of 1 150 CEAs, Ballotta et al. [10] reported a 30-day mortality rate of 0.3%, and a stroke rate of 0.9%, with a combined mortality and stroke rate of 1.2%. The incidence of late occlusion and recurrent stenosis 70% or greater was 0.6% and 0.5%, respectively, with a combined occlusion and restenosis rate of 1.1%. The rate of freedom from occlusion, restenosis 70% or greater, and combined occlusion and restenosis 70% or greater at 12 years was 99.4%, 99.5%, and 98.8%, respectively. All cases of occlusion and restenosis developed asymptomatically. Of 600 CEAs, including 47% performed for treating asymptomatic stenosis, Scavée et al. [11] observed a combined 30-day stroke and death rate of 0.9%. In this series, endarterectomies were performed with temporary shunting and arteriotomies were closed by vein patch angioplasties. Archie et al. [12] reported a series of 1 360 CEAs performed on 1 133 patients, including 514 (37.8%) with 70% or greater asymptomatic stenosis. The combined 30-day stroke and death rate was 2.1%. The 30-day ipsilateral major stroke or mortality rate was 1.2% and the 30-day rate of ipsilateral major stroke or death from stroke was 0.4%. The cumulative mortality rate was 13% at 5 years and 31% at 10 years. The cumulative stroke rate was 7% at 5 years and 14% at 10 years. The 50% or greater restenosis rate was higher in women than in men at 5 years (9% versus 5%; p = 0.02,), but tended to equalize later. Chiesa et al. [13] reported their results in a total of 8 403 CEA performed from 1992 to 2008 on 6 151 patients. The > 60% stenoses were deemed asymptomatic in 4 538 (54%) cases. Peri-operative mortality was 0.32%, whereas peri-operative neurological morbidity was 1.04%. Despite an evident increasing trend, there was no significant difference in the combined ipsilateral stroke and peri-operative death rate between octogenarians and younger patients (2.1% vs. 1.2%, p > 0.05).

Results issued from database analyses are consistent with those from single center studies. The 2009 report of the National Surgical Quality Improvement Program [14] showed among patients without any neurologic symptoms (2 245 from 3 949 patients) a 1.3% 30-day stroke rate, a 0.5% death rate and a 1.7% combined stroke/death rate. In this global series, the criteria for "high risk", as defined by the SAPPHIRE study [15], were met by 30% of the patients and 19% were octogenarians. After review of 3 259 CEAs from the Society for Vascular Surgery carotid vascular registry, including 58% for asymptomatic disease, Sidawy et al. [16] reported 30-day stroke/death/myocardial infarction rate of 3.75% in symptomatic patients and 1.97% in asymptomatic patients (p = 0.05). Even larger contemporary series consistently demonstrate excellent peri-operative outcomes after CEA. In the Nationwide Inpatient Sample (NIS) database , which includes results for 122 984 CEAs performed in 2005, Timaran et al. [17] reported in-hospital mortality rate of 0.6% and stroke rate of 1.1%. It should be underlined that the vast majority of patients (92.3%) were operated for asymptomatic disease with excellent postoperative stroke (1%) an in-hospital mortality (0.5%) rates. From the same NIS database including results for 245 000 CEAs performed in 2003 and 2004, among which 92% were for asymptomatic disease, McPhee et al. [18] already reported a stroke rate of 0.4% and an in-hospital mortality rate of 0.9%. Obviously, these excellent results compare favourably with those coming from large RCTs. Effectively, for asymptomatic disease only, ACAS [1] showed a 30-day procedural death/stroke risk of 2.3% (including a 1.2% rate of angiographic complications) and ACST [2] showed a 3.1% risk.

Moreover, despite it has been thought for several years that CEA's results have reached its limits, several studies demonstrated improving outcomes during recent years of practice. Matsen et al. [19] reported an in-hospital stroke/rate death of 1.3% among nearly 24 000 CEAs, including 84.8% for asymptomatic disease, performed between, 1993 and 2003. During the study period, they observed that stroke rate improved from 2.12% in 1994 to 0.29 to 0.65% from 1996 to 2003. Similarly, Kragsterman et al. [20] reviewed outcomes of 671 asymptomatic patients undergoing CEA in Sweden between 1994 and 1998 (330 patients) and 1999 and 2003 (341 patients). They demonstrated that stroke/death rate, of 2.1% during the entire period, improved from 3.3% to 0.9% between the first and the second period of the study. Possible explanations of this improvement not only include improvements in surgical techniques and anesthetic management but also advancements in medical treatment against hypertension and hyperlipidemia. Then, since large RCTs were published, one must recognize that excellent early results are now achieved in contemporary practice with CEA, and this not only in tertiary care centers.

Risk factors for peri-operative death and stroke after CEA were recently assessed by the NYCASS Study [21], a population-based cohort of 9 308 CEA performed on Medicare patients from January 1998 through June 1999 in New York State. Patients were asymptomatic in 6653 cases (71.5%). The 30-day rate of death or stroke was 2.71% among 5 200 asymptomatic patients with no history of stroke/transient ischemic attack (TIA). It reached 4.06% among 1 453 asymptomatic patients with a distant history of stroke/TIA, 5.62% among those operated on for carotid TIA, 7.89% of those with stroke, and 13.33% in those with crescendo TIA/stroke-in-evolution. Significant multivariable predictors of death or stroke included age ≥ 80 years (OR, 1.30), nonwhite (OR, 1.83), admission from the emergency department (OR, 1.95), asymptomatic but distant history of stroke/TIA (OR, 1.40), TIA as an indication for surgery (OR, 1.81), stroke as the indication (OR, 2.40), crescendo TIA/stroke-in-evolution (OR, 3.61), contralateral carotid stenosis ≥ 50% (OR, 1.44), severe disability (OR, 2.94), coronary artery disease (OR, 1.51), and diabetes on insulin (OR, 1.55). Another recent study [22], using data collected as part of the Vascular Study Group of Northern New England, aimed to investigate risk factors for stroke and death after CEA. This group reviewed 2 714 patients undergoing 3 092 primary CEAs at 11 hospitals from 2003 to 2007. Thirty-day stroke and death rate was 1.8%. In multivariate analyses, emergency CEA (OR, 7.0), contralateral internal carotid artery occlusion (OR, 2.8), pre-operative ipsilateral cortical stroke (OR, 2.4), congestive heart failure (OR, 1.6), and age > 70 (OR, 1.3) were associated with postoperative stroke or death. Pre-operative antiplatelet therapy was protective (OR, 0.4). In the subgroup of asymptomatic patients (56%), multivariate analysis showed that contralateral ICA occlusion (OR, 3.7) and age > 70 years (OR, 2.9) were associated with an increased risk of 30-day stroke or death. The predicted patient risk of stroke or death varied from < 1% in patients with no risk factors to nearly 4% in patients aged > 70 years with a contralateral ICA occlusion.

Is the spontaneous risk of the disease so high?

It is now widely recognized that CEA is a low-risk procedure for treating severe symptomatic and asymptomatic carotid disease, with excellent long-term durability [23]. However, some opinion leaders consider that the real benefit of surgery is largely counterbalanced by a low spontaneous risk of the disease [3]. In fact, their argument is not limited to a medical one but rather includes an economical one.

Regarding the spontaneous risk of the disease, it is admitted that the absolute risk reduction of any stroke and death after CEA is small. More precisely, it might not exceed 3% over three years for the outcome of any stroke. However, it is possible that the studies included in reviews providing this evaluation are biased against surgery, since patients in the medical arm were often allowed to cross over to CEA after presenting a TIA. In a recent and mathematically speaking outstanding demonstration, Ross Naylor [3] finally demonstrated that, although it is stated that CEA will reduce the risk of stroke in asymptomatic patients by 50%, a strategy aimed at treating all asymptomatic patients could only prevent 5% of all strokes destined to occur. Furthermore, he affirmed that this 5% rate is an overestimate and that several years would be needed to treat all patients by CEA or CAS screened with a 60%-99% asymptomatic stenosis, depending on the number of yearly operated cases.

Apart from this logistical problem, the same author questioned elsewhere the financial aspect of such a policy [24]. Commenting the 2005 Mc Phee [18] analysis, in which 91% of cases treated by CEA and 9% of cases treated by CAS were asymptomatic cases, he stated that the annual cost to the US Health Services would equate to 21 billion dollars for "unnecessary interventions". It is noticeable that this analysis led to an estimated cost needed for preventing one "any stroke" at five years of about $370 provided procedural risk was 2.3%. This cost might reach about $ 428 in case of a 3.8% procedural risk. The Cochrane review [25] of CEA for asymptomatic carotid stenosis gave an estimation of cost effectiveness of the procedure in Australia in 1997. It was concluded that the public health impact of operating on all patients with asymptomatic disease was likely to be small, especially that the incidence of asymptomatic 60% to 99% stenosis is relatively low.

At last, one must recognize with Naylor [24] that improvements in what now constitutes the optimal medical therapy may have reduced the spontaneous risk of stroke at a lower level than that observed in ACAS and ACST. In ACST [3], the progressive increase in the proportion of patients receiving statin therapy ranged from 17% during the 1993 to 1996 period to more than 90% by the end of 2003. During the same periods of the study, the 5-year risk of any stroke decreased from 17.5 % in ACAS to 11.8% in ASCT. This accounts for a 33% relative risk reduction during the period. Also, there were proportional reductions in the 5-year risk of any major stroke (down 33% from 9.1% in ACAS to 6.1% in ACST) and in ipsilateral stroke (down 52% from 11.0% in ACAS to 5.3 % in ACST). The 10-year data presented by ACST support the evidence of a sustained decline in the annual rate of ipsilateral and any stroke over the last two decades. Indeed, in the second 5-year period of the study, the 5-year risk of ipsilateral stroke felt to 3.6%. This declining stroke risk might be mainly attributed to improvements in medical therapy.

But may some intrinsic factors of the patient influence the spontaneous risk of stroke? The investigators of the ACSRS "natural history" study followed-up 1 115 asymptomatic patients treated with medical therapy [26]. They identified significant differences in patients' subgroups with respect to stroke and death risk. In the highest risk group, which included patients with 82%-99% stenosis (NASCET criteria) and history of contralateral TIA and serum creatinine level > 0.085 mmol/L, the annual ipsilateral stroke rate was 4.3% compared with 0.7% in the lowest risk group. Patients with a 90%-99% stenosis plus the two caveats faced a 6.5% annual risk of stroke. As Naylor remarked [24], the number of patients fulfilling all three of these conditions actually seems quite low in clinical practice. However, even though it is an overall weaker relation than that observed in symptomatic carotid stenosis, there is a relationship between severity of the stenosis and the risk of ipsilateral ischemic stroke. The weakness of this relationship is well illustrated by the lack of association between stenosis severity and CEA benefit in ACAS and ACST. Moreover, there is evidence that progression of carotid stenosis could be associated with an increased risk of ischemic stroke.

Current results of carotid artery stenting

As proposed above for evaluating CEA, estimates of the current results of CAS can be obtained from single center publications, large registries and collective studies and RCTs. However, only few data concern asymptomatic disease.

In their review of the literature published in 2004, Higashida et al. [27] collected the results of 11 large CAS series reported since 1996 which included a total of 1 311 patients. From 10 series, it could be estimated that the mean proportion of asymptomatic disease was 46.3% (range, 27% to 72%). Despite comparative analysis of these reports was made difficult by inconsistencies in the sample populations, lesion characteristics, endovascular techniques and outcome data, the overall reported rate of technical success was > 95%. Procedure-related mortality rates, including cardiac deaths, were 0.6% to 4.5%. Minor stroke rates were 0% to 6.5% and restenosis rate was < 5%. However, studies representing very high-risk cohorts were excluded. In a clinical update, Goodney et al. [28] summarized the results of 27 case-series including more than 24.000 patients and reported between 1996 and 2005. The mean proportion of asymptomatic disease was 47.3% (range, 23 to 92%). Embolic protection devices had been widely used since 2002. The 30-day stroke rates varied from 1% to 8%, with a trend towards lower rates as experience increased with time. Overall, the average 30-day stroke rate was 3% across all studies (range, 1.1% to 7.8%) and the average combined 30-day rate of stroke, myocardial infarction, or death was 4% (range, 0% to 10.9%). Early restenosis rates, only reported in half of the studies, ranged from 1% to 8%.

Recently the early and long-term results of a retrospective study were published involving 3 178 CAS procedures performed at four European carotid high volume centers [29]. The asymptomatic population included 1 861 patients (58.5%). The type of stroke or peri-operative deaths rate was 7.4% at 5 years. Stroke-related mortality rates were 0.9%, 2%, 3.3%, 4.8% and 6.1% at year 1, 2, 3, 4 and 5, respectively. All neurological complications rates were 3.3%, 5.4%, 7%, 10.1% and 10.6% at year 1, 2, 3, 4 and 5, respectively. These rates were considered by the authors as comparable to those of RCTs for asymptomatic patients.

In their 2006 clinical update, Goodney et al. [28] reported the results of 8 industry-sponsored trials, yet never published in peer-reviewed journals, which included 37% to 83% of asymptomatic patients. A total of 2 827 patients underwent a CAS procedure. The overall 30-day stroke rate ranged from 1.4% to 4.4% and the death rate ranged from 0.4% to 5.8%. Recently, an amalgamated registry [30] of high risk for surgery patients undergoing CAS presented data from two large prospective postmarket surveillance stenting studies. In all, 6 320 patients either enrolled in EXACT (2 145 patients) or in CAPTURE 2 (4 175 patients) were available for outcome analysis. For the combined asymptomatic population (5 559 patients, 88%), the 30-day death and stroke rate was 3.2%. Thirty-day death and major stroke rate was 1.3%. For the nonoctogenarian asymptomatic group (4 282 patients), the 30-day death and stroke rate was 2.9%. Most (75%) of the strokes were minor. For the octogenarian asymptomatic group (1 277 patients), the 30-day death and stroke rate was 4.4%. The 30-day rate of death and stroke for the 371 asymptomatic patients with anatomic high-risk features was 2.7%. Again, most (78%) of the strokes were minor. The 30-day rate of death and stroke for the 4 603 asymptomatic patients with physiological factors unfavorable for surgery was 3.3%. The actual definition of high surgical risk still remains a matter of debate. However, the results of this combined study bring a significant achievement for the practice of CAS in patients deemed high-risk for surgery, especially that in the comparable population, they met the AHA standards and recommendations.

The number of RCTs comparing CEA and CAS in patients with asymptomatic disease exclusively is limited [31,33]. Thus, only low to moderate quality evidence is available. CAVATAS-2001 included only 16 asymptomatic patients among 504 patients. KENTUCKY-2004 included 85 asymptomatic patients randomized into CAS in 43 cases and surgery in the 42 remaining cases. No post-operative event occurred in both groups. The SAPPHIRE trial [15] included 238 asymptomatic patients among 334 deemed high risk for surgery, 167 of whom were treated with CAS. However, the results were not reported separately for the asymptomatic cohort. Also, the cumulative incidence of major cardiovascular event (stroke, death and myocardial infarction rate) at one year following the procedure was lower in the stenting groups (12.2% vs. 20.1%) but no difference remained when only stroke and death rates were compared.

Four large ongoing trials, ACT-1, ACST II, TACIT and SPACE II, intend to make a randomized comparison between CAS en CEA in asymptomatic patients [3]. Details on these trials are available on following sites for ACT-1 (www.act1trial.com), ASCT II (www.acst.org.uk), TACIT (TACIT@SIR-Foundation.org) and Space II (Neurologie@med-uni-heidelberg.de). In all, the number of patient intended to be enrolled in these trials is about 13 000. This implies the inclusion of moderate stenoses (≥ 50% in TACIT and SPACE II), although the spontaneous neurological risk of such lesions seems really low. On the contrary, ACT-1 aims to randomize low-risk patients with severe (80% to 99%) carotid artery stenosis. Despite a comparison of interventional therapies against best medical treatment is nowadays fully justified, no medical arm is included in ACT-I and ACST II. In the four studies however, all patients are supposed to receive a dual antiplatelet therapy. Only 540 patients out of 3 640 are planned to receive medical treatment alone in SPACE II. It is questioned whether this sample of population will provide a sufficiently powered statistical analysis. Naturally, continued effort and the eventual completion of these trials will improve the understanding of the relative indications and contraindications of CAS and CEA.

Attention has recently been focused on the identification of patients at greater risk for adverse outcome during and after CAS in an effort to refine the indications for its use. The higher rate of adverse outcomes in octogenarians has become evident after the CREST trial [34] which reported a 30-day stroke and death rate of 12.1% for octogenarians compared with 3.23% among nonoctogenarians. This rate was not influenced by symptom status, lesion severity or use of distal embolic protection devices. The increased risk with age actually starts at 75 and accelerates over 80. Anatomic factors such as adverse arch anatomy, arch elongation, vessel tortuosity, calcification have been associated with increased risk of CAS and seem to be more prevalent in the elderly. A scoring system might there be useful to categorize expected difficulty on CAS and aid case selection [35]. Recently, Faggioli et al. [36] suggested the existence of a pathogenetic association between the degree of atherosclerotic changes of the aortic arch and the risk of peri-procedural embolism, at least in patients with complex aortic arch anatomy and carotid tortuosity in whom catheterization maneuvers are likely to be prolonged. It was also suggested that high aortic arch calcium content and type II arches may be markers of increased potential for embolization during arch catheterization maneuvers. More recent reports than CREST suggest that CAS can be performed with low complication rates in elderly patients [37,38]. However, it remained uncertain whether asymptomatic elderly patients derive benefit from carotid revascularization because, in addition to periprocedural risks, longevity following the procedure has to be considered. Recently, Chiam et al. [37] reported the outcome of 142 elderly patients (≥ 80 years) undergoing 153 CAS procedures. In the subgroup of 114 (72%) asymptomatic patients, the any stroke and death rate was 2.6%. Independent predictors of mortality in this subgroup were smoking history, previous ipsilateral or contralateral carotid endarterectomy, hemoglobin level and increasing age. Finally, a proportion of 85% and 76% of elderly patients survived 2 and 3 years, respectively. These results suggest that if the periprocedural event rates are within the AHA guidelines standards (< 3%), as was the case for this series, the benefit-to-risk ratio may favor carotid revascularization in the asymptomatic elderly subgroup. But this retrospective study only analyzed highly selected patients, with suitable clinical and anatomic criteria, in order to exclude patients at high stent risk. More over, no comparative group exists with medical therapy or CEA. The results should thus be determined more conclusively and data from ongoing randomized trials such as CREST appears of major importance in this domain.

The safety and efficacy of CAS in women as compared to men is another concern which remained to be adequately investigated in asymptomatic patients [38]. In fact, the SAPPHIRE trial did not separately analyse outcomes for women, who represented one third of the patients. Less than 30% of patients were women in the SPACE trial and this subgroup suffered a large difference in periprocedural complication rates between CAS and CEA (1.71%) than men (0.04%). Also, the EVA-3S trial enrolled < 30% females and did not make any gender-specific observations. Recently, Goldstein et al. [39] compared the outcome of 93 women and 135 men undergoing 97 and 141 CASs, respectively. Fifty-four (55,7%) women and 92 (65.3%) men were asymptomatic. The combined 30-day stroke, death and myocardial infarction rate was 5.7% for males compared to 5.4% for females. There were no differences observed in the long-term survival, stroke-free survival, or restenosis rates between genders. In the lack of randomized trials to answer questions regarding the impact of gender on CAS, the results of this retrospective study suggest equivalent outcomes in women when compared to men.

At last, one can wonder about the results of CAS according to operator specialty. In their review of the 2005 to 2006 state In-Patient database from New York and Florida, Steppacher et al. [40] analyzed the outcome of 4 001 procedures performed by vascular surgeons (1 350 cases) or non vascular surgeons (interventional cardiologists and radiologists, 2 651 cases). Despite the fact that during this period CAS was supposed to be exclusively offered to patients deemed at high risk for CEA, the proportion of asymptomatic disease was very high in both groups (92.3%). Fortunately, peri-operative rates of stroke and death appeared quite low and consistent with the widely admitted "3% rule" [41], except that outcomes were not analyzed after discharge. Anyway, a propensity score matching for more than 12 covariates, including pre-operative neurological status, showed no difference between vascular surgeons and non-vascular surgeons in-hospital stroke (1.1% vs. 1.7%) and mortality (0.9% vs. 0.5%) rates.

How might we identify threatening carotid asymptomatic disease?

Identification of asymptomatic patients who are at increased risk of stroke despite medical treatment would improve the yield of prophylactic invasive treatment [42]. Potential ways to identify these high risk patients include an epidemiological and demographical approach (patient features), an anatomic and pathological approach (carotid plaque features) and a hemodynamical approach (intracranial features).

Patient features

Some of the main epidemiological and demographical data have already been addressed above and can be resumed as following. The risk of ipsilateral stroke in patients with asymptomatic severe carotid stenosis increases with age. For a given age group, unstable asymptomatic plaques as well as stroke rates are higher in men.

Other general vascular disease risk factors, such as hypertension or cardiac disease, are common among vascular patients and in isolation are poor predictors of stroke. Blood inflammatory markers (blood white cells, C-reactive protein, homocystein levels...), although useful in general vascular risk disease stratification, are not effective in stratifying ipsilateral stroke risk.

Carotid plaque features

Although this relation exists [43], the relation between asymptomatic carotid stenosis severity and the risk of ipsilateral ischemic stroke is weaker than that observed in symptomatic stenosis. This probably explains why ACAS and ACST failed to demonstrate a relation between stenosis severity and CEA benefit. However, progression of carotid stenosis and irregular carotid plaque surface [44] may be associated with an increased risk of ischemic stroke. In addition, the carotid plaque composition may represent an independent risk factor for ischemic stroke. Several observational ultrasound studies have suggested that increased plaque echolucency, a marker of plaque lipid and hemorrhage content, is associated with higher risks of stroke or TIA distal to a carotid stenosis [45]. Contrast agent microbubbles enhancement, which is correlated with carotid plaque neovascularization, appears more intense in symptomatic patients [46].

However, the reproducibility of these techniques remains questioned. A systematic review [47] of dedicated observational studies even failed to demonstrate a statistical correlation between carotid intraplaque hemorrhage, diagnosed on CEA specimens, and clinical symptoms. Determination of the Gray Scale Median (GSM) using high resolution B-mode echographic images combined with a quantitative computer-assisted measurement of plaque echogenicity, has been proposed as an alternative method to evaluate plaque morphology. After examination of almost 300 plaques, Sabetai et al. [48] showed that hypoechoic plaques are more likely to be symptomatic than hyperechoic ones. Accordingly, the ICAROS study [49] demonstrated that low GSM plaques (≤ 25) were independent predictors of stroke complicating CAS. However, there are no available studies which aimed to determine whether the GSM technique could be a useful predictor of stroke in a medically treated cohort of patients with asymptomatic carotid artery stenosis. In vivo high-resolution magnetic resonance imaging (MRI) appears to be a promising technique capable to measure the volume of carotid plaques and characterize their components [50]. In fact, histological studies have observed that stable plaques are characterized by a low grade chronic inflammatory infiltrate, whereas unstable and symptomatic plaques are characterized by an active inflammation. Carotid ultrasound investigation may allow identification of microvessels with neoangiogenesis at the base of unstable plaques [51]. With MRI, inflammatory activity of carotid plaques can be investigated using ultrasmall particles of iron oxide as targeted contrast agent [44]. Asymptomatic plaques have less incidence of fibrous cap rupture and juxta-luminal hemorrhage while arteries with thin or ruptured fibrous caps, intraplaque hemorrhage, larger maximum % lipid-rich/necrotic core and larger maximum wall thickness are associated with the occurrence of subsequent cerebrovascular events [50]. Severity of white matter ischemia has been shown to be an independent predictor of stroke risk. However, the number of prospective data demonstrating a relationship between plaque morphology or rupture on MRI and risk of ipsilateral ischemic event in asymptomatic patients is limited. Several other novel techniques, such as Fluorine -18-labelled fluorodeoxyglucose positron emission tomography (FDG-PET), optical coherence tomography (OCT) and time-resolved laser-induced fluorescence spectroscopy (TR-LIFS) have also been used for the characterisation of vulnerable carotid plaques [52]. However, although pathological features associated with plaque instability, such as ulceration, plaque hemorrhage, plaque rupture or lumen thrombus may be encountered in about 20%-50% of symptomatic patients, they may also be seen in about 15%-45% of asymptomatic patients. FDG-PET has been furthermore used to monitor the therapeutic effect of statins on the stabilization of vulnerable atherosclerotic plaques.

Intra-cranial features

Based on pathophysiological considerations, the hemodynamic impairment resulting from a carotid artery stenosis may be a useful adjunct to identify high-risk patients [53]. However, most studies which assessed impaired cerebrovascular reactivity, relative cerebral hypoperfusion or metabolic changes on MRI as predictors of stroke risk suffer from methodological problems. In most cases, these studies have mixed pathologies (complete occlusions, intracranial disease) or symptomatic status. Secondly, evidence of cerebral impairment by one method is not always correlated with abnormal results by another. Lastly, assessment of outcomes often relies on a retrospective study design, subsequently biased by lost to follow-up patients, lack of blinding approach or censoring of patients who were finally treated surgically.

On the opposite, a well designed study [54] showed a link between cerebrovascular reactivity to hypercapnia (measured by transcranial ultrasonography and calculated by the breath-holding index values in the middle cerebral arteries) and the risk of ischemic events ipsilateral to severe asymptomatic carotid stenosis. In two studies [55,56], absence of micro-embolic signals detected by transcranial Doppler examination was associated with a low risk of subsequent stroke or TIA. On the contrary, stroke related arteries (acute or in the past) are associated with a higher presence of micro-embolic signals. Despite these facts, detection of micro-embolic signals is not of proven use for risk stratification, choice of medical therapy or choice of intervention. According to Ritter et al. [57], micro-embolic signal detection would be ready for the clinical routine in symptomatic patients only.

Is there a place for medical therapy?

Medical treatment has improved substantially since the randomized trials of surgery versus medicine for carotid stenoses were completed. Newer antiplatelet agents are available and more aggressive and effective management of risk factors associated with carotid artery disease, such as hypercholesterolemia, is a rule. It is now widely considered that intensive medical treatment may have reduced the natural history risk of stroke to levels below that observed in ACAS and ACST.

Antihypertensive treatment aims to maintain blood pressure consistently under 140/90 mmHg. In patients with diabetes or chronic renal failure, the target is lowered to 130/80 mmHg. It is demonstrated that a 5-6 mmHg lowering of the systolic blood pressure or 2-3 mmHg of the diastolic blood pressure leads to a 40% relative risk reduction for stroke [58]. This result is independent of age and form of hypertension and even holds true in patients over 80 year old or suffering from isolated systolic hypertension. In the absence of definitive recommendation, the choice between antihypertensive agents may be guided by the presence of co-morbid conditions and by the cost.

Amarenco and Labreuche [59] recently reported a meta-analysis of statins for stroke prevention. Over 165 000 high-risk patients were pooled from 24 randomized trials with at least 1 000 patients each. A consistent 18% reduction of all strokes was demonstrated in patients randomized to statins. Each 1 mmol/L (39 mg/dL) reduction of LDL cholesterol by statins was correlated to a 21.1% reduction of relative risk for stroke. The lower the LDL cholesterol concentration, the greater was the risk reduction for both primary and secondary prevention of stroke. However, the incidence of fatal stroke was reduced by 13% but this didn't reach the statistical significance. The incidence of hemorrhagic stroke did not increase but caution was recommended when considering statin therapy in patients with prior cerebral hemorrhage. It is now admitted that in case of carotid artery disease, lipid-lowering therapy should include a statin and aims to achieve a LDL-cholesterol value of less than 100 mg/dL. In case of associated coronary artery disease or in patients with multiple vascular risk factors, this target should be lowered to a value of less than 70 mg/dL. Statins produces a relative risk reduction for stroke of approximately 26% over a follow-up period of 4.7 years. Another advantage of statins may be related to secondary effects that might contribute to carotid plaque regression or at least delay plaque progression, although the benefit derived from pleiotropic effects of statin therapy remains unclear. In ACST, the most important change in medical practice during the 10 years that the study recruited was an increase in the proportion of patients receiving statin therapy [24]. Although only 17% of patients received statin therapy during the first three years of inclusion (1993-1996), 70% and more than 90% were respectively taking statins by the end of 2003 and by 2008. However, fewer than 40% of patients were taking statins by the midpoint of the trial duration (1997) and prior to 2002, a significant proportion of female patients did not receive statin therapy at all. More importantly, the doses of statin commonly used during the first five years of the study were by far lower than those currently recommended.

Smoking cessation is imperative. Necessary psychological or medical assistance should be given in order to obtain it. Patients should be advised to reduce alcohol intake. They should be screened for diabetes and treated if any. Antiplatelet therapy should be administered all life long, either using a single treatment (aspirin or clopidogrel) or a dual antiplatelet therapy in patients with concomitant symptomatic coronary artery disease, recent coronary stenting and severe peripheral arterial occlusive disease. However, there is very little evidence that antiplatelet therapy is beneficial for preventing stroke and a long-tem protective effect of aspirin therapy has not been clearly demonstrated yet. Associated measures include modifications in lifestyle such as a regular program of aerobic exercise along with a diet low in saturated fat. Most of all, patients with asymptomatic carotid disease should be instructed about neurological symptoms and how to seek for medical attention if one of them occur.

Despite the lack of any conclusive grade I evidence supporting the benefit of medical treatment alone, there is a recent trend to advocate it for prevention of stroke associated with asymptomatic severe carotid stenosis. In her systematic review and analysis of 11 studies isolated among 67 [60], Anne L. Abbott intended on demonstrating that medical "intervention" is now best than CEA or CAS, mainly because high risk patients who may benefit from these two techniques cannot be identified. The key findings of her review included falls in reported average annual rates of ipsilateral and any territory stroke with isolated medical intervention since the mid 1980s. Moreover, she indicated that from 2001, average annual rates of ipsilateral strokes among patients treated with medical intervention alone fell below those of patients treated by CEA during ACAS. She also found current medical intervention alone as being in Australia at least 3 to 8 times more cost-effective than surgery and medical therapy. Naturally, her conclusions are not supported by a specifically dedicated randomized control study. The demonstration totally relies on statistical tests retrospectively applied to data issued from studies supposed to share fundamental criteria for sound methodology. However, the same method was not used to estimate the potential fall of these rates in the surgical arm of the studies. There were no "dynamic" comparisons between medical and surgical therapies, for specific periods of the studies. Considerations on the experience of surgeons participating to the trials are lacking. Sample sizes were heterogeneous. Data extracted from four studies involved author personal communications rather than fully published and peer reviewed material. Two studies (ECST and NASCET) designed to determine outcome of symptomatic disease were even though included. At last, absence of raw data in some studies led to take into account Kaplan Meier estimates rather than observed values for average annual stroke rates. For all these reasons, we consider that the caveat against surgery contained in this review should be taken very cautiously. Recommendations and guidelines issued from scientific societies or public health administrations appear to us of a greater value.

Guidelines for dealing with asymptomatic carotid surgery

The management of patients with asymptomatic carotid disease remains controversial. The literature on this subject abounds in studies with often discordant results and conclusions regarding the interest of CEA, CAS or medical treatment. Some opinion leaders try to convince the whole medical world that their point of view is the one to follow. Scientific societies and public health administrations may help to make a decision by appointing committees of experts in order to formulate evidence-based clinical guidelines. Mainly because both surgery and medical therapy may have devastating consequences, it appears logical that physicians make the final decision, specifically tailored to the patient they face. Below are detailed the available guidelines focused on asymptomatic carotid disease.

French guidelines from the "Haute Autorité de Santé" (HAS, 2007) [www.has-santé.fr]

- Asymptomatic patients with low-grade carotid stenosis (< 60%) should not be offered carotid surgical revascularization;
- asymptomatic patients with carotid stenosis (≥ 60%) should be offered carotid surgical revascularization if the 30-day stroke /death rate is < 3%;
- there are no valid indications for CAS in asymptomatic patients with carotid stenosis; however, in case of stenosis ≥ 60%, if a carotid artery revascularization is deemed necessary and if the surgeon estimates conventional surgery as being contra-indicated, CAS may exceptionally be proposed after a multidisciplinary discussion with written conclusions.

North American guidelines from the Society for Vascular Surgery (SVS, 2008)

- Asymptomatic patients with low-grade carotid stenosis (< 60%) should be offered optimal medical therapy rather than revascularization (Grade I recommendation, high quality evidence);
- asymptomatic patients with moderate to severe carotid stenosis (≥ 60%) should be offered CEA plus medical therapy as long as the operative risk is low (Grade I recommendation, high quality evidence);
- CAS is inappropriate for asymptomatic patients with ≥ 60% carotid stenosis. Possible exceptions may include patients with acceptable medical risk who present with severe carotid artery stenosis (≥ 80%) and high anatomic risk for CEA but with compelling anatomy for CAS (Grade I recommendation, low quality evidence). High anatomical risk defined as previous CEA with recurrent stenosis; prior ipsilateral irradiation to neck with permanent skin changes; previous ablative neck surgery; common carotid artery stenosis below the clavicle; contralateral vocal cord paralysis; and presence of a tracheotomy stoma [61].

European guidelines from the European Society for Vascular Surgery (ESVS, 2009)

- CEA is recommended in asymptomatic men < 75 year-old with 70%-99% stenosis if the peri-operative stroke/death risk is < 3% (Grade A);
- the benefit of CEA in asymptomatic women with

carotid stenosis is significantly less than in man (Grade A). CEA should therefore be considered only in younger fit women (Grade A);
- it is advisable to offer CAS in asymptomatic patients only in high-volume centers with documented low peri-procedural stroke and death rates or within well-conducted clinical trials (Grade C);
- for medical patients at extremely high-risk (severe medical co-morbidities at the same time), best medical treatment might be the best option instead of invasive intervention (Grade C);
- CAS should not be offered to asymptomatic "high-risk" patients if the peri-interventional complication rate is > 3% (Grade C);
- CAS is indicated in case of contralateral laryngeal nerve palsy, previous radical nerve dissection, cervical irradiation, restenosis from prior CEA, high bifurcation or intracranial extension of a carotid lesion, provided that the peri-interventional stroke or death rate is higher than accepted for CEA (Grade C);
- CAS is not advisable in patients with extensive aortic and supra-aortic vessel plaques, calcification and tortuosity, unless performed in high volume centres with documented low peri-procedural stroke and death rate (Grade C).

These guidelines and especially those emanating from the SVS and the ESVS reveal transatlantic consensus in major areas of the decision making algorithm. The grade system used by the SVS is not only based on data but also on prevailing values and preferences. The grade system used by the ESVS only takes into account the quality of supporting data. The threshold degree of stenosis for intervention in asymptomatic patients varies between 60% for the SVS and HAS guidelines, based on ACAS, and 70% for the ESVS guidelines, based on ACST. In the three documents, a caveat regarding expected low peri-operative risk is included. ESVS document adds a gender-related caveat which seems appropriate, based on available RCTs, and an age-related caveat which is not totally supported by available data. The role of CAS is considered variably in the three documents, mainly because numerous uncertainties regarding its interest and results preclude the achievement of a consensus [62].

What is "our current best practice" for asymptomatic carotid disease?

Despite all that has been written since the publication of randomized trials, management of patients with asymptomatic carotid disease remains a matter of controversy. As concluded by Hobson et al. [61] on behalf of the Society for Vascular Surgery, "practice guidelines can be only as robust as their evidence basis". In the absence of high quality, reliable data, clinical decisions must be based on lower quality data and on clinical experience, judgment, values, and preferences". Interpretation and weighting of these data may differ from a specialist to another. Most neurologists have concluded that, despite many results could favour surgery, asymptomatic patients should not be routinely offered revascularization or even screened for carotid stenosis, but instead should be informed about the benefits and risks of medical treatment versus surgery. Most surgeons estimated that the trial data provided ample justification for surgery at centers with a proven low complication rate. What is more paradoxical is the attitude of some others who became progressively opinion leaders despite the fact that the message they delivered was a deliberate and insistent non operative pleading in case of asymptomatic disease. Using mostly statistical or economical arguments rather than medical evidence, they aimed to demonstrate that prophylactic surgery even being the probably safest approach in skilled hands, was nor medically justified nor cost-effective for public savings. Despite that message, several registries have shown a proportion of revascularized asymptomatic patients being higher than 90% [38,40]. This proportion exceeds by far the one we observe in our current practice, usually comprised between 55% and 70%. Fortunately, surgical results were almost constantly good if not excellent in asymptomatic trials and the "3% rule" [41], recommending a procedural risk < 3% in asymptomatic patients, was most frequently validated. Attention was thus focused on extra-cerebral complications, i.e. medical complications or cranial nerve injuries, although it must be underlined that in the vast majority of cases more than 90% of nerve palsies disappear completely within the first postoperative year. Partisans of CAS including cardiologists who perform more than 60% of these procedures in United States have seen here an opportunity to extend the indications of CAS. Results from the SAPPHIRE trial, which only included patients deemed high-risk for surgery, sounded like an additional evidence to behave this way. We are now informed that reasonable indications for CAS are probably extremely limited in the field of asymptomatic carotid disease. Also, unless in case of hostile anatomy (tracheotomy stoma, burnt skin from irradiation), we never propose CAS for asymptomatic patients.

What about the patient himself? As an individual, the patient never considers himself as being part of statistical estimates. He understands that his brain is threatened by a severe carotid stenosis, no matter what the overall percentage of this threat actually is. He realizes that he will (100%) or not (0%) develop a neurological complication as mid-term or long-term evolution of his disease. He expects from his surgeon a clear-cut answer to his personal problem. We are convinced that, as normal surgeons, we should not operate all patients with asymptomatic carotid stenosis and especially those with < 70% stenosis. But as experts in that domain, we should rely on strong, though not necessarily fully evidence-based, arguments and draw our own conclusions about the case of our specific patient. A case by case patient assessment and selection is required, at the end of which expert surgeons should not feel ashamed to offer a revascularization if they sincerely think it worth it. For that reason, it is essential that patients should only be referred to surgeons with a large experience and with very low complication rates. We must give the patients clear and understandable information on these complications and convince them, as deeply as we are, to take a small immediate risk in exchange for a long-term benefit. Patients who do not opt for surgery should be educated about the symptoms of TIA, amaurosis fugax and stroke. They should be advised to seek medical attention urgently in the case these symptoms arise in the future. Naturally, they should be aware of the absolute necessity of observing rigorously the best medical treatment all life long. They should also understand that denying surgery equates being exposed all life long to a cumulative risk of cerebrovascular event. They should realize that in case their carotid stenosis is very severe, irregular, or progressive, the usual frequency of annual ultrasound evaluation (once a year) will become insufficient and that operation would become urgent to consider once symptoms appear. At last, they should question about their quality of life and be prepared to answer this simple dilemma: does a three-day hospitalization for a potentially unnecessary successful carotid surgery will impair their quality of life more than dreading all life long the occurrence of an ipsilateral cerebrovascular event. There is in the literature a cruel lack of data that remains to be assessed.

REFERENCES

1 Anonymous. Endarterectomy for asymptomatic carotid artery stenosis. Executive Committee for the Asymptomatic Carotid Atherosclerosis Study. *JAMA* 1995; 273: 1421-1428.

2 Anonymous. Asymptomatic Carotid Surgery Trial (ACST) Collaborative Group Prevention of disabling and fatal strokes by successful carotid endarterectomy in patients without recent neurological symptoms: randomised controlled trial. *Lancet* 2004; 363: 1491-1502.

3 Naylor R. When and how to treat asymptomatic carotid disease? In: Branchereau A, Jacobs M (eds). *Innovative Cardiovascular Procedures*. Turin: Edizioni Minerva Medica; 2009. pp : 119-132.

4 Donnan GA, Fisher M, Macleod M et al. Stroke. *Lancet* 2008; 371: 1612-1623.

5 Liapis CD, Bell PR, Mikhailidis D et al. ESVS guidelines. Invasive treatment for carotid stenosis: indications, techniques. *Eur J Vasc Endovasc Surg* 2009; 37(4 Suppl): 1-19.

6 Feigin VL, Lawes CM, Bennett DA et al. Stroke epidemiology: a review of population-based studies of incidence, prevalence, and case-fatality in the late 20th century. *Lancet Neurol* 2003; 2: 43-53.

7 Asplund K, Karvanen J, Giampaoli S et al. MORGAM Project. Relative risks for stroke by age, sex, and population based on follow-up of 18 European populations in the MORGAM Project. *Stroke* 2009; 40: 2319-2326.

8 Abbott AL. Medical (nonsurgical) intervention alone is now best for prevention of stroke associated with asymptomatic severe carotid stenosis: results of a systematic review and analysis. *Stroke* 2009; 40: e573-583.

9 AbuRahma AF. Processes of care for carotid endarterectomy: surgical and anesthesia considerations. *J Vasc Surg* 2009; 50: 921-933.

10 Ballotta E, Da Giau G, Ermani M et al. Early and long-term outcomes of carotid endarterectomy in the very elderly: an 18-year single-center study. *J Vasc Surg* 2009; 50: 518-525.

11 Scavée V, Viejo D, Buche M et al. Six hundred consecutive carotid endarterectomies with temporary shunt and vein patch angioplasty: early and long-term results. *Cardiovasc Surg* 2001; 9: 463-468.

12 Archie JP Jr. A fifteen-year experience with carotid endarterectomy after a formal operative protocol requiring highly frequent patch angioplasty. *J Vasc Surg* 2000; 31: 724-735.

13 Chiesa R, Melissano M, Castellano R et al. Carotid endarterectomy: experience in 8403 cases. In: Kieffer E, Goëau-Brissonnière O (eds). *Carotid revascularisation in 2008*. Neuilly: GMS Santé; 2008. pp 68-80.

14 Kang JL, Chung TK, Lancaster RT et al. Outcomes after carotid endarterectomy: is there a high-risk population? A National Surgical Quality Improvement Program report. *J Vasc Surg* 2009; 49: 331-338.

15 Yadav JS, Wholey MH, Kuntz RE et al. Protected carotid-artery stenting versus endarterectomy in high-risk patients. *N Engl J Med* 2004; 7; 351: 1493-501.

16 Sidawy AN, Zwolak RM, White RA et al. Outcomes Committee for the Society for Vascular Surgery. Risk-adjusted 30-day outcomes of carotid stenting and endarterectomy: results from the SVS Vascular Registry. *J Vasc Surg* 2009; 49: 71-79.

17 Timaran CH, Veith FJ, Rosero EB et al. Intracranial hemorrhage after carotid endarterectomy and carotid stenting in the United States in 2005. *J Vasc Surg* 2009; 49: 623-628.

18 McPhee JT, Schanzer A, Messina LM et al. Carotid artery stenting has increased rates of postprocedure stroke, death, and resource utilization than does carotid endarterectomy in the United States, 2005. *J Vasc Surg* 2008; 48: 1442-1450.

19 Matsen SL, Chang DC, Perler BA et al. Trends in the in-hospital stroke rate following carotid endarterectomy in California and Maryland. *J Vasc Surg* 2006; 44: 488-495.

20 Kragsterman B, Pärsson H, Lindbäck J et al. Outcomes of carotid endarterectomy for asymptomatic stenosis in Sweden are improving: Results from a population-based registry. *J Vasc Surg* 2006; 44: 79-85.

21 Halm EA, Tuhrim S, Wang JJ et al. Risk factors for perioperative death and stroke after carotid endarterectomy: results of the new york carotid artery surgery study. *Stroke* 2009; 40: 221-229.

22 Goodney PP, Likosky DS, Cronenwett JL; for the Vascular Study Group of Northern New England. Factors associated with stroke or death after carotid endarterectomy in Northern New England. *J Vasc Surg* 2008; 48: 1139-1145.

23 Sebesta P, Sedivy P, Klika T et al. Résultats à long terme de l'endartériectomie carotidienne. In Branchereau A, Jacobs M, editors. *Chirurgie conventionnelle ou endovasculaire. Comment choisir?* Oxford: Paris Consultants Ltd; 2007. pp. 39-56.

24 Naylor AR, Gaines PA, Rothwell PM. Who benefits most from intervention for asymptomatic carotid stenosis: patients or professionals? *Eur J Vasc Endovasc Surg* 2009; 37: 625-632.

25 Chambers BR, Donnan G. Carotid endarterectomy for asymptomatic carotid stenosis. Cochrane Database of Systematic Review 2005, Issue 4. Art. No.: CD001923.DOI: 10.1002/14651858.CD001923.pub2.

26 Nicolaides AN, Kakkos SK, Griffin M et al. Severity of asymptomatic carotid stenosis and risk of ipsilateral hemispheric ischaemic events: results from the ACSRS study. *Eur J Vasc Endovasc Surg* 2005; 30: 275-284.

27 Higashida RT, Meyers PM, Phatouros CC et al. Reporting standards for carotid artery angioplasty and stent placement. *Stroke* 2004; 35: e112-134.

28 Goodney PP, Schermerhorn ML, Powell RJ. Current status of carotid artery stenting. *J Vasc Surg* 2006; 43: 406-411.

29 de Donato G, Setacci C, Deloose K et al. Long-term results of carotid artery stenting. *J Vasc Surg* 2008; 48: 1431-1440.

30 Gray WA, Chaturvedi S, Verta P et al. Thirty-day outcomes for carotid artery stenting in 6320 patients from 2 prospective, multicenter, high-surgical-risk registries. *Circ Cardiovasc Intervent* 2009; 2: 159-166.

31 Luebke T, Aleksic M, Brunkwall J. Meta-analysis of randomized trials comparing carotid endarterectomy and endovascular treatment. *Eur J Vasc Endovasc Surg* 2007; 34: 470-479.

32 Jeng JS, Liu HM, Tu YK. Carotid angioplasty with or without stenting versus carotid endarterectomy for carotid artery stenosis: a meta-analysis. J *Neurol Sci* 2008; 270: 40-47.

33 Ederle J, Featherstone RL, Brown MM. Randomized controlled trials comparing endarterectomy and endovascular treatment for carotid artery stenosis: a Cochrane systematic review. *Stroke* 2009; 40: 1373-1380.

34 Hobson RW 2nd, Howard VJ, Roubin GS et al. Carotid artery stenting is associated with increased complications in octogenarians: 30-day stroke and death rates in the CREST lead-in phase. *J Vasc Surg* 2004; 40: 1106-1111.

35 Macdonald S, Lee R, Williams R et al. Towards safer carotid artery stenting: a scoring system for anatomic suitability. *Stroke* 2009; 40: 1698-1703.

36 Faggioli G, Ferri M, Rapezzi C et al. Atherosclerotic aortic lesions increase the risk of cerebral embolism during carotid stenting in patients with complex aortic arch anatomy. *J Vasc Surg* 2009; 49: 80-85.

37 Chiam PT, Roubin GS, Panagopoulos G et al. One-year clinical outcomes, midterm survival, and predictors of mortality after carotid stenting in elderly patients. *Circulation* 2009 ; 119: 2343-2348.

38 Vogel TR, Dombrovskiy VY, Haser PB et al. Outcomes of carotid artery stenting and endarterectomy in the United States. *J Vasc Surg* 2009; 49: 325-330.

39 Goldstein LJ, Khan HU, Sambol EB et al. Carotid artery stenting is safe and associated with comparable outcomes in men and women. *J Vasc Surg* 2009; 49: 315-323.

40 Steppacher R, Csikesz N, Eslami M et al. An analysis of carotid artery stenting procedures performed in New York and Florida (2005-2006): procedure indication, stroke rate, and mortality rate are equivalent for vascular surgeons and non-vascular surgeons. *J Vasc Surg* 2009; 49: 1379-1385.

41 Roubin GS, Iyer S, Halkin A et al. Realizing the potential of carotid artery stenting: proposed paradigms for patient selection and procedural technique. *Circulation* 2006 25; 113: 2021-2030.

42 Lanzino G, Rabinstein AA, Brown RD Jr. Treatment of carotid artery stenosis: medical therapy, surgery, or stenting? *Mayo Clin Proc* 2009; 84: 362-387.

43 AbuRahma AF, Wulu JT Jr, Crotty B. Carotid plaque ultrasonic heterogeneity and severity of stenosis. *Stroke* 2002; 33: 1772-1775.

44 Kwee RM, van Oostenbrugge RJ, Hofstra L et al. Identifying vulnerable carotid plaques by noninvasive imaging. *Neurology* 2008; 70: 2401-2409.

45 Mathiesen EB, Bønaa KH, Joakimsen O. Echolucent plaques are associated with high risk of ischemic cerebrovascular events in carotid stenosis: the tromsø study. *Circulation* 2001; 103: 2171-2175.

46 Xiong L, Deng YB, Zhu Y et al. Correlation of carotid plaque neovascularization detected by using contrast-enhanced US with clinical symptoms. *Radiology* 2009; 251: 583-589.

47 Gao P, Chen ZQ, Bao YH et al. Correlation between carotid intraplaque hemorrhage and clinical symptoms: systematic review of observational studies. *Stroke* 2007; 38: 2382-2390.

48 Sabetai MM, Tegos TJ, Nicolaides AN et al. Hemispheric symptoms and carotid plaque echomorphology. *J Vasc Surg* 2000; 31: 39-49.

49 Biasi GM, Froio A, Diethrich EB et al. Carotid plaque echolucency increases the risk of stroke in carotid stenting: the Imaging in Carotid Angioplasty and Risk of Stroke (ICAROS) study. *Circulation* 2004; 110: 756-762.

50 Takaya N, Yuan C, Chu B et al. Association between carotid plaque characteristics and subsequent ischemic cerebrovascular events: a prospective assessment with MRI. Initial results. *Stroke* 2006; 37: 818-823.

51 Giannoni MF, Vicenzini E, Citone M et al. Contrast carotid ultrasound for the detection of unstable plaques with neoangiogenesis: a pilot study. *Eur J Vasc Endovasc Surg* 2009; 37: 722-727.

52 U-King-Im JM, Young V, Gillard JH. Carotid-artery imaging in the diagnosis and management of patients at risk of stroke. *Lancet Neurol* 2009; 8: 569-580.

53 Touzé E. Natural history of asymptomatic carotid artery stenosis. *Rev Neurol* 2008; 164: 793-800.

54 Silvestrini M, Vernieri F, Pasqualetti P et al. Impaired cerebral

vasoreactivity and risk of stroke in patients with asymptomatic carotid artery stenosis. *JAMA* 2000; 283: 2122-2127.

55 Abbott AL, Chambers BR, Stork JL et al. Embolic signals and prediction of ipsilateral stroke or transient ischemic attack in asymptomatic carotid stenosis: a multicenter prospective cohort study. *Stroke* 2005; 36: 1128-1133.

56 Spence JD, Tamayo A, Lownie SP et al. Absence of microemboli on transcranial Doppler identifies low-risk patients with asymptomatic carotid stenosis. *Stroke* 2005; 36: 2373-2378.

57 Ritter MA, Dittrich R, Thoenissen N et al. Prevalence and prognostic impact of microembolic signals in arterial sources of embolism. A systematic review of the literature. *J Neurol* 2008; 255: 953-961.

58 Ederle J, Brown MM. The evidence for medicine versus surgery for carotid stenosis. *Eur J Radiol* 2006; 60: 3-7.

59 Amarenco P, Labreuche J. Lipid management in the prevention of stroke: review and updated meta-analysis of statins for stroke prevention. *Lancet Neurol* 2009; 8: 453-463.

60 Abbott AL. Medical (nonsurgical) intervention alone is now best for prevention of stroke associated with asymptomatic severe carotid stenosis: results of a systematic review and analysis. *Stroke* 2009; 40: e573-e583.

61 Hobson RW 2nd, Mackey WC, Ascher E et al. Management of atherosclerotic carotid artery disease: clinical practice guidelines of the Society for Vascular Surgery. *J Vasc Surg* 2008; 48: 480-486.

62 Liapis CD, Bell PR, Mikhailidis D et al. ESVS guidelines. Invasive treatment for carotid stenosis: indications, techniques. *Eur J Vasc Endovasc Surg* 2009; 37(4 Suppl): 1-19.

4

BEST PRACTICE FOR SYMPTOMATIC CAROTID DISEASE

ROSS NAYLOR

Stroke is the leading cause of death and permanent neurological disability in the western world. However, despite popular opinion, the majority of strokes will not be attributable to symptomatic carotid disease. Out of every 100 strokes destined to occur, 20 will be hemorrhagic (intra-cranial, subarachnoid). Of the 80 ischemic strokes remaining, 20 will affect the vertebrobasilar territory, while 60 will affect the carotid territory. Of the 60 ischemic, carotid territory strokes, 30 will follow thrombo-embolism from atherosclerotic disease in the internal carotid artery (ICA), but about 66% of these will only have mild/moderate ipsilateral disease. Fifteen will be secondary to small vessel intra-cranial disease (usually affecting the lenticulostriate arteries), 9 will be cardio-embolic, 3 will be hematological and 3 will be due to miscellaneous etiologies (dissection, aneurysm, arteritis). Accordingly, the proportion of patients with strokes attributable to significant carotid disease (i.e. appropriate for reconstruction) is probably about 10%. This should be borne in mind in any discussion about the best use of resources.

This chapter will deal primarily with the evidence supporting the optimal management of patients whose symptoms are attributable to thrombo-embolism from atherosclerotic disease at the origin of the internal carotid artery. It will not deal with the management of acute stroke (e.g. thrombolysis) and it will not provide evidence or recommendations regarding technical aspects of carotid endarterectomy (CEA) (e.g. shunting, patching, anesthesia) or carotid artery stenting (CAS) (e.g. open/closed stents, protection devices).

It has become traditional to grade the level of recommendation according to the quality of evidence. In order to maintain consistency, each recommendation has been graded using the criteria adopted for the recently published European Society of Vascular Surgery Guidelines [1] which were derived from the US Agency for Healthcare Research and Quality [2]. A Grade

A Recommendation denotes evidence from at least one good quality randomized trial as part of a body of literature of overall good quality and consistency. Grade B Recommendations are derived from well conducted clinical studies in the absence of good quality randomized clinical trials. Grade C Recommendations are based upon expert committee reports or opinions and/or the clinical experiences of "respected authorities".

Clinical symptoms

The three "classical" carotid territory symptoms include; 1) hemisensory/motor loss; 2) transient or permanent monocular blindness; and 3) higher cortical dysfunction (dysphasia, visuospatial neglect). Typical vertebrobasilar symptoms include bilateral sensory/motor loss, bilateral blindness, dysarthria, ataxia, unsteadiness of gait and balance problems and should not be attributed to carotid disease unless there is evidence of developmental anomalies of the circle of Willis (e.g. persistence of the foetal configuration where the ICA is the principle source of blood to the posterior cerebral artery). Similarly, non-hemispheric symptoms (isolated diplopia, isolated vertigo, isolated dizziness, syncope and presyncope) should not be attributed to carotid disease, unless they co-exist with one or more "classical" carotid territory symptoms. Most transient ischemic attacks (TIAs)/minor strokes attributable to extra-cranial carotid disease follow thrombo-embolism. Only a minority follow hemodynamic failure. Examples of clinical symptoms suggestive of a hemodynamic etiology include those precipitated by ingestion of food or emerging from a hot bath.

Recommendations

1) All patients reporting carotid territory symptoms should be referred to dedicated cerebral vascular clinics in order that they can be investigated and treated as soon as possible (Grade A);
2) referral should never be influenced by the presence or absence of a carotid bruit (Grade B);
3) isolated non-hemispheric symptoms should not be attributed to extracranial ICA disease (Grade B).

Investigation

Since the landmark randomized trials reported in 1991 (see later), there has been a major change in practice within health systems towards expedited investigation and treatment in patients with symptomatic cerebral vascular disease. Accordingly, the 2008 Guidelines issued by the European Stroke Organisation (ESO) [3] recommend that Governments should undertake a systematic review of practice/education to ensure that 1) patients understand the importance of reporting symptoms rapidly to their family doctor; 2) that family doctors (and hospitals) should now recognise that TIA/minor strokes are emergencies (just as they do for heart attacks or unstable angina); and that 3) emergency services should rapidly triage and direct symptomatic patients either to dedicated stroke units or to rapid access TIA clinics [3].

The evidence underpinning the move towards expedited intervention will be discussed later. However, the ESO makes the following recommendations regarding investigations in recently symptomatic patients presenting with TIA or minor stroke.

Recommendations

1) All patients with a suspected TIA/minor stroke should undergo expedited baseline investigations including; full blood count, biochemical screen (to include urea/electrolytes, glucose, liver function tests, cholesterol), ECG and a chest X-ray (Grade A);
2) in patients with a suspected TIA or minor stroke, urgent computed tomography (CT) or magnetic resonance imaging (MRI) is recommended in order to exclude hemorrhage (Grade A);
3) all patients presenting with a suspected TIA/minor stroke should undergo expedited carotid imaging by Duplex ultrasound, CT angiography or MR angiography (Grade A);
4) routine intra-arterial catheter angiography (mandatory in the original international trials) is now considered unnecessary because of the risk of procedural stroke (Grade A). [3]

There has been much debate about which "non-invasive" imaging modality should become the new "gold standard". In reality, the choice will depend upon availability/access to CT angiography (CTA) or MR angiography (MRA), institutional preferences, the experience of vascular sonographers and whether CAS is being considered. In order to address this issue, the UK Health Technology Assessment (HTA) undertook a systematic review and meta-analysis [4] of studies comparing the accuracy of ultrasound, MRA (including contrast enhanced MRA [CEMRA]) and CTA [but not multi-detector CTA, MDCTA]).

The HTA concluded that while CEMRA was the most accurate imaging modality overall (sensitivity 94%, specificity 93% for diagnosing a 70%-99% stenosis), its generalizability was limited by inaccessibility and delays. As a consequence, the HTA recommended that Duplex ultrasound should remain the "first line" modality for diagnosing 70%-99% ICA stenoses because of 1) low cost; 2) the higher number of strokes prevented in the long term because patients would be undergo CEA more quickly than if other imaging modalities were used; 3) its overall robustness in sensitivity analyses; and 4) its ability to be performed within "single visit clinics". The HTA [4] did, however, highlight concerns about the reliability of Duplex ultrasound in patients with 50%-69% stenoses. Here the specificity remained high (0.91), but the sensitivity fell to 0.36. This compares with a sensitivity of 89% and a specificity of 84% for diagnosing 70%-99% stenoses.

It is, however, essential that surgeons and vascular sonographers know which stenosis measurement is being used in their institution (ECST or NASCET). In the UK there is some confusion over practice (most centers are probably using the NASCET measurement method) [5]. In general, a 50% NASCET stenosis is approximately equivalent to a 75% ECST, while a 70% NASCET stenosis equates to an 85% ECST lesion.

Based largely upon the evidence from the HTA systematic review, a number of recommendations/suggestions regarding the optimal investigation of recently symptomatic patients with TIA/minor stroke can now be made.

Recommendations

1) Duplex ultrasound is the first line imaging modality for the majority of patients presenting with a suspected TIA/minor stroke (Grade A);
2) centers, surgeons and sonographers must know whether the stenosis measurement method used in their hospital is NASCET or ECST based. This is crucial to ensure that inappropriate management decisions are avoided (Grade B);
3) where possible (and especially if there is doubt about the accuracy of the ultrasound scan), some form of corroborative imaging should be considered (MDCTA, CEMRA); this should not, however, lead to significant delays in planned interventions (Grade A);
4) patients being considered for CAS require expedited CEMRA or MDCTA (in addition to Duplex ultrasound) in order to provide additional information; e.g. extent of aortic arch disease, vessel tortuosity/calcification, integrity of the circle of Willis (Grade B);
5) if the surgeon plans to undertake CEA on the basis of ultrasound alone, it would be preferable if a second sonographer repeated the scan to confirm the presence of a 70%-99% stenosis. This also ensures internal validation of vascular laboratory performance (Grade B);
6) in light of the lower specificity of ultrasound in the diagnosis of 50%-69% stenoses, the HTA advises performing corroborative CEMRA or MDCTA studies in patients with 50%-69% stenoses in whom > 4 weeks has elapsed since the index event. However, if two (independent) Duplex scans were performed within 4 weeks of the index event, the HTA felt it reasonable to proceed to CEA (on the basis of US alone) as the number of strokes prevented through rapid access to CEA was likely to exceed the risk of patients with < 50% stenoses undergoing inappropriate surgery (Grade B).

Best medical therapy

When the randomized trials started recruiting in the mid-1980s, the concept of "best medical therapy" was rudimentary compared to what would now be considered acceptable. Accordingly, Table I summarizes recommendations made by the 2008 ESO regarding what should now be considered best practice [3].

In summary, all patients should have optimization of risk factors (hypertension, hypercholesterolemia), lifestyle modification (smoking cessation, weight loss, diet, alcohol and exercise), cessation of hormone replacement therapy in post-menopausal women and the introduction of antiplatelet and statin therapy. At present most guidelines recommend long term aspirin therapy (alone) in patients undergoing carotid endarterectomy. Dual antiplatelet therapy (aspirin and dipyridamole)

Table I SUMMARY OF 2008 EUROPEAN STROKE ORGANISATION RECOMMENDATIONS FOR WHAT CONSTITUTES 'BEST MEDICAL THERAPY' IN PATIENTS WITH SYMPTOMATIC CAROTID DISEASE [3]

Treatment	*Level of recomendation*
BP < 140/90 mmHg or < 130/80 mmHg in diabetics	Grade A
Glycemic control to prevent other diabetic complications	Grade C
Statin therapy	Grade A
Stop smoking	Grade B
Avoid heavy consumption of alcohol	Grade B
Regular physical activity	Grade B
Low salt, low saturated fat, high fruit and vegetable diet rich in fibre	Grade B
If Body Mass Index elevated, reduce weight	Grade B
Heart rate should not be used for stroke prevention in women	Grade A
Anti-oxidant vitamin supplements are not recommended	Grade A
Aspirin (long term after carotid endarterectomy)	Grade A
Aspirin and dipyridamole (non-operated patients)	Grade A
Aspirin and clopidogrel (after carotid artery stenting)	Grade B

should be offered to patients with symptomatic carotid disease not undergoing CEA, while clopidogrel is usually reserved for patients unable to tolerate aspirin or dipyridamole. The 2008 ESO Guidelines [3] state that combination aspirin and clopidogrel is not recommended in patients with recent ischemic stroke except in specific circumstances (unstable angina, non-Q wave myocardial infarction [MI], recent coronary stenting). However, in patients undergoing CAS, it is recommended that aspirin and clopidogrel be started pre-operatively and then be continued for three months post-intervention.

In the past, it has been assumed that there must be a significant "lag phase" for medical therapy to take effect. This assumption has, however, been challenged by the EXPRESS trial. This study looked at the effect of changing practice within cerebral vascular clinics and, in particular, whether the very rapid introduction of anti-platelet agents, anti-hypertensives and statins reduced the early risk of stroke [6]. The first phase of the study examined outcomes in existing cerebrovascular services between April 2002 and September 2004. During this time, the primary care doctor faxed a referral to the hospital. The patient was then triaged and allocated to the next available appointment within a dedicated TIA clinic (which only ran during week days). The patient was seen by a consultant with an interest in stroke where an urgent CT scan, ECG and carotid Duplex scan was ordered. A full assessment of the patient's risk factors was undertaken and a treatment plan faxed back (within 24 hours) to the primary care physician. The patient was not issued with prescription medications. Instead, the choice and dosage was documented in the faxed treatment plan with a request for the doctor to prescribe the medications when the patient sought an appointment.

In the second phase (October 2004 to March 2007), the primary care physician now sent the patient to an open access TIA clinic which ran every day of the week. This ensured that the patient was seen much quicker than previously. More importantly, the patient was issued with a four week supply of anti-platelet, statin and anti-hypertensive medications within the clinic. The treatment plan was then faxed (as before) to the primary care physician.

The 90-day stroke risk during phase 1 was 10.3%. This fell by 80% to 2.1% in phase II. The implications for practice from this large study are clear. Patients presenting with TIA/minor stroke need rapid access to specialist clinics and they need to be issued with appropriate medications when they attend.

Recommendations

1) All patients presenting with carotid territory symptoms showed be commenced on "best medical therapy" (Table I). Responsibility for who implements this should be clarified within individual units and medical therapy should be started as soon as possible after onset of symptoms (Grade A);
2) whenever possible, patients should be issued with medications at the clinic (Grade B).

CEA

The European Carotid Surgery Trial (ECST), the North American Symptomatic Carotid Endarterectomy Trial (NASCET) and the Veterans Affairs (VA) trials randomized patients with recent carotid territory symptoms (within 6 months) and who had varying degrees of carotid stenosis. Because there were two methods for measuring stenosis severity, two definitions of the "30-day risk" and differing end points (ipsilateral/any stroke), there have been many interpretations of the data. As a consequence, the Carotid Endarterectomy Trialists Collaboration (CETC) undertook an individual patient meta-analysis of > 6 000 patients randomized within ECST, NASCET and VA, having first re-measured the degree of stenosis using the NASCET measurement method [7-9].

Table II details the 5-year risks of "any stroke" and "ipsilateral stroke" in the CETC. Recently symptomatic patients with 70%-99% stenoses gained the maximum benefit from CEA (156 ipsilateral and 159 "any" strokes prevented at 5 years per 1 000 CEAs). Less clinical benefit (but still statistically significant) was observed in recently symptomatic patients with 50%-69% stenoses (78 ipsilateral strokes and 46 "any" strokes prevented at 5 years per 1 000 CEAs). No benefit (in terms of late stroke prevention was observed in recently symptomatic patients with < 50% stenoses.

Recommendations

Although now considered somewhat historical (but unlikely ever to be repeated), the CETC data support the following recommendations:

1) CEA is recommended in otherwise fit patients who present with carotid territory symptoms within the past 6 months and who have an ipsilateral 50%-99% carotid stenosis (Grade A);
2) CEA is not recommended in recently symptomatic patients who have an ipsilateral carotid stenosis < 50% (Grade A).

CLINICALLY IMPORTANT SUBGROUP ANALYSES FROM THE RANDOMIZED TRIALS

Because of the very large number of patients within the CETC database, it is now possible to identify subgroups of patients who have more (or less) to gain from surgical intervention. Clinical and imaging characteristics that were associated with significantly increased benefit from CEA (i.e. patients had a greater risk of stroke if treated medically) include: 1) males vs. females; 2) increasing age, especially > 75 years; 3) patients presenting with hemispheric vs. ocular symptoms; 4) patients presenting with cortical vs. lacunar stroke; 5) patients with increasing medical co-morbidity; 6) patients undergoing early surgery, especially the first two weeks; 7) patients with irregular vs. smooth plaques; 8) increasing degree of stenosis severity, but not subocclusion; 9) contralateral occlusion; 10) tandem intracranial disease; and 11) those unable to recruit intracranial collaterals.

Although one has to be cautious about over-interpreting subgroup analyses, a number of important observations are worthy of mention.

TIME TO INTERVENTION

It has become customary to retain the 6-month threshold used in the randomized trials as the accepted definition of being "recently symptomatic". However, this "one size fits all" policy has recently been challenged.

Most surgeons are taught that the early risk of stroke (after presenting with a TIA or minor stroke) is only about 1%-2% at 7 days, increasing to 2%-4% at 30 days. This, in conjunction with a perception that the procedural risk increases with expedited intervention, has meant that there has been little impetus to change practice.

Table II COMBINED ENDARTERECTOMY TRIALISTS COLLABORATION (CETC) INDIVIDUAL PATIENT META-ANALYSIS OF DATA FROM ECST, NASCET AND THE VA STUDY*

1) Any stroke at five years (including 30-day stroke/death)								
		30-day	*5-year risk*				*CVA prevented*	
Trial	*Stenosis*	*CEA risk*	*Surgery*	*Medical*	*ARR*	*RRR*	*NNT*	*Per 1 000 CEAs*
CETC	< 30%		18.36%	15.71%	- 2.6%	n/b	n/b	None at 5 years
CETC	30%-49%	6.7%	22.80%	25.45%	+2.6%	10%	38	26 at 5 years
CETC	50%-69%	8.4%	20.00%	27.77%	+7.8%	28%	13	78 at 5 years
CETC	70%-99%	6.2%	17.13%	32.71%	+15.6%	48%	6	156 at 5 years
CETC	String	5.4%	22.40%	22.30%	- 0.1%	n/b	n/b	None at 5 years
2) Ipsilateral stroke at five years (including 30-day stroke/death)								
		30-day	*5-year risk*				*CVA prevented*	
Trial	*Stenosis*	*CEA risk*	*Surgery*	*Medical*	*ARR*	*RRR*	*NNT*	*Per 1 000 CEAs*
CETC	< 30%		12.05%	9.78%	- 2.2%	n/b	n/b	None at 5 years
CETC	30%-49%	6.7%	14.78%	18.06%	+ 3.2%	18%	31	32 at 5 years
CETC	50-69%	8.4%	13.61%	18.18%	+ 4.6%	25%	21	46 at 5 years
CETC	70%-99%	6.2%	10.36%	26.24%	+15.9%	61%	6	159 at 5 years
CETC	String	5.4%	16.82%	15.15%	- 1.7%	n/b	n/b	None at 5 years

(*) adapted from Combined Endarterectomy Trialists Collaboration[7-9]. This is an overview of the combined data from ECST, NASCET and the VA Study with all angiograms being remeasured according to NASCET criteria. n/b: no benefit demonstrated, ARR: absolute risk reduction; RRR: relative risk reduction; NNT: number need to treat to prevent one stroke.
CEA: carotid endarterectomy; CVA: cerebrovascular accident

Evidence from meta-analyses of population based natural history studies using "face to face" follow-up have now shown that the two day risk of stroke is almost 7%, increasing to 10% at 7 days and 13% at 30 days [10]. These early risks are much greater than was previously taught and suggest that, in practice, the majority of "high risk" symptomatic patients probably suffer their stroke before they have any chance of undergoing either CEA or CAS.

The second challenge to contemporary practice (regarding early stroke risk) came from the CETC [7-9]. Table III shows how delay to surgery impacts upon the benefit conferred to patients (in terms of strokes prevented), both for the overall cohort within the CETC and then stratified for gender (see below). Note that patients with 70%-99% stenoses secured a declining benefit from CEA the longer it was delayed. If surgery was performed within 2 weeks, 230 strokes would be prevented at 5 years per 1 000 CEAs. However, if 12 weeks or more elapsed before surgery was performed, only 74 ipsilateral strokes would be prevented at 5 years. If one now analyses the benefit accruing to a patient with a 50%-69% stenosis, it is apparent that the number of strokes prevented decreases even more steeply. In particular, if CEA was deferred by > 12 weeks in a patient with a 50%-69% stenosis, the CETC data suggest that no benefit was forthcoming.

Table III ABSOLUTE RISK REDUCTION (ARR) CONFERRED BY CEA IN THE 5 YEAR RISK OF IPSILATERAL CAROTID TERRITORY STROKE (INCLUDING THE PERI-OPERATIVE RISK) IN PATIENTS WITH A NASCET 50%-69% AND 70%-99% STENOSIS, STRATIFIED FOR 1) DELAY FROM INDEX EVENT TO RANDOMIZATION AND 2) GENDER*

	50%-69% stenosis			*70%-99% stenosis*		
(1) All patients	*ARR*	*NNT*	*CVA/1000*	*ARR*	*NNT*	*CVA/1000*
< 2 weeks	14.8%	7	148	23.0%	4	230
2-4 weeks	3.3%	30	33	15.9%	6	159
4-12 weeks	4.0%	25	40	7.9%	13	79
> 12 weeks	-2.9%	nb	nb	7.4%	14	74
(2) Males						
< 2 weeks	15.2%	7	152	23.3%	4	233
2-4 weeks	6.8%	15	68	23.8%	4	238
4-12 weeks	5.0%	20	50	18.3%	5	183
> 12 weeks	6.3%	16	63	20.4%	5	204
(3) Females						
< 2 weeks	13.8%	7	138	41.7%	2	417
2-4 weeks	-5.7%	nb	nb	6.6%	15	66
4-12 weeks	-2.2%	nb	nb	-2.2%	nb	nb
> 12 weeks	-21.7%	nb	nb	-2.4%	nb	nb

(*) data derived from the CETC [7-9]. with all pre-randomization angiograms remeasured using NASCET method.

ARR: absolute risk reduction (%) conferred by surgery over best medical therapy; NNT: number of CEAs needed to be performed to prevent one stroke at 5 years; CVA/1 000: number of ipsilateral strokes prevented at five years by performing 1 000 CEAs; nb: no benefit conferred by CEA

BENEFIT ACCORDING TO GENDER?

Table III also shows that the benefit accruing to the patient (relative to delay to surgery) also varied between males and females [9]. Note that while the number of strokes prevented in males undergoing CEA diminished as the delay increased (especially in patients with 50%-69% stenoses), the benefit conferred in males with 70%-99% stenoses did appear to be maintained. Contrast this with the data observed in females. While considerable benefit accrued to female patients with 70%-99% stenoses who underwent CEA < 2 weeks, the benefit diminished precipitously with any ensuing delay and, by four weeks, females did not appear to gain any benefit from intervention, even if they had more severe disease.

SUBOCCLUSION CARRIES A LOW RISK OF STROKE

It has long been assumed that patients with "subocclusion" faced a very high risk of stroke if left untreated. Sub occlusion (or the string sign) is defined as being present when there is no opening out of the ICA beyond the stenosis and there is only a small, thready channel extending high

Table IV ABSOLUTE RISK REDUCTION IN THE TWO YEAR RISK OF IPSILATERAL STROKE IN PATIENTS RANDOMIZED WITHIN NASCET, STRATIFIED FOR AGE (*)

	< 50% stenosis		*50%-69%*		*70%-99%*	
Age	*ARR*	*NNT*	*ARR*	*NNT*	*ARR*	*NNT*
>75	7.3	14	17.3	6.0	28.9	3
65-74	1.1	91	5.3	19	15.1	7
< 65	1.4	71	-1.2	n/a	9.7	10

(*) data derived from Alamowitch [11].

ARR: absolute risk reduction in ipsilateral stroke conferred by CEA at 2 years; NNT: number needed to treat to prevent one ipsilateral stroke at 2 years

into the neck. By contrast, a critical stenosis with no subocclusion (or string sign) opens out into a normal caliber vessel.

The CETC have shown that the absolute risk reduction in stroke at 5 years conferred by CEA in patients with 90%-95% stenoses *without* subocclusion was approximately 35% (a massive reduction). By contrast, Table II shows that there was no evidence that CEA conferred benefit (in terms of late stroke prevention) in the recently symptomatic patient with subocclusion [7-9].

Do elderly patients gain less benefit from CEA?

It has been assumed (by some) that the procedural risk following CEA in recently symptomatic, elderly patients is higher than in other patient subgroups and that this is likely to cancel out any long term benefit. In fact, secondary analyses from NASCET have shown the exact opposite to be true (Table IV). Patients aged > 75 years gained consistently greater benefit from CEA across all stenosis categories and, most particularly, in patients with 70%-99% stenoses where only three CEAs needed to be performed to prevent one ipsilateral stroke at two years [11].

Recommendations

1) It is no longer acceptable to simply treat all patients who report symptoms within the preceding six months as being the same. They face significantly different risks if intervention is delayed (Grade A);
2) health systems need to change referral and investigative practices in order to ensure that patients who present with carotid territory symptoms undergo CEA within 2 weeks of onset of symptoms (Grade A);
3) the deleterious effect of delay to CEA is most marked in females, especially those with 50%-69% stenoses. Delay beyond 4 weeks means that they face all of the risks of surgery with little prospect of benefit. Females must be fast-tracked for intervention if they are to gain benefit (Grade A);
4) patients with subocclusion and a string sign do not seem to gain significant benefit from CEA. There is no need for emergency intervention (Grade A);
5) patients should not be denied consideration for CEA on the basis of age. Elderly patients (aged > 75 years) gained more benefit from CEA than any other age group (Grade A).

CAS

CAS has emerged as an alternative to CEA in the treatment of patients with carotid disease. Potential advantages include: no incision, no risk of cranial nerve injury and possibly less physiological stress. However, unlike the seminal randomized trials evaluating the roles of CEA and medical therapy two decades earlier, there remains (as yet) no consensus regarding which intervention is safer in symptomatic patients.

The literature contains a huge number of single center studies and registries citing the benefits of CAS, but this is really no different to the parallel situation in the 1980s when surgeons were challenged (by neurologists) to use randomized

Table V THIRTY-DAY PROCEDURAL RISKS IN RECENTLY SYMPTOMATIC PATIENTS RANDOMIZED WITHIN TRIALS COMPARING CEA WITH CAS

Trial	*Year*	*n*	*30-day risk of death/stroke*	
			CAS	*CEA*
Leicester	1998	23	5/11 (45%)	0/12 (0.0%)
WALLSTENT	2001	219	13/107 (12.1%)	5/112 (4.5%)
Kentucky I	2001	104	0/ 53 (0.0%)	1/51 (2.0%)
CAVATAS	2001	504	25/251 (10%)	25/253 (9.9%)
EVA-3S	2006	527	25/265 (9.4%)	10/262 (3.8%)
SPACE	2006	1 196	42/607 (6.9%)	38/589 (6.4%)
BACASS	2006	20	0/10 (0.0%)	1/10 (10%)
ICSS	2009	1 710	71/828 (8.5%)	42/821 (5.1%)

trial evidence to determine optimal practice. To date, 11 randomized trials comparing CEA with CAS have either published or released preliminary data [12]. These include; the Leicester Trial (1998), WALLSTENT (2001), Kentucky I (2001), CAVATAS (2001), Kentucky II (2004), SAPPHIRE (2004), EVA-3S (2006), SPACE (2006), BACASS (2006), TESCAS-C (2006) and ICSS (2009). CREST is due to report in 2010.

For the purposes of comparing outcomes in symptomatic patients, three trials (Kentucky II, SAPPHIRE, and TESCAS-C) have to be excluded. This is because they either randomized asymptomatic patients (Kentucky II) or contained symptomatic and asymptomatic patients (SAPPHIRE, TESCAS-C). Table V summarizes the procedural risks following CEA and CAS in 8 studies that randomized recently symptomatic patients. Overall, CAS was associated with a near twofold excess risk of death/stroke within the first 30-days (OR 1.8 (95% CI 1.4-2.3).

However, advocates of CAS could (reasonably) argue that much has changed since Leicester, WALLSTENT and CAVATAS published their data, especially regarding dual antiplatelet therapy, dedicated carotid stents and cerebral protection devices. Accordingly, is it still reasonable to include such historical data within contemporary meta-analyses? In view of this potentially confounding issue, Table VI only includes procedural risks from randomized trials with > 100 patients who published outcomes after 2005. In this pooled series of 3 372 patients, the procedural risk was 8.1% following CAS versus 5.4% after CEA. The largest of these three contemporary randomized trials (ICSS) released its procedural risks in May 2009. Addressing the European Stroke Conference [13], Professor Martin Brown (PI) reported that the early procedural risk after CAS (8.5%) was significantly higher than after CEA (5.1%) and that (in a substudy) new ischemic lesion on MR were significantly more common after CAS (46%) than after CEA (14%). Professor Brown concluded that ICSS "*provided strong evidence that CEA was safer than CAS in the primary intention to treat analysis and also in the per-protocol analysis, where twice as many strokes were associated with stenting as with endarterectomy*". He finished with the observation that "*carotid endarterectomy was still the treatment of choice for suitable patients with a recently symptomatic carotid artery stenosis.*"

Notwithstanding contemporary randomized trial evidence showing higher procedural risks after CAS, is there any evidence that late outcomes are significantly different? In the past, observers speculated that patients undergoing CAS would probably incur a higher rate of restenosis and

Table VI 30-DAY PROCEDURAL RISKS IN RECENTLY SYMPTOMATIC PATIENTS RANDOMIZED WITHIN TRIALS COMPARING CEA WITH CAS WHICH PUBLISHED AFTER 2005

Trial	*Year*	*n*	*30-day risk of death/stroke*	
			CAS	*CEA*
EVA-3S	2006	527	25/265 (9.4%)	10/262 (3.8%)
SPACE	2006	1196	42/607 (6.9%)	38/589 (6.4%)
ICSS	2009	1710	71/828 (8.5%)	42/821 (5.1%)
Total			138/1 700 (8.1%)	90/1 672 (5.4%)

that this could translate into a higher risk of late stroke. In fact, one of the key findings from CAVATAS, SAPPHIRE, EVA-3S and SPACE is that following a *successful* CAS procedure (i.e. no procedural stroke), the risk of late stroke was no different to that observed following CEA. This observation was a consistent finding across all four of the studies and important to document [14-17].

The 2009 Cochrane Review [12] (which published before release of the ICSS data) concluded that "*the results do not support a change in clinical practice away from recommending carotid endarterectomy as the treatment of choice for suitable carotid artery stenosis*". For obvious reasons, this recommendation will not change when the ICSS data are included. Accordingly, established CAS practitioners (especially those who participated in the most recent trials), those less experienced CAS practitioners wishing to increase their experience and those "novices" wishing to start CAS face a dilemma [18]. At present, level I evidence does not support a move towards the uncritical use of CAS in otherwise "standard risk" patients with recently symptomatic disease. If, however, an interventionist or surgeon wishes to offer CAS to "standard risk" symptomatic patients, they must ensure that their patients are investigated and treated quickly (i.e. within 2 weeks of the index event) and with a procedural risk < 6%. If neither of these caveats can be met, it would be safer to offer the patient an expedited CEA. In particular, delaying any intervention in order to achieve lower procedural risks is not acceptable practice.

In the long term, however, it is highly likely that selected patient subgroups will benefit from CAS (e.g. perhaps the younger symptomatic patient as was observed in the SPACE study). Once CREST releases its preliminary data in 2010, it is intended that EVA-3S, SPACE, ICSS and CREST will combine their data and perform an individual patient meta-analysis. With > 5 000 randomized "recently symptomatic" patients, it should be possible to identify patient subgroups who might be best treated by CAS.

Recommendations

1) In otherwise "standard risk" recently symptomatic patients with a 50%-99% carotid stenosis, CEA remains the preferred and safer intervention (Grade A);
2) surgeons or interventionists who intend to offer CAS to "standard risk" symptomatic patients must ensure that; 1) CAS is performed within 2 weeks of the presenting event (as required for CEA) and that 2) the 30-day risk of death/stroke is audited and maintained < 6% (Grade C).

"High risk" for CEA symptomatic patients

SAPPHIRE was the first randomized trial to evaluate the role of CAS in patients deemed "high risk for CEA" [15]. The rationale was that a less invasive intervention such as CAS might prove safer than surgery. SAPPHIRE undoubtedly aroused considerable controversy following its publication and while many believe it was compromized by a number of methodological and other slightly less

Table VII 30-DAY RATES OF DEATH/STROKE IN THE "HIGH RISK FOR CEA" CAS REGISTRIES, STRATIFIED FOR NEUROLOGICAL SYMPTOM STATUS

Registry	*Year*	*30-day death/stroke*		
		Overall	*ASYMP*	*SYMP*
CABERNET	2005	4.0%	3.3%	6.4%
ARCHeR	2006	6.6%	5.4%	11.6%
CREATE	2006	4.5%	2.9%	11.3%
CAPTURE I	2007	5.7%	4.9%	10.6%
BEACH	2007	5.3%	4.1%	7.7%
CAPTURE II	2008	5.2%	4.7%	9.1%
EXACT	2008	4.5%	4.0%	8.6%
CAPTURE II < 80	2009	3.8%	3.1%	6.0%
EXACT < 80	2009	4.0%	3.0%	7.3%

palatable issues, it did identify an important clinical question to be addressed.

One of the reasons SAPPHIRE suspended recruitment (and was therefore underpowered especially in symptomatic patients) was because of the emergence of a myriad of "high risk for CEA" CAS Registries. Each was funded by Industry (with their own propriety stent and protection device to promote), relatively few have published in peer reviewed journals and most contained predominantly asymptomatic patients. In order to interpret the available data, it is important to ascertain what the term "high risk for CEA" actually means, especially in symptomatic patients. The criteria can be classified as; 1) medical features (e.g. age > 80 years, significant pulmonary disease, positive stress test, recent MI, unstable angina, cardiac failure, contralateral recurrent laryngeal nerve palsy); 2) imaging features (e.g. contralateral occlusion); and 3) operative features (e.g. awaiting coronary bypass, recurrent stenosis after CEA, radiation arteritis, high bifurcation).

In order to qualify for being "high risk for CEA", the patient had to be recently symptomatic (< 6 months), he/she had to have a 50%-99% ipsilateral ICA stenosis and then display one or more of the adverse features listed above. Crucial (thereafter) to understanding the relevance of the published data is awareness that while most of the "high risk for CEA" features do not increase the natural history risk of stroke in asymptomatic individuals [19] the opposite is true in patients with symptomatic carotid disease; i.e. most of the factors that are defined as being "high risk for CEA" are also "high risk for stroke". Accordingly, on occasions it may be appropriate to increase the accepted threshold of procedural risk from < 6%.

Table VII details the 30-day rates of death/stroke in a number of "high risk for CEA" CAS Registries, where outcomes were stratified for symptom status. The largest of these (the combined EXACT and CAPTURE Registries) performed subgroup analyses in patients aged < 80 years and > 80 years. The authors concluded that "*outcomes in non-octogenarian, high surgical risk patients have improved since the pivotal Food and Drug Administration approval trials and have achieved American Heart Association (AHA) standards in both symptomatic and asymptomatic lesions*" [20]. Interestingly, the procedural risks in patients aged > 80 years were considerably higher than the AHA recommended thresholds of risk, stressing the importance of being careful in patient selection and interpretation of the data.

Accordingly, there is evidence that CAS is now

meeting accepted thresholds of risk in "high risk for CEA" patients, but it is important that patients are not (again) treated on a "one size fits all" strategy. Earlier in this chapter, a number of clinical and imaging features were highlighted as being predictive of increased benefit from CEA. By inference, it is likely that the same will apply to CAS. However, this also means that certain patients are going to be relatively low risk for stroke in the long term (e.g. females, 50%-69% stenoses, delayed cases, subocclusion, retinal symptoms) and after due consideration, it may be preferable to treat these patients conservatively. Finally, it still has to be determined what should be the revised acceptable threshold of risk in symptomatic "high risk for CEA" patients. If it exceeds 10% (as was apparent in a number of the studies in Table VII), it is unlikely that any long term benefit will accrue to the patient.

One important issue to have received relatively little attention in the "high risk for CEA" CAS Registries is the effect of delay to intervention upon outcome in symptomatic patients. Only CAPTURE [21] has published data on the effect of expedited CAS and they observed that CAS when performed within 2 weeks of the most recent symptom (but not necessarily the presenting symptom) was associated with a statistically significant 2.5 fold excess risk of death/stroke (95%CI 1.3-4.8). As a consequence of this, some interventionists (like their surgical counterparts) may prefer to delay CAS in order to achieve lower procedural risks. It should be borne in mind that while such a strategy may make the Interventionist (or surgeon) look better, it will be to the ultimate cost of the patient.

Guidelines

1) Non-octogenarian, recently symptomatic patients with 50%-99% stenoses who are considered "high risk" for CEA may be considered for CAS provided that procedural risks are audited and maintained < 8% (Grade B);
2) octogenarian, recently symptomatic patients with 50%-99% stenoses who are considered "high risk" for CEA face a higher procedural risk with CAS. Consideration should be given to whether the patient also reports clinical or imaging features that make them higher risk for stroke if left untreated. Otherwise, many might benefit from being reconsidered for CEA or conservative management (Grade C);
3) interventionists considering "high risk for CEA" patients for CAS should remain cognizant of the fact that the maximum benefit will be conferred to the patient if they are treated quickly. If it is felt that the risk of CAS in the early period may be too high, the patient should be reconsidered for CEA (Grade B).

REFERENCES

1 Liapis CD, Bell PR, Mikhailidis D et al. ESVS Guidelines. Invasive treatment for carotid stenosis : indications, techniques. *Eur J Vasc Endovasc Surg* 2009; 37: S1-S19.

2 Anonymous. AHPC. United States Department of Health and Human Services. Agency for Health Care Policy and Research. Acute pain management: operative on medical procedures and trauma. p 107. Rockville MD: AHPCR; 1993.

3 Anonymous. European Stroke Organisation (ESO) Executive Committee; ESO Writing Committee. Guidelines for the management of ischaemic stroke and transient ischaemic attack 2008. *Cerebrovasc Dis* 2008; 25: 457-507.

4 Wardlaw JM, Chappell FM, Stevenson M et al. Accurate, practical and cost-effective assessment of carotid stenosis in the UK. *Health Technol Assess* 2006; 10:iii-iv, ix-x, 1-182.

5 Walker J, Naylor AR: Ultrasound based diagnosis of 'carotid stenosis >70%': An audit of UK practice. *Eur J Vasc Endovasc Surg* 2006; 31: 487-490.

6 Rothwell PM, Giles MF, Chandratheva A et al. Effect of urgent treatment of transient ischaemic attack and minor stroke on early recurrent stroke (EXPRESS study): A prospective population based sequential comparison. *Lancet* 2007; 370: 1432-1442.

7 Rothwell PM, Eliasziw M, Gutnikov SA et al. Analysis of pooled data from the randomised controlled trials of endarterectomy for symptomatic carotid stenosis. *Lancet* 2003; 361: 107-116.

8 Rothwell PM, Eliasziw M, Gutnikov SA et al. Endarterectomy for symptomatic carotid stenosis in relation to clinical subgroups and timing of surgery. *Lancet* 2004; 363: 915-924.

9 Rothwell PM, Eliasziw M, Gutnikov SA et al. Sex difference in the effect of time from symptoms to surgery on benefit from carotid endarterectomy for transient ischaemic attack and minor stroke. *Stroke* 2004; 35: 2855-2861.

10 Giles MF, Rothwell PM. Risk of stroke after transient ischaemic attack: a systematic review and meta-analysis. *Lancet Neurol* 2007; 6: 1063-1072.

11 Alamowitch S, Eliasziw M, Algra A et al. Risk, causes and prevention of ischaemic stroke in elderly patients with symptomatic internal carotid artery stenosis. *Lancet* 2001; 357: 1154-1160.

12 Ederle J, Featherstone RL, Brown MM. Randomized controlled trials comparing endarterectomy and endovascular treatment for carotid artery stenosis: A Cochrane Review. *Stroke* 2009; 40: 1373-1380.

13 Anonymous. European Stroke Conference 2009. ICSS: Carotid endarterectomy superior to stenting, at least in the short term [Internet] Available at *www.medscape.com/viewarticle/703471* (cited 2009, Jul 29).

14 McCabe DJ, Pereira AC, Clifton A et al. Restenosis after carotid angioplasty, stenting or endarterectomy in the Carotid and

Vertebral Artery Transluminal Angioplasty Study (CAVATAS). *Stroke* 2005; 36: 281-286.

15 Eckstein HH, Ringleb P, Allenberg JR et al. Results of the Stent-Protected Angioplasty versus Carotid Endarterectomy (SPACE) study to treat symptomatic stenoses at 2 years: a multinational, prospective, randomised trial. *Lancet Neurol* 2008; 7: 893-902.

16 Mas JL, Trinquart L, Leys D et al. Endarterectomy Versus Angioplasty in Patients with Symptomatic Severe Carotid Stenosis (EVA-3S) trial: results up to 4 years from a randomised, multicentre trial. *Lancet Neurol* 2008; 7: 885-892.

17 Gurm HS, Yadav JS, Fayad P et al. Long term results of carotid stenting versus endarterectomy in high-risk patients. *N Engl J Med* 2008; 358: 1572-1579.

18 Naylor AR. ICSS and CAPTURE/EXACT: More questions than answers. *Eur J Vasc Endovasc Surg* 2009; 38: 397-538.

19 Naylor AR. Is surgery still generally the preferred option in patients with carotid artery disease? *Surgeon* 2008; 6: 6-12.

20 Gray WA, Chaturvedi S, Verta P. Thirty-day outcomes for carotid artery stenting in 6320 patients from two prospective, multicentre, high-surgical-risk Registries. *Circ Cardiovasc Intervent* 2009; 2: 159-166.

21 Gray WA, Yadav JS, Verta P et al. The CAPTURE Registry: Predictors of outcomes in carotid artery stenting with embolic protection for high surgical risk patients in the early post-approval setting. *Catheter Cardiovasc Interv* 2007; 70: 1025-1033.

5

CRUROPEDAL RECONSTRUCTIONS IN PERIPHERAL ARTERIAL OCCLUSIVE DISEASE

EIKE SEBASTIAN DEBUS, HOLGER DIENER,
MARTIN WINKLER, AXEL LARENA-AVELLANEDA

Surgical intervention in the therapy for peripheral arterial occlusive disease (PAOD) is mainly dependent on the extent and location of the arterial lesion. The use of invasive therapeutic measures in advanced symptomatic stages of PAOD is agreed upon, while surgical intervention in early stages (such as IIb in the Fontaine classification) should be used more restrictive, depending on the extent of the individual strain. A reduction of pain-free walking distance of under 100 meters in above knee occlusions is considered such a tremendous limitation in mobility that most of these patients prefer invasive treatment when possible. The critically ischemic extremity (stage III-IV in the Fontaine classification) is defined as a diminished vascular perfusion to the extent of impending amputation [1]. The danger to tissue vitality in these cases is principally reversible but nonetheless critical and on the verge of irreversible damage. Skeletal muscles tolerate ischemia for about 6 hours and are therefore the tissue most sensitive to decreased blood supply. Hence, the time period to irreversible tissue damage is determined by this 6-hour interval. With regard to the acuteness of ischemia development, we can differentiate between acute and chronic critical ischemia of extremities. Acute ischemia is defined by a rapid progress or sudden onset of diminished vascular perfusion with either a relevant aggravation of pre-existing symptoms or an abrupt start of first-time symptoms. The development from claudication to resting pain and further to tissue loss (ulcus arteriosum) may appear stepwise and most often marks the end-point of this progressing arterial occluding process.

Critical ischemia

An overall agreement exists with regard to the expected prognosis of patients who within 6-12 months after symptom onset require amputation because of irreversible damage to perfusion [2]. These patients frequently show a lowered ankle pressure between 50-70 mmHg as well as lowered $tcpO_2$ levels < 30-50 mmHg. Further on, acute critical ischemia always is characterized by sudden onset of critically diminished peripheral perfusion, consisting of diminished or lost motor and or sensory functions. Immediate treatment is then required without any time loss. Complete loss of function requires therapy within 6 hours of onset, otherwise amputation of the extremity is suspected. For reasons of time sparing, diagnostic angiography may be transferred into the operation theatre. Duplex sonography usually is sufficient as pre-operative diagnostic work up. Surgical embolectomy is required as early as possible, unless loss of function is not complete. In these cases, intra-arterial fibrinolysis or thrombus aspiration may be an option. Intra-arterial thrombolysis can be performed safely by ultrasound guidance; after completed thrombolysis the underlying condition (stenosis) can be detected and aimed recanalized [3]. The prognosis of patients with chronic critical limb ischemia (CLI) is harder to assess and depends on a multitude of indicators. The evaluation of spontaneous progress is difficult because these patients are most often in need of comprehensive therapy that cannot be denied simply for study purposes. There is, however, a considerable difference between patients with CLI and claudication: the fait of claudicants is determined mainly by cardio- and cerebrovascular incidents, whereas the risk of critical leg ischemia remains low, with a risk of amputation of 2% within 10 years [4]. Those patients with CLI and standard therapy show that as early as one year after diagnosis and adequate therapy, approximately 40% will lose their leg within 6 months, and up to 20% will die. Studies on the prevalence of cardiovascular disease in patients with peripheral artery disease (PAD) show that the history, clinical examination and electrocardiogram identify a prevalence of coronary artery and cerebral artery disease in 40% to 60% of such patients. In the PARTNERS study [5], 13% of subjects screened had an Ankle Brachial Index (ABI) of ≤ 0.90 and no symptomatic coronary artery disease (CAD) or cerebral artery disease, 16% had both PAOD and symptomatic coronary artery or cerebral artery disease, and 24% had symptomatic coronary artery and cerebral artery disease and a normal ABI. However, the link between PAOD and cerebral artery disease seems to be weaker than that with CAD: by Duplex examination, carotid artery disease occurs in 26% to 50% of patients with symptomatic PAD, but only about 5% of patients with PAD will have a history of any cerebrovascular event. There is a range of overlap in disease in the cerebral, coronary and peripheral circulations reported in the REACH survey [6]. Of those patients identified with severe symptomatic PAOD, 4.7% had concomitant CAD, 1.2% had concomitant cerebral artery disease and 1.6% had both. Thus, in this survey, about 65% of patients with PAOD had clinical evidence of other vascular disease. However, in one prospective study of 1886 patients aged 62 or over only 37% of subjects had no evidence of disease in any of the three territories [7]. The prevalence of renal artery stenosis of 50% or over ranges from 23% to 42%. Although it has not been studied specifically it is very likely that renal artery stenosis is also a partly independent risk factor for mortality in patients with PAOD, since renal artery stenosis of 50% or over is associated with a 3.3-fold higher mortality rate than in the general population. The short-term mortality of patients presenting with acute ischemia is 15% to 20%. Once they have survived the acute episode, their pattern of mortality will follow that of the claudicant or patient with chronic CLI, depending on the outcome of the acute episode. There is a strong correlation between ABI, as a measure of the severity of the PAOD, and mortality. A number of studies, using different ABI "cut-off" points have demonstrated this relationship. For instance, in a study of nearly 2000 claudicants, patients with an ABI < 0.50 had twice the mortality of claudicants with an entry ABI of > 0.50. The Edinburgh Artery Study [8] has also shown that the ABI is a good predictor of non-fatal and fatal cardiovascular events as well as total mortality, in an unselected general population. It has also been suggested that there is an almost linear relationship between ABI and fatal and non-fatal cardiovascular events; each decrease in ABI of 0.10 being associated with a 10% increase in relative risk for a major vascular event. In a study of patients with type 2 diabetes, the lower the ABI the higher the 5-year risk of a cardiovascular event [9].

Basic principles of surgery

SUTURE MATERIAL

For aseptic vascular suture, it is recommended to use a non-absorbable suture material with minimal foreign-body reaction. In order to endure the constant strain exercised by the pulse wave, the suture should not display any tendency of plasticity. Polypropylene is a suture material that meets these demands. On the other hand, a reversible elongation might be desirable. Some vascular surgeons prefer polybutester (Novafil®, Vascufil®) under the conception of a pulse synchronized elastic elongation of the suture. Monofilament suture poses the best option for vascular suture because of minimal tissue trauma. Braided suture material must be avoided since it presents a rough tissue drag and therefore may lead to increased intimal hyperplasia. In case of infection, absorbable synthetic monofilament suture may be used, but insufficiency of the suture due to early bacterial resorption remains a risk [10]. To minimize this risk, the use of long-term absorbable suture like polydioxanon is recommended in these cases. It is believed that the use of non-absorbable suture in the presence of infection may cause a persistent foreign-body reaction with a permanent host for bacteria and therefore fuel the infection. This hypothesis is not yet proven for monofilament polypropylene suture material. The vascular suture is accomplished by the use of atraumatic needle-suture combinations.

SUTURE TECHNIQUES

The goal of every vascular suture is to achieve complete hemostasis by an exact adaptation of vessel edges. At the same time, the integrity of the vessel wall must be restored. This can be achieved by using an everting suture technique in which the vessel intima lies exactly upon the other. For this purpose, the following techniques may be applied:

1) interrupted suture: this type is obligatory in sutures of infantile and juvenile vessels. Because of the expected growth of the young patient, the vessel growth also needs to be taken into account. The interrupted suture allows for an adequate adaption of the anastomosis suture to a certain degree.
2) Running suture: this is a standard technique and can always be used except in the case of infantile/juvenile vessels.
3) Running mattress suture: the advantage of this technique lies in the secure and exact hemostasis due to a broad adaptation of intima. A disadvantage may be the possibility of constriction of the vessel lumen and should therefore be reserved for vessels with a large diameter.
4) Non-eversion-transluminal suture (parachute-suture): this technique may be used in case of difficult access to the posterior wall.

All running sutures imply the risk of causing unintentional gathering of tissue, as intended in using the tobacco pouch suture technique, leading to constriction of the anastomosis. This problem might be avoided by the use of the opposing four-point technique in which double-armed sutures are used for a running opposite suture. Both threads are tied with themselves at the corners of the anastomosis. Then each needle is used to run the suture line in a simple over and over fashion to the middle of the anastomosis and then tied together. Therefore the anastomosis will be suspended at four points, reducing the possibility of tissue gathering to a maximum of one-fourth of the total suture line (Fig. 1A-D).

BYPASS MATERIAL

Autologous material (veins, arteries), xenogenous grafts (bovine) and alloplastic prostheses are used in peripheral reconstructive vascular surgery. The alloplastic materials (polyethylenterephtalate [PET], formerly Dacron and polytetrafluorethylene [PTFE]) are derived from polymers used in the textile industry. The polyester material is woven or knitted, and the differing manufacturing techniques show various advantages and disadvantages. The woven structures are altogether denser, but when remodeling and cutting of bypass ends is needed, the material shows a tendency to fray and therefore seldom is used in cruropedal reconstructions. Porous knitted prostheses or patches, on the other hand, show a better healing and incorporation of material but display a higher tendency to dilate. Because of its porous property, this material is coated with (bovine) collagen, albumin, or gelatin. The healing and incorporation process of PET-webs may be optimized by using a velour coating. By further impregnation with silver ions, an antibacterial effect is aimed for. The pore size of PTFE materials can range between 1 and 100 µm. Due to this micro-porous structure, a higher density as well as an improved incorporation process can be achieved.

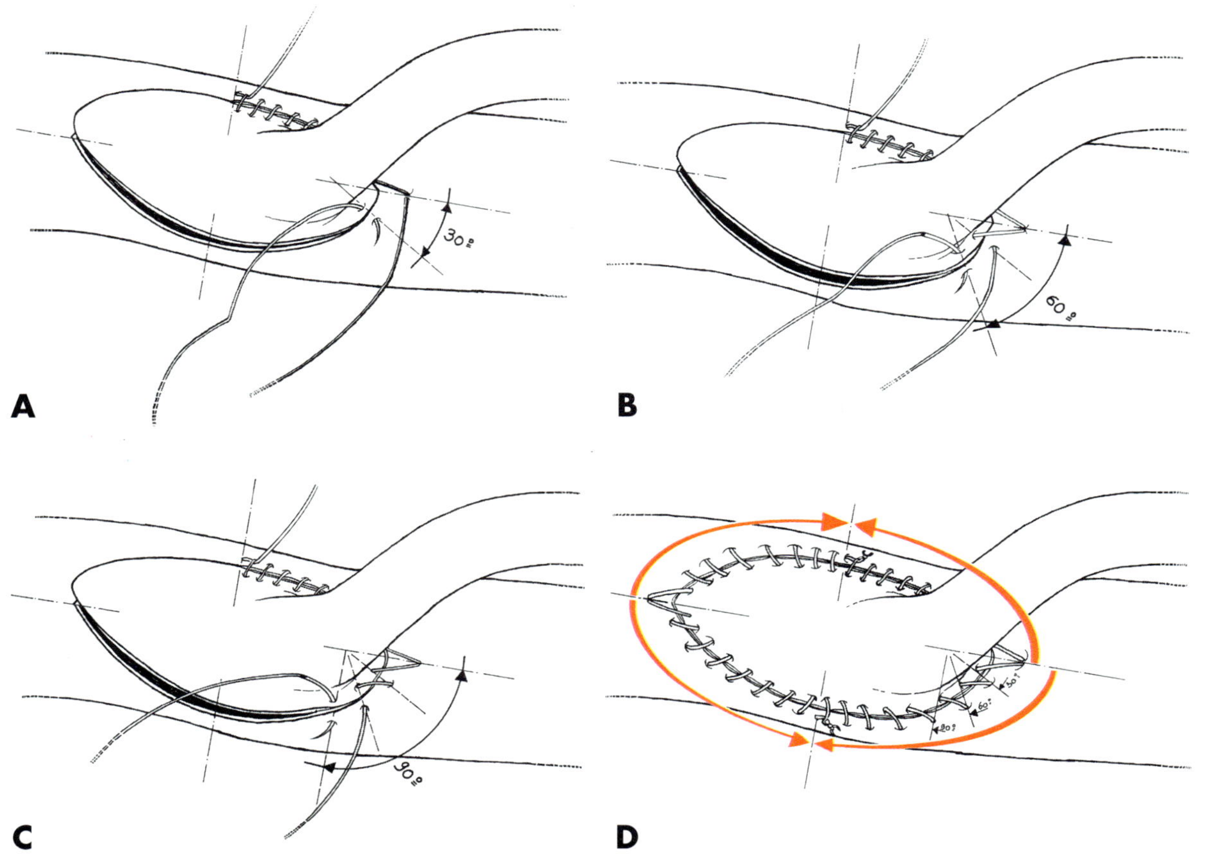

FIG. 1 A-D: Opposing four-point technique. Double-armed sutures are used for a running opposite suture. Both threads are tied with themselves at the corners of the anastomosis. Then each needle is used to run the suture line to the middle of the anastomosis.

Operative quality control

Following the reconstruction process, some sort of technical quality check should be performed. Various techniques are used to accomplish adequate quality control. The most commonly used techniques are angiography, operative flow recording, and color-coded Duplex sonography. Alternatively, a post-operative color-coded Duplex sonography may be performed. The Duplex is the most widespread method with utmost clinical importance. There are no risks and complications associated with this method. Duplex gives excellent hemodynamic informations and therefore is especially useful as an intra-operative tool for quality control. On the other hand, this technique is operator dependent and time consuming. Calcified segments are difficult to assess. In these cases, arteriography is of the distal arterial tree may give important additional information, so that both techniques should be available in the operative setting. Intra-operative angiography is of major value in localizing an obstruction and visualizing the distal arterial tree. It also assists in distinguishing patients who will benefit from additional endovascular treatment of (remained) inflow or outflow stenosis above and/or below the reconstructed arterial segment. Computed tomographic angiography (CTA) and magnetic resonance (MR) angiography may also be used in this setting as a postoperative control. MR imaging of the vasculature can be cumbersome and time-consuming. The advantages of CTA include its speed, convenience and ability for cross-sectional imaging of the vessel. The main disadvantage of CTA is its dependence on iodinated contrast media. In patients with impaired renal function, this added load of contrast might increase the risk of renal injury. In general, the intra-operative controls are preferred since they allow immediate adjustment, if needed.

Table MORPHOLOGICAL CLASSIFICATION OF LESIONS IN THE FEMOROPOPLITEAL REGION (ACCORDING TO TASC II)

Type of lesion	*Morphology*	*Treatment of choice*
Type A lesion	Single stenosis ≤ 10 cm in length Single occlusion ≤ 5 cm in length	Endovascular
Type B lesion	Multiple lesions (stenoses or occlusions), each ≤ 5 cm Single stenosis or occlusion ≤ 15 cm not involving the infra geniculate popliteal artery Single or multiple lesions in the absence of continuous tibial vessels to improve inflow for a distal bypass Heavily calcified occlusion ≤ 5 cm in length Single popliteal stenosis	Endovascular. The patient's co-morbidities, fully informed patient preference and the local operator's long-term success rates must be considered when making treatment recommendations
Type C lesion	Multiple stenoses or occlusions totaling >15 cm with or without heavy calcification Recurrent stenoses or occlusions that need treatment after two endovascular interventions	Open surgery in good risk patients. The patient's co-morbidities, fully informed patient preference and the local operator's long-term success rates must be considered when making treatment recommendations
Type D lesion	Chronic total occlusions of CFA or SFA (>20 cm, involving the popliteal artery) Chronic total occlusion of popliteal artery and proximal trifurcation vessels	Open surgery

CFA: common femoral artery; SFA: superficial femoral artery

Surgical therapy of PAOD

Basic principles

The following guiding principles hold true for infra-inguinal reconstruction:
- distal anastomosis should be placed upon the biggest and least calcified recipient artery;
- autologous material should be used in infra-inguinal bypasses;
- the bypass length should be kept as short as possible (the donor artery does not always have to be the common femoral artery).

The bypass length does not seem to be as important as the quality of the distal recipient artery in terms of patency rate. A longer bypass may be tolerated to reach a better artery located in a more distal area. The choice of surgical procedure is dependent on location and extent of the lesions (Table).

Management of accompanying infra-inguinal occlusion processes

About 50% of all patients needing surgery because of stenosis of the infra-inguinal and infragenicular region display relevant accompanying aorto-iliac occlusion processes. The need for additional vascular or endovascular reconstruction is estimated at 20%-25%, according to the own practice. In most cases, revascularizing interventions at the proximal end sufficiently improve blood influx. In the following situations, a simultaneous proximal reconstruction will be necessary:
- whenever the proximal lesion shows relevant hemodynamic disturbance;
- stenosis of the profunda region;
- occlusion or relevant hemodynamic stenosis of the femoral superficial artery in the popliteal segment;
- existence of distal tissue necrosis.

Although this poses a relevant clinical problem, there is little literature available.

Open desobliteration and eversion

The open desobliteration presents a classic surgical method in the treatment of PAOD. This technique was established by Jean Cid Dos Santos in 1946. It is important to extend the arteriotomy about 1-2 cm distal and proximal of the lesion in order to guarantee sufficient management of the landing point. Subsequently, an adequate dissection layer is chosen in the media layer in order to ensure a safe and easy extraction of the sub-intimal plaque. In case of a subtle plaque tail, luminal vascular reconstruction is finished at this point. Most of the time, the plaque seems to carry on to the periphery and to central regions, making a transverse cut in the media region necessary. In this case, a fixating suture of the plaque tail in the direction of blood flow is recommended to prevent distal dissection. This can be accomplished by using running sutures. Before closure of the arteriotomy using a patch plasty, it is of utmost importance to check for a clean, detritus-free desobliteration layer to prevent local thrombus formation with further embolization and early occlusion of the vessel. The patch should be placed in "over-pass technique", so that the patch end is not located directly opposite to the intimal running suture, preventing an iatrogenic stenosis. In very few cases, the eversion desobliteration technique might be of use. In this technique, the artery is opened by transverse or diagonal cut, a circular dissection of the layer between media and serosa is performed, and the vascular serosa is everted over the calcified plaque until the plaque is completely everted. An advantage of this technique is definitely the missing stenosis factor compared to a longitudinal arteriotomy. However, a disadvantage is the lack of sufficient handling of the distal plaque tail with risk of dissection.

Patch plasty

This technique is a common reconstructive method. It can be used by itself as well as in combination with desobliterating procedures. The idea behind this method is to avoid a constricting longitudinal suture after arteriotomy in areas of vulnerable vascular status. The most frequently used patches in the cruropedal region are autologous venous patches (greater or lesser saphenous vein) as well as xenogenous patches made from denaturized bovine pericardium (Vascuguard®). Alloplastic materials are avoided, since the advantages of autologous and xenogenous material are superior healing and incorporation, excellent patency rates, and little susceptibility to infection. Xenogenous material combines the advantages of biomaterial (infection resistance, compliance match, excellent openness rates) with those of alloplastic materials (unlimited availability).

Bypass

Infra-inguinal bypass procedures need to arise from a patent and uncompromized inflow artery, although the actual level (common femoral artery versus superficial femoral or popliteal artery) does not correlate with patency. If the infra-inguinal bypass is constructed following an inflow procedure, patency is improved by making the proximal anastomosis to a native artery rather than the inflow graft [11]. The quality of the outflow artery is a more important determinant of patency than the actual level where the distal anastomosis is performed. Herefore, a distal vessel of the best quality should be used for the distal anastomosis.

Femoropopliteal bypasses

Alloplastic prostheses have become an accepted alternative to autologous vein bypass in the femoropopliteal region; however, the greater saphenous vein (GSV) is more and more favored for this region. Comparative meta-analysis studies have showen better results for the autologous vein bypass above the knee joint. The 5-year patency rate for GSV was reported to be 66% followed by PTFE with 47%. Below the knee joint, the difference becomes more evident. Here, the 5-year patency rate was reported to be 77% for reversed GSV, 68% for in-situ GSV, 60% for human umbilical vein (HUV), and only 40% for PTFE. Several randomized studies have shown equal patencies for PTFE and Dacron. The HUV initially showed a tendency towards better patency rates, but in the course of the study, it also tended to display late degenerating processes with secondary formation of aneurysms [12]. A recent study, however, demonstrated similar long term results of graft patency, when femoropopliteal HUV bypasses are compared to PTFE conduit [13].

Conduit

Vein has better long-term patency than prosthetic material in the infra-inguinal region [14].

A meta-analysis suggests much less satisfactory results of PTFA-coated grafts to the infrapopliteal arteries (5-year patency: primary 30.5%, secondary 39.7%) [15]. The consequences of a prosthetic graft occlusion may be more severe than a vein graft occlusion [16]. A recent study questioned the wisdom of using a prosthetic graft when acceptable vein was available in order to "save the vein". Using this strategy, up to 33% of subsequent secondary bypass grafts did not have adequate vein available at that time. The GSV, either in a reversed or in-situ configuration offers the best match of size and quality. In its absence, other venous tissue including contralateral long saphenous vein, lesser saphenous vein, femoral vein and arm vein have been used. Venous grafts all have better results than prosthetic materials.

Secondary revascularization procedures

Secondary patency results from the salvage of an occluded bypass and assisted patency results from pre-occlusion intervention. The non-tolerance of vein grafts to thrombosis and the success of assisted patency support the recommendations that all venous bypass grafts be followed by a regular regime of Duplex scanning with set parameters for intervention including angioplasty (open or transluminal) or short segment interposition. However, this recommendation has recently been questioned by a randomized, controlled trial showing no cost benefit of such an approach [17]. In the presence of an occluded but established graft, thrombolysis may be indicated in the very early stages to remove clot and reveal the cause of the thrombosis. When limb salvage is assessed following failure of an infra-inguinal bypass the original indication for surgery is an important factor. The 2-year limb salvage rates for occluded grafts done for claudication is 100%, for rest pain is 55% and when done for tissue loss is 34%. The early occlusion of a graft (< 30 days occlusion) led to a very poor 2-year limb salvage rate of 25% [18].

Cruropedal lesions

There is no objective evidence to preferentially select either tibial or peroneal artery. The results of femoral crural bypass have not been subjected to meta-analysis yet. Five-year assisted patency rates in grafts constructed with vein approach 60% and those constructed with prosthetic material are usually less than 35%. Reports have documented the suitability of constructing bypass grafts to plantar arteries with reasonable success rates. Patients with cruropedal lesions usually have few options in developing collateral vessels to compensate for reduced blood flow. Hence, these patients display faster progression to stage III and IV in the Fontaine classification, where intervention is advised. The earlier stages should be treated by conservative means. Patients with CLI should be treated as an emergency since any time delay in treatment has to be avoided. However, the majority of patients are still not treated in specialized centers. Patients displaying chronic resting pain seem to be less in danger of amputation compared to those who display signs of tissue loss. Patients with signs of CLI should be referred to a specialized center where ideally all disciplines necessary for the holistic therapy of vascular patients are available.

Cruropedal vascular reconstruction

The revascularization of peripheral vascular vessels is still discussed critically on the one hand due to the demanding technical effort and high occlusion rates at an early stage on the other. Which surgical technique is applicable depends on the location and extent of the lesions. In the last few years, excellent long-term results were published for femorocrural bypass surgery with a reported patency rate of 83% over a 5-year period [19-23], resulting in a "boom" of crural vascular surgery [24,25]. In particular, bypass anastomosis on the peroneal artery (PA) is rarely performed because this vessel often displays slender lumina, and operative dissection is technically demanding. Several authors have postulated that the PA, in contrast to the other two arteries, only takes part in the perfusion of the pedal area via collateral vessels and therefore is confronted with too high of a peripheral efflux resistance, accounting in turn for early bypass occlusion. Furthermore, the poor results of revascularization compared to those of anterior or posterior tibial bypass revascularization often have led to considerations of primary amputation instead of PA reconstruction. On the other hand, studies have shown that the PA often seems to be spared by arteriosclerosis [26]. This phenomenon accounts for the term "peroneal leg". This shows that in many cases of PAOD with distal affection, the PA poses the only vessel available for anastomosis, leaving the revascularization technique of the PA as the last chance to prevent amputation. Compared to bypasses onto the tibial arteries, the PA bypass nowadays shows equal results for patency, limb salvage, and mortality. The operative access to the PA is technically more demanding and presents a far greater trauma to the patient due to extensive tissue damage. The preparation of the PA, similar to the preparation of the tibial vessels, is mainly performed via medial access. Alternatively, the lateral access may be of use where a resection of the fibula bone of several centimeters is required to reveal the PA. Both of these access points are traumatizing for the patient, leading to an increased amount of wound healing complications and edema, limiting patients postoperatively in their mobility. The newly described dorsolateral access allows for preparation of the PA without fibula bone resection and hence with far less tissue trauma (Fig. 2) [27].

Venous bypass: in-situ versus reversed

The long-term patency of in-situ bypass reconstruction has been compared to the reversed venous bypass technique. Studies have shown a clear advantage in favor of the reversed technique after a 5-year study interval (46.2% vs. 68.8%) [28]. This is mainly attributed to the technically more demanding effort of the in-situ technique. These bypasses require frequent secondary intervention, most notably due to "forgotten" side branches. The secondary patency rate, on the other hand, shows no relevant difference compared to the reversed bypass technique (71.6% vs. 79.4%). Differences in outcome will depend upon indications for surgery, the quality of the vessels, and co-morbidities.

Isolated popliteal segment

In some cases, the bypass reconstruction onto an isolated segment of the popliteal region may be reasonable under the circumstances of good distal collateralization [29]. The long-term patency rates for such bypasses has proven to be of lower quality compared to that of free distal perfusion in the popliteal segment and crural bypass; however, the overall patency is 55%-74% [30].

Arteriovenous fistula

When a prosthetic bypass graft is placed into the below-knee popliteal or distal artery adjunct procedures, such as arteriovenous fistula (AV) at or distal to the bypass and the use of a vein interposition/cuff, have been suggested. The AV fistula is a mean to enhance the patency in patients with poor efflux by reducing the peripheral outflow by partially bridging into the venous low pressure system. There is little reliable data concerning this technique, but so far it appears that the AV fistula technique cannot significantly improve the results in comparison to direct anastomosis techniques. Randomized studies have shown a patency rate for AV fistulas of 55.2% over a one-year period, whereas the control group achieved an openness rate of 53.4% [31].

Venous cuff

Distal interposition venous cuffs have been described to optimize outcome of synthetic grafts. Based on their results with vein cuffs in 42 patients, Pappas et al. [32] concluded that this reconstruction is an acceptable alternate conduit in patients with

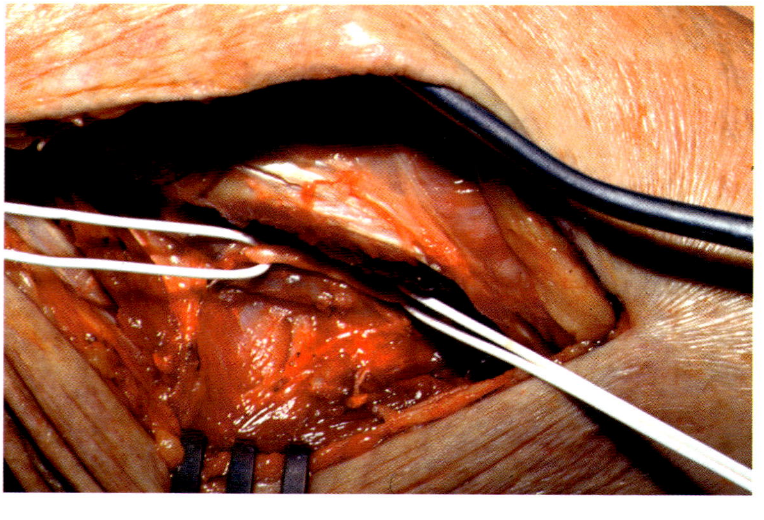

FIG. 2 Dorso-lateral approach to the PA without resection of the fibula.

CLI when autologous saphenous vein is absent. Various venous cuff techniques have been introduced in order to face the compliance mismatch between rigid synthetic bypass material and elastic vessels at the distal anastomosis region. Randomized studies of venous cuff techniques applied to regions above the knee joint have shown no relevant improvement compared to direct suture techniques. However, applying this technique in regions below the knee joint has shown a significant advantage regarding the venous cuff technique with a two-year patency rate of 57% versus 29% [33]. Combination of venous cuff and arteriovenous fistula may have additive effects [34]. Further studies are required to support the current study results.

Surveillance programs following revascularization

Patients are considered successfully treated when peripheral perfusion is restored to a point where claudication symptoms or resting pain has vanished or ischemic tissue necrosis shows a relevant healing tendency with the formation of granulating tissue. However, these patients cannot be considered completely cured with respect to the underlying disease since a progression of disease is very likely and relapse conditions (CLI) are common. Those patients receiving reconstructive surgery therefore need regular post-operative checkups in order to reveal bypass occlusion at an early point.

The importance of the healing process in ischemic tissue often seems underestimated. Any sign of stagnation of the healing process and of course any type of tissue damage progression should lead to the presumption of bypass occlusion or overall progression of the underlying disease and requires immediate further diagnostic measurements. Following construction of an autogenous bypass graft, it has been recommended in the past that a program of regular graft review with Duplex scanning should be undertaken [35]. The purpose of this is to identify lesions that predispose to graft thrombosis and allow their repair prior to graft occlusion. A recent multicenter, randomized, controlled trial has shown that Duplex surveillance after venous femoral distal bypass grafts leads to no significant clinical benefit or quality of life improvement at 18 months. The previous recommendation of routine Duplex scanning following autogenous lower extremity bypass has proven to be not cost-effective according to this study. In practice, many surgeons continue a program of vein graft surveillance awaiting further confirmation of the findings of this trial. According to the TASC II document [2], patients undergoing bypass graft placement in the lower extremity for the treatment of claudication or limb-threatening ischemia should be entered into a clinical surveillance program. This program should consist of interval history (new symptoms), vascular examination of the leg with palpation of proximal, graft and outflow vessel pulses, periodic measurement of resting and, if possible, post-exercise ankle brachial indices. Clinical surveillance programs should be performed in the immediate post-operative period and at regular intervals (usually every 6 months) for at least two years. In addition, the whole vascular status of the patient should be examined to reveal early signs of limiting cardiovascular co-morbidities.

Discussion

The PTFE or knitted polyester (Dacron) graft has been used alternatively to the GSV, but earlier reports on plain synthetic grafts showed poor results. Improving patency was attempted by adjunctive procedures at distal anastomosis and conduits that incorporated a thin wall, an external support, or a tapered end. These changes, along with other factors, are associated with better results [35, 36]. Before implanting a synthetic graft some authors prefer using the arm veins, spliced veins, human umbilical veins, or cold stored venous allografts [37, 38]. Comparative studies have shown similar results for limb salvage and patency [39], although the operation of a complex autologous conduit is more difficult and longer and associated with a significantly increased rate of re-intervention [40, 41]. The use of a synthetic graft is definitely justified to avoid limb amputation, but below knee alloplastic reconstructions are still mostly abandoned, despite recently reported improved results. Despite aggressive therapeutic measures, patients with distal ischemia experience significantly reduced life expectancy. Three years after successful intervention, less than 60% are still alive [42]. Therapeutic measures should not exclusively focus on limb salvage but also take into account the overall health condition of the patient. Therefore, quality of life is another relevant end point [43]. Impaired wound healing, readmission, and re-operations significantly reduce the quality of life in patients following infra-inguinal bypass.

The time to heal exceeded three months in 54% of the patients. This is of particular importance as life expectancy of these patients is low and the operative trauma of a vein graft is more intense than of a synthetic graft [44]. This aspect is of greater importance if arm veins, spliced veins, or human umbilical veins are used because the number of re-operations is much higher. Therefore, the use of alloplastic materials even for below knee reconstruction might be considered in a well defined population characterized by severely impaired life expectancy. The ideal therapy therefore consists of restoration of extremity function, optimization of life expectancy by treatment of the underlying disease and its risk factors, and the best possible social reintegration of the patient. The extent and radicalness of reperfusion measurements is dependent on the overall clinical constitution of the patient as well as the expected revascularization prognosis. The fact, that patients displaying symptoms of CLI are in need of surgery or interventional treatment to reduce the risk of amputation is not a subject of discussion. However, the process of deciding on intervention, technique, and extent is a complex process that cannot be solved by solely applying textbook knowledge. Even though it is of utmost importance to form individually based therapeutic decisions, certain basic principles need to be taken into account. Mortality, morbidity, and co-morbidity, as well as risk factors and life expectancy, need to be evaluated regarding prognosis and long-term results of each intervention technique applied. Ideally the patient should be treated with the method posing the least risk of intervention while at the same time offering the best initial success rate and long-term openness prognosis. In many cases, multiple lesions are found, rendering a combination of interventional and surgical techniques the better option that may significantly enhance the outcome. In the crural region, studies have shown that the autologous vein displays a better outcome compared to alloplastic bypass material. This led to the consensus of favoring venous bypass even if the GSV is not available. Only in cases where there is no side branch vein (small saphenous vein or veins of the arm) is the use of a synthetic bypass recommended [45]. Randomized studies of venous bypass material in this region have shown a patency rate of 72%-83% over a 5-year period. The patency rate of PTFE material, on the other hand, only averages a 17% rate after a 4-year period. However, heparin-bonded PTFE may be associated with favorable long-term results [46,47]. Composite bypass grafts (partly alloplastic, partly autologous) in the infra-inguinal region display a patency rate of 61% over a 4-year interval but require up to 20% secondary intervention to maintain sufficient function. The superficial femoral vein may also serve as an adequate bypass option. The resection of this vein may lead to initial edema. The success rate of this bypass alternative is comparable to that of GSV. It is commonly accepted that the integrity of plantar perfusion is a major predictor of the patency success rate of cruropedal reconstructions [48]. The patency rate of pedal bypass reconstruction is not significantly different from that of proximal crural bypasses.

REFERENCES

1 Fontaine R, Kim M, Kieny R. Surgical treatment of peripheral circulation disorders. *Helv Chir Acta* 1954; 21: 499-533.

2 Norgren L, Hiatt WR, Dormandy JA et al. Inter-society consensus for the management of peripheral arterial disease (TASC II). Eur J Vasc Endovasc Surg 2007; 33 (Suppl 1): S1- S75.

3 Wissgott C, Richter A, Kamusella P et al. Treatment of critical limb ischemia using ultrasound-enhanced thrombolysis (PARES Trial): final results. J Endovasc Ther 2007; 14: 438-443.

4 Lawall H, Diehm C, Pittrow P. Leitlinien zur Diagnostik und Therapie der peripheren arteriellen Verschlusskrankheit (PAVK). *Vasa* 2009; 38: S75.

5 Hirsch AT, Criqui MH, Treat-Jacobson D et al. Peripheral arterial disease detection, awareness, and treatment in primary care. JAMA 2001; 286: 1317-1324.

6 Bhatt D, Steg P, Ohman E et al. International prevalence, recognition, and treatment of cardiovascular risk factors in outpatients with atherothrombosis. *JAMA* 2006; 295: 180-189.

7 Aronow WS, Ahn C. Prevalence of coexistence of coronary artery disease, peripheral arterial disease, and atherothrombotic brain infarction in men and women > or = 62 years of age. *Am J Cardiol* 1994; 74: 64-65.

8 Fowkes FG, Housley E, Cawood EH et al. Edinburgh Artery Study: prevalence of asymptomatic and symptomatic peripheral arterial disease in the general population. *Int J Epidemiol* 1991; 20: 384-392.

9 Mehler PS, Coll JR, Estacio R et al. Intensive blood pressure control reduces the risk of cardiovascular events in patients with peripheral arterial disease and type 2 diabetes. *Circulation* 2003; 107: 753-756.

10 Larena-Avellaned A, Debus ES, Diener H et al. Species-dependent premature degradation of absorbable suture materials caused by infection – impact on the choice of thread in vascular surgery. *Vasa* 2004; 33: 165-169.

11 Lam E, Landry G, Edwards J et al. Risk factors for autogenous infrainguinal bypass occlusion in patients with prosthetic inflow grafts. *J Vasc Surg* 2004; 39: 336-342.

12 Shah DM, Leather RP, Darling RC et al. Long term results of using in situ saphenous vein bypass. *Adv Surg* 1996; 30: 123-140.

13 Neufang A, Espinola-Klein C, Dorweiler B et al. Femoropopliteal

prosthetic bypass with glutaraldehyde stabilized human umbilical vein (HUV). *J Vasc Surg* 2007; 46: 280-288.

14 Scharn DM, Dirven M, Barendregt WB et al. Human umbilical vein versus heparin-bonded polyester for femoropopliteal bypass: 5-year results of a prospective randominzed multicentre trial. *Eur J Vasc Endovasc Surg* 2008; 35: 61-67.

15 Klinkert P, van Dijk PJ, Breslau PJ. Polytetrafluoroethylene femorotibial bypass grafting: 5-year patency and limb salvage. *Ann Vasc Surg* 2003; 17: 486-491.

16 Albers M, Battistella V, Romiti M et al. Meta-analysis of polytetrafluoethylene bypass grafts to infrapopliteal arteries. *J Vasc Surg* 2003; 37: 1263-1269

17 Jackson MR, Belott TP, Dickason T et al. The consequences of a failed femoropopliteal bypass grafting: comparison of saphenous vein and PTFE grafts. *J Vasc Surg* 2000; 32: 498-505.

18. Davies AH, Hawdon AJ, Sydes MR et al. Is duplex surveillance of value after leg vein bypass grafting?: Principal results of the Vein Graft Surveillance Randomised Trial (VGST). *Circulation* 2005; 112: 1985-1991.

19 Baldwin Z, Pearce B, Curi M et al. Limb salvage following infrainguinal bypass graft failure. *J Vasc Surg* 2004; 39: 951-957.

20 Faries PL, Logerfo FW, Arora S et al. A comparative study of alternative conduits for lower extremity revascularization: all-autogenous conduit versus prosthetic grafts. *J Vasc Surg* 2000; 32: 1080-1090.

21 Kreienberg PB, Darling RC 3rd, Chang BB et al. Early results of a prospective randomized trial of spliced vein versus polytetrafluoroethylene graft with a distal vein cuff for limb-threatening ischemia. *J Vasc Surg* 2002; 35: 299-306.

22 Parsons RE, Suggs WD, Veith FJ et al. Polytetrafluoroethylene bypasses to infrapopliteal arteries without cuffs or patches: a better option than amputation in patients without autologous vein. *J Vasc Surg* 1996; 23: 347-354.

23 Pereira CE, Albers M, Romiti M et al. Meta-analysis of femoropopliteal bypass grafts for lower extremity arterial insufficiency. *J Vasc Surg* 2006; 44: 510-517.

24 Pereira CE, Albers M, Romiti M et al. Meta-analysis of femoropopliteal bypass grafts for lower extremity arterial insufficiency. *J Vasc Surg* 2006; 44: 510-517.

25 Sandford RM, Bown MJ, Sayers RD et al. Is infrainguinal bypass grafting successful following failed angioplasty? *Eur J Vasc Endovasc Surg* 2007; 34: 29-34.

26 Raftery KB, Belkin M, Mackey WC et al. Are peroneal bypass grafts hemodynamically inferior to other tibial artery bypass grafts? *J Vasc Surg* 1994; 19: 964-968.

27 Debus ES, Larena A, Sailer MA et al. Dorsolateral peroneal bypass grafting – introduction of an approach to the peroneal artery and first clinical experiences. *Gefässchirurgie* 2002; 7: 89-93.

28 Watelet J, Soury P, Menard JF et al. Femoropopliteal bypass: in situ or reversed vein grafts? Ten year results of a randomized prospective study. *Ann Vasc Surg* 1997; 11: 510-519.

29 Barral X, Salari GR, Toursakission B et al. Bypass to perigenulate collateral vessels. A useful technique for limb salvage: preliminary report on 22 patients. *J Vasc Surg* 1998; 27: 928-935.

30 Kram HB, Gupta SK, Veith FJ et al. Late results of two hundred seventeen femoropopliteal bypasses to isolated popliteal artery segments. *J Vasc Surg* 1991; 14: 386-390.

31 Hamsho A, Nott D, Harris PL. Prospective, randomized trial of distal arteriovenous fistula as an adjunct to femoro-infrapopliteal PTFE bypass. *Eur J Vasc Endovasc Surg* 1999; 17: 197-201.

32 Pappas PJ, Hobson RW 2nd, Meyers MG et al. Patency of infrainguinal polytetrafluoroethylene bypass grafts with distal interposition vein cuffs. *Cardiovasc Surg* 1998; 6: 19-26.

33 Griffiths GD, Nagy J, Black D, Stonebridge PA. Randomized clinical trial of distal anastomotic interposition vein cuff in infrainguinal polytetrafluoethylene bypass grafting. *Br J Surg* 2004; 91: 560-562.

34 Neville RF, Dy B, Singh N et al. Distal vein patch with an arteriovenous fistula: a viable option for the patient without autogenous conduit and severe distal occlusive disease. *J Vasc Surg* 2009; 50: 83-88.

35 Visser K, Idu MM, Buth J et al. Duplex scan surveillance during the first year after infrainguinal autologous vein bypass grafting surgery: costs and clinical outcomes compared with other surveillance programs. *J Vasc Surg* 2001; 33: 123-130.

36 Robinson BI, Fletcher JP, Tomlinson P et al. A prospective randomized multicentre comparison of expanded polytetrafluoroethylene and gelatin-sealed knitted Dacron grafts for femoropopliteal bypass. *Cardiovasc Surg* 1999; 7: 214-218.

37 Smeets L, Ho GH, Tangelder MJ et al. Outcome after occlusion of infrainguinal bypasses in the Dutch BOA Study: comparison of amputation rate in venous and prosthetic grafts. *Eur J Vasc Endovasc Surg* 2005; 30: 604-609.

38 Halloran BG, Lilly MP, Cohn EJ et al. Tibial bypass using complex autologous conduit: patency and limb salvage. *Ann Vasc Surg* 2001; 15: 634-643.

39 Hôlzenbein TJ, Pomposelli FB Jr, Miller A et al. Results of a policy with arm veins used as first alternative to an unavailable ipsilateral greater saphenous vein for infrainguinal bypass. *J Vasc Surg* 1996; 23: 130-140.

40 Kreienberg PB, Darling RC 3rd, Chang BB et al. Early results of a prospective randomized trial of spliced vein versus polytetrafluoroethylene graft with a distal vein cuff for limb-threatening ischemia. *J Vasc Surg* 2002; 35: 299-306.

41 Goshima KR, Mills JL Sr, Hughes JD. A new look at outcomes after infrainguinal bypass surgery: traditional reporting standards systematically underestimate the expenditure of effort required to attain limb salvage. *J Vasc Surg* 2004; 39: 330-335.

42 Panneton JM, Gloviczki P, Bower TC et al. Pedal bypass for limb salvage: impact of diabetes on long-term outcome. *Ann Vasc Surg* 2000; 14: 640-647.

43 The ICAI group (Gruppo di studio dell ischemia cronica degli arti inferiori). Long-term mortality and its predictors in patients with critical leg ischemia. *Eur J Vasc Endovasc Surg* 1997; 14: 91-95.

44 Hallin A, Bergqvist D, Fugl-Meyer K et al. Areas of concern, quality of life and life satisfaction in patients with peripheral vascular disease. *Eur J Vasc Endovasc Surg* 2002; 24: 255-263.

45 Kent KC, Bartek S, Kuntz KM et al. Prospective study of wound complications in continuous infrainguinal incisions after lower limb arterial reconstruction: incidence, risk factors, and cost. *Surgery* 1996; 119: 378-383.

46 Daenens K, Schepers S, Fourneau I et al. Heparin-bonded ePTFE grafts compared with vein grafts in femoropopliteal and femorocrural bypasses: 1- and 2-year results. *J Vasc Surg* 2009; 49: 1210-1216.

47 Loesel-Sadée H, Alefelder C. Heparin-bonded expanded polytetrafluoroethylene graft for infragenicular bypass: five-year results. *J Cardiovasc Surg* 2009; 50: 339-343.

48 Schweiger H, Klein P, Lang W. Tibial bypass grafting for limb salvage with ringed polytetrafluorethylene prostheses: results of primary and secondary procedures. *J Vasc Surg* 1993; 18: 867-874.

6

HOW TO PERFORM ENDOVASCULAR REVASCULARIZATIONS

MAURO GARGIULO, FEDERICA GIOVANETTI, FRANCESCA FRATESI, ANTONIO FREYRIE, NATASCIA MUCCINI, GIANLUCA FAGGIOLI, FILIPPO MAIOLI, ANDREA STELLA

Critical limb ischemia (CLI) is defined as a condition in which peripheral arterial occlusive disease (PAOD) has resulted in leg or foot pain at rest or in the development of ulcers or gangrene with ankle or toe systolic pressures less than 50 or 30 mmHg, respectively. Without revascularization, patients with CLI are at risk for leg amputation and potentially fatal complications due to the progression of gangrene and infection and ultimately sepsis.

Endovascular therapy is the treatment of choice for CLI in patients with arterial stenosis or short arterial occlusion [1]. The procedural and clinical goals of this therapy are limb revascularization by restoration of straight-line pulsating blood flow to the foot, and to relieve CLI to achieve wound healing, avoiding major amputation.

The selection of the appropriate endovascular technique must be considered in the light of many variables: the extension and location of the PAOD, the nature of the occlusive disease (stenosis/occlusion, calcified plaque) and therefore, in the algorithm for treatment of CLI, the first step is to confirm ischemic etiology of the leg symptoms and the second step is to define the extend and severity of the obstructive disease.

Assessment of CLI

After the clinical diagnosis of CLI is established, more specific vascular tests must be performed and among objective criteria for the diagnosis of arterial occlusive disease the use of Ankle Brachial Index (ABI), toe systolic pressure (TSP) and transcutaneous oxygen tension ($TcPO_2$) has been suggested. A resting ABI of < 0.4 strongly suggests CLI; in diabetics the ABI may be unreliable due to significant calcification of the media layer, making the tibial arteries incompressible [2]. A Toe Systolic Pressure of ≤ 30 mmHg suggests the presence of CLI; in patients with forefoot gangrene the TSP is often impossible to measure due to the presence of a lesion [2]. For all these reasons, frequently, in clinical practice the $TcPO_2$ at the dorsum of the foot is required to objectively confirm the diagnosis of CLI; on the basis of the Faglia's data, $TcPO_2 < 40$ mmHg indicated a CLI and a need for revascularization [3].

Once CLI has been confirmed, specific vascular investigations must be performed to assess the length and morphology of the arterial occlusive disease. In patients with CLI, multi-level arterial occlusive disease is commonly present; for the revascularization strategy it is important to assess all major vessels including abdominal aorta, iliac arteries, infra-inguinal vessels, infrapopliteal vessels and foot arteries. Duplex scanning (DS) is an excellent technique to determine the exact location and severity of PAOD [4,5] and it is ideal for predicting access sites for interventions. There are some limitations to be considered when evaluating this technique: the procedure is operator-dependent, the method is inconclusive in patients with arterial wall or plaque calcification and in patients with leg edema, tandem lesions may be underestimated in case of poor run-in. As a result of limitations to DS, in patients with equivocal examinations, arteriography is required to assess the extension of arterial disease and both techniques must be used to supplement each other [6].

After assessment of the arterial occlusive disease we can decide on the type of endovascular revascularization. If we look at the history of endovascular therapy, the first endovascular arterial procedure was performed in 1963 by Dotter and Judkins; they treated focal distal superficial femoral artery stenosis with a coaxial system in a patient with severe ischemia [7]. In 1974 Gruentzig and Hopff first described the clinical application of a double lumen balloon catheter [8]; this catheter had one lumen for a guidewire and one lumen for inflation of the balloon. The original balloons were made of PVC and were excessively compliant; in 1979 the polyethylene balloons (less trackability, lower compliance and profile than PVC balloons) were introduced in the market. Now percutaneous transluminal angioplasty (PTA) with balloon catheter is the gold standard among percutaneously applied technology in the treatment of PAOD; it can be used alone or associated with other endovascular procedures (stents or endografts implantations, debulking techniques etc). Whatever the choice of endovascular technique, the first step in endovascular therapy is the choice of vascular access.

Vascular access

A key issue in the successful completion of a complex endovascular interventions is selection of the appropriate vascular access. Access to blood vessels can be achieved by means of direct puncture (Seldinger technique) or surgical vessel exposure. The Seldinger technique was first described in 1953 by a Swedish radiologist to perform angiography [9]. The artery is punctured percutaneously with a sharp hollow needle (Seldinger needle) maintaining a 45° angle as compared to the ideal center-line of the target blood vessel (Fig. 1). After puncture, the needle is pushed upwards and a 0.035" floppy-angled guidewire is inserted. Following, the needle is withdrawn and the artery is compressed to avoid bleeding. A sheath is threaded over the wire and inserted into the artery. The choice of sheath diameter and length depends on the diameter of the endovascular equipment that will be required to complete the intervention and the extend of the arterial disease. In specific cases (graft in the puncture site, obesity, hybrid procedures etc.) the percutaneous approach is not possible and surgical exposure of the artery is required (Fig. 2). The endovascular approach to the arteries could be antegrade or retrograde. The stand-

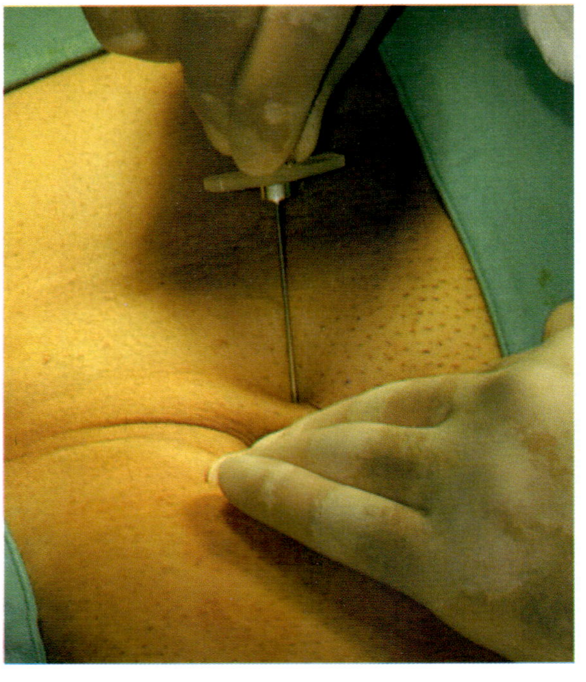

FIG. 1 Percutaneous antegrade access to the common femoral artery with a sharp hollow needle.

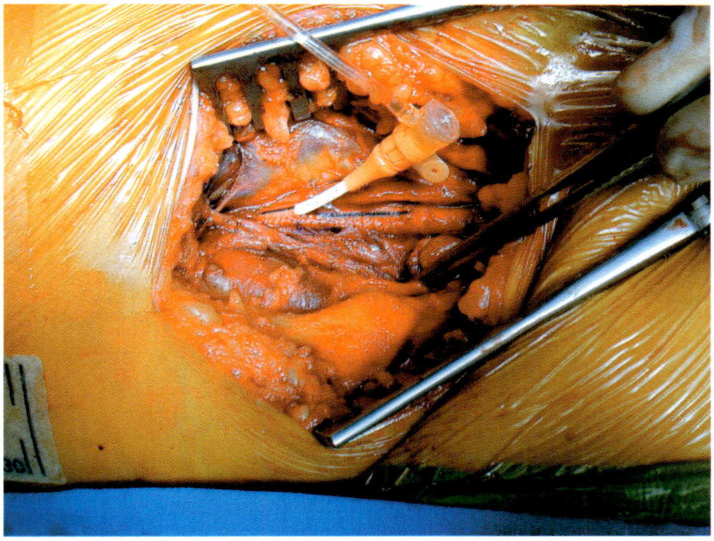

FIG. 2 Surgical access to the femoral artery in a patient with PAOD undergoing a hybrid procedure: endarterectomy, patch plasty and angioplasty.

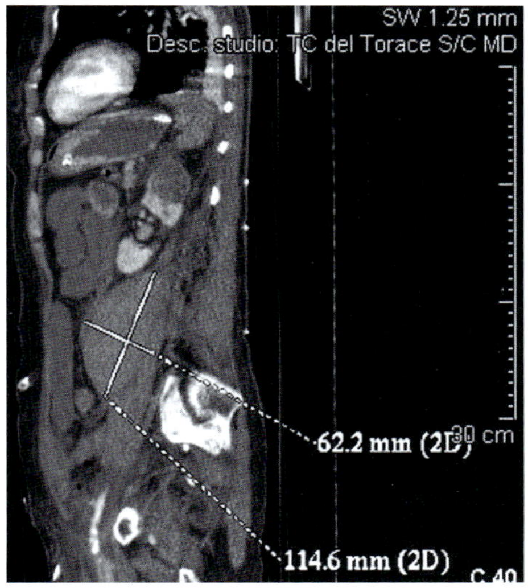

FIG. 3 Retroperitoneal hematoma due to antegrade puncture of the common femoral artery and inadequate manual compression.

ard access to blood vessels is the common femoral artery (CFA) approached in retrograde (first choice in the treatment of aortic lesions, ipsilateral iliac lesions, contralateral iliac and infra-inguinal lesions) or antegrade (ipsilateral infra-inguinal lesions) manner.

The retrograde CFA access is a commonly used approach to treat contralateral iliac and proximal superficial femoral artery (SFA) disease. In patients with an acute angle at the aortic bifurcation or significant iliac tortuosity or in patients requiring popliteal and/or infrapopliteal endovascular treatment, the retrograde CFA access can be replaced by the antegrade, ipsilateral CFA approach; indeed in these patients the endovascular procedure with contralateral approach could be difficult and time consuming. In the ipsilateral and antegrade approach, CFA punctures may be performed below the groin crease because of the lower risk of retroperitoneal hemorrhage due to external iliac artery puncture (Fig. 3). Those puncture sites ensure a safer vessel compression at the end of the endovascular procedure.

Another alternative to the CFA access is the retrograde approach using direct puncture of the popliteal [10] or pedal arteries [11] and the combined antegrade and retrograde approach ("Safari" technique) [12]. These accesses have recently been suggested in cases of inability to cross the SFA, popliteal and tibial artery occlusions. However, these techniques require a long training and learning-curve. Also the antegrade approach from the upper extremity arteries (brachial or axillary arteries) can be considered in patients with CFA approach contra-indications; it is only suitable in patients with aorto-iliac or proximal-mid SFA disease.

CONTRALATERAL RETROGRADE CFA ACCESS

The Seldinger technique is used for access in the CFA contralateral to the target lesion. A diagnostic catheter is then advanced in the ipsilateral iliac artery in a retrograde fashion over a 0.035 wire to the aorta and used to engage the contralateral common iliac artery (CIA) (Fig. 4). To reach the CIA contralateral to the CFA, peculiar-shaped curved catheters are available such as "Pig-tail", "Simmons", "J-curved", "Cobra" and "Hooh". A soft hydrophilic guidewire (0.035 inch) is navigated through the guiding catheter and advanced into the femoral artery and the diagnostic catheter is positioned in the artery. Following, the floppy wire is exchanged for a stiff-angled 0.035" guidewire and the diagnostic catheter is pushed forward to achieve a stable access to the contralateral CFA. The stiff guidewire opens the angle of the aortic bifurcation and facilitates the placement of the appropriate crossover sheath. To provide optimal support for the recanalization procedure, a crossover sheath is threaded over the wire and/or the catheter to the contralateral CFA ostium.

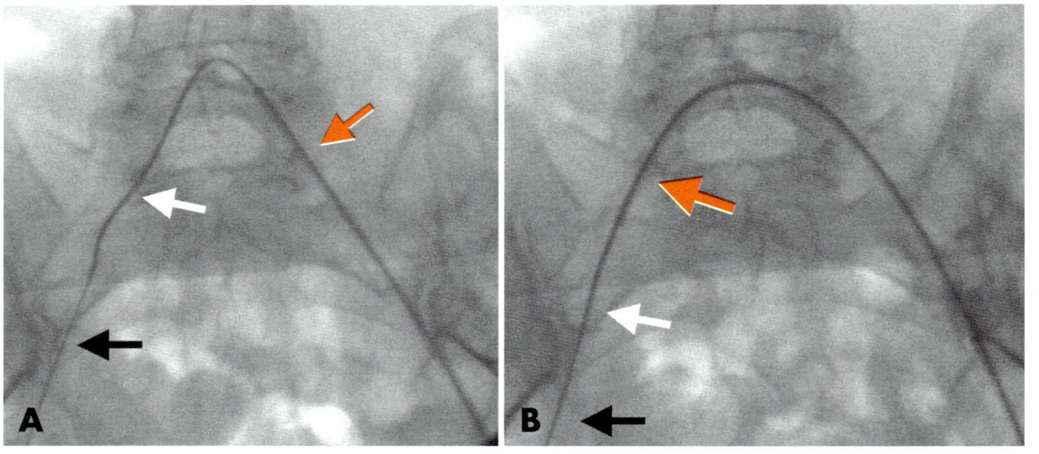

FIG. 4 Left common femoral artery retrograde access to treat a proximal lesion of the right superficial femoral artery. Black arrows: 0.035 stiff guidewire; white arrows: pig tail catheter; red arrows: 45 cm sheath. A) The sheath (length 45 cm) is in the ipsilateral left iliac axis; B) The sheath has made the cross-over over the stiff guide wire and the catheter and is in the right iliac axis.

Ipsilateral antegrade CFA access

The Seldinger technique is used for access in the CFA ipsilateral to the target lesion. Supra-inguinal puncture should be avoided due to the high risk of retroperitoneal hemorrhage. Particular attention should be given to the lenght of the sheath considering the level of the lesion to treat. The standard sheath used in this access is short (11 cm), enabling diagnostic angiography and endovascular procedures in the femoro-popliteal axis with a stable access. In patients who need treatment of isolated popliteal and/or tibial arteries lesions, we use a long sheath (> 30 cm). A long sheath is also helpful in multisegmental atherosclerotic disease because, after the treatment of the proximal lesion, the sheath can be threaded into the SFA to perform the distal treatment without sheath changing.

Ipsilateral retrograde popliteal or pedal access

This type of approach is indicated in patients with SFA, popliteal or tibial arteries obstruction. The first step is a antegrade or retrograde CFA access with the patient in the supine position. Following, the patient is placed in the prone position to reach the popliteal fossa. In particular cases a road-map arteriography can be performed from the CFA access to visualize the popliteal artery. Due to the small diameter of the popliteal artery (6 mm approximately), the sheath diameter of choice ranges from 4 F to 6 F. The first-choice guidewire used in this access is a 0.018" or 0.014" stiff hydrophilic wire. The retrograde pedal artery approach was first described by Iyer in 1990 using a cutdown of the pedal arteries [13]. To perform the dorsalis pedis or plantar artery access we need a road-mapping arteriography or a fluoroscopy of the foot. A 20 G needle is used to puncture the artery and a 4 F sheath to introduce guidewires and balloon catheters. In order to limit vascular trauma the application of a sheath can be abandoned. The first-choice guidewire used in this type of access is a 0.014" stiff hydrophilic wire [14].

In both retrograde popliteal and tibial approach, when recanalization is achieved, the wire is pushed from the distal puncture site further into the antegrade sheath. Over this wire, from the antegrade access, a guiding-catheter or balloon catheter is inserted to assure the antegrade access to the lesion and peripheral retrograde access is removed.

A specific type of retrograde approach for recanalization of below knee artery occlusion is the trans-collateral loop technique (Fig. 5), which has been suggested by Fusaro et al. [15] in patients with challenging infrapopliteal occlusion.

Antegrade brachial access

Brachial artery puncture, using the Seldinger technique, is performed with the wrist extended and the hand in supine position. The landmark for the puncture site is the wrist crease. The small size

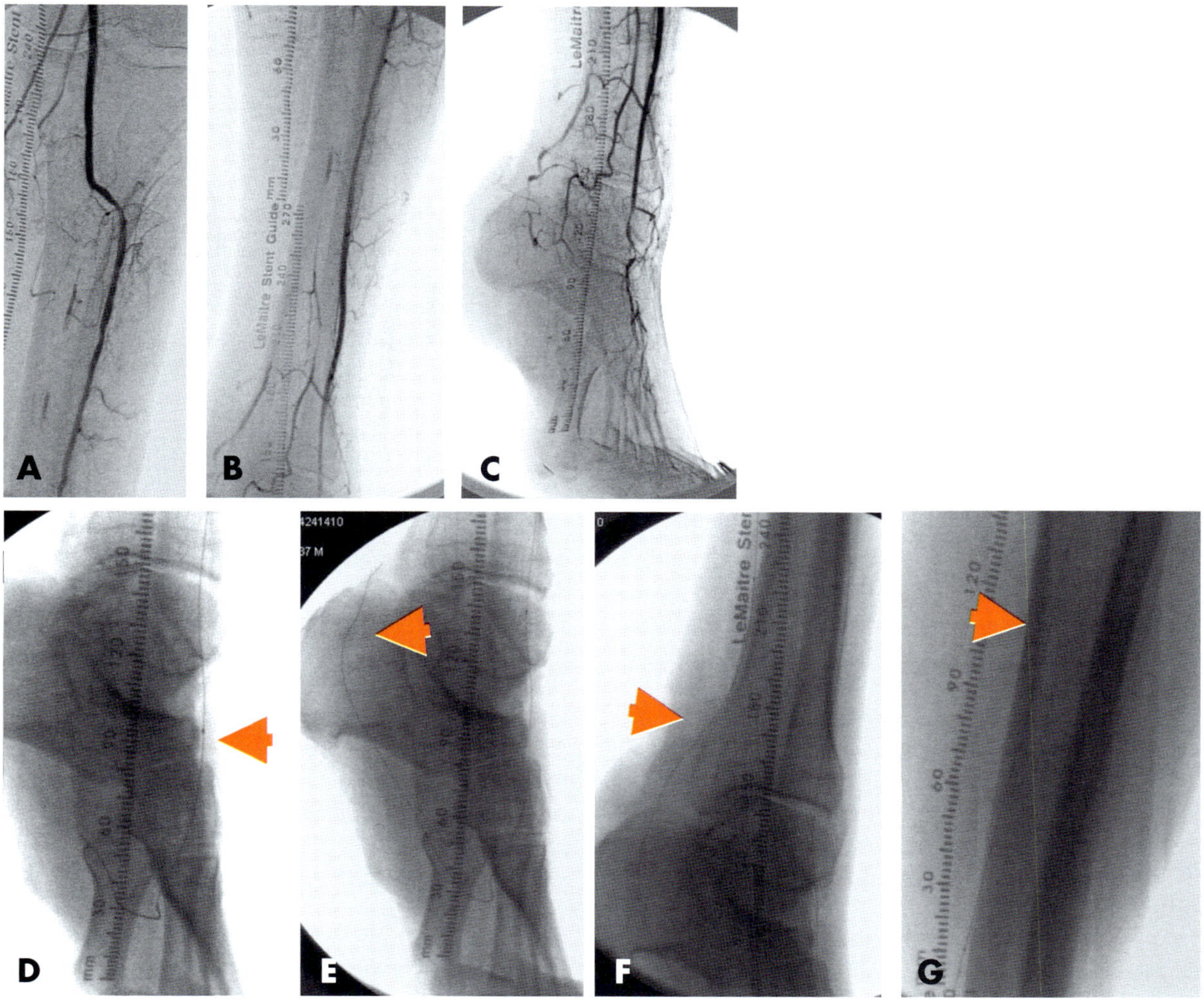

FIG. 5 Tibial artery disease in diabetic patients. Long obstruction of the posterior tibial artery and multiple obstructions of the peroneal artery (A-C). Recanalization of the proximal segment of the posterior tibial artery by a 0.014 guidewire introduced into the anterior tibial artery. The guidewire (red arrow), supported by a low-profile balloon-catheter is in the dorsalis pedis (D), in the plantar artery (E) (the loop technique), in the distal segment of the posterior tibial artery (F) and in the proximal segment of posterior tibial artery (G).

of this artery (4-5 mm approximately) only allows the use of a small size sheath (4 F, 5 F). This fact, matched with the length of the interventional devices, limits the indications of this access. However, this approach offers the advantage of early ambulation and lowers the risk of bleeding complications but increases the risk of ischemic complications, due to spasm or thrombosis of the access artery. A serious complication is cerebral embolism due to the wire crossing in the aortic arch; the risk can be reduced using the left arm. After arterial access and positioning of the sheath, intra-arterial heparin is given as a matter of routine between 3 000 and 5 000 units and the diagnostic arteriogram is performed; the angiography provides the basis for selection of the guidewire and balloon catheters and to define the PTA technique.

PTA technique

The PTA technique involves the use of a balloon catheter to dilate the arterial segment affected by obstructive lesions. A wide variety of balloon catheters are available; all have opaque markers at the proximal and distal ends of the balloon to facilitate accurate positioning. Balloon catheters are described by a series of numbers which indicate balloon diameter, balloon length, catheter French size and catheter length. With regard to balloon diameter, most operators choose a balloon width equal to the measured calibre of a normal portion of the vessel adjacent to the arterial lesions; this is a good option for stenosis whereas it is better to underestimate the balloon diameter in arterial occlusions because overdilatation could increase the risk of arterial rupture and flow limiting dissection. In general the range of balloon sizes for the aorta, iliac, femoro-popliteal and infrapopliteal arteries varies between 9 to 18 mm, 6 to 9 mm, 4 to 6 mm and 1.5 to 4 mm, respectively.

The balloon length must be longer than the segment to be dilated and the balloon compliance must be defined according to the morphology of the arterial lesion. Compliance is a measure of the degree to which a balloon stretches in response to increasing inflation pressure. Compliant balloons are more likely to stretch beyond their maximal diameter and therefore have a lower burst pressure and supply a lower dilating force; in low-compliance balloons, the diameter will increase linearly with the pressure until the maximum diameter is achieved and the maximal diameter will not change significantly in response to additional pressure. The third group of balloons is the "high-pressure" balloon which are the least compliant. Today we use high-pressure balloons for heavily calcified arterial lesions and low-compliance balloons for all other arterial lesions.

PTA is a simple and effective technique in the treatment of arterial stenosis of non-calcified plaque or short occlusion; it presents considerable technical difficulties in patients with arterial long occlusion or arterial stenosis by calcified plaque. In the latter cases the critical point is to pass the arterial lesion with a hydrophilic guidewire (straight or J, floppy or stiff), the diameter of which varies according to the arterial segment to be treated (range: 0.035-0.014 inch) and the operator experience. In order to support the guidewire the use of an angiographic catheter (straight or angled, 4 or 5 Fr) or a low-profile balloon catheter can be considered; in these cases the guidewire should kept at least several centimeters ahead of the tip of the catheter. The diseased segment is probed and the operator should be guided both by feel and fluoroscopy. At this point, arterial recanalization may be effected by intraluminal or intentional subintimal technique.

Intraluminal technique

The ease with which an occluded arterial segment is crossed by intraluminal technique is dependent on the age of the thrombus and on the severity of the occlusive lesion. The guidewire (J or straight) is advanced into the initial segment of the occlusion until it buckles or resistence is encountered. The degree of buckling and resistance to advancement offers an indication of the extent of the thrombus and the severity of occlusive disease. If the resistance is high at this point it is necessary to advance a straight catheter to give further support to the guidewire. During these maneuvers it is necessary to inject small boluses of contrast medium to be sure of being in the lumen of the vessel and not in the subintimal space (unintentional subintimal recanalization). After the occluded segment is passed there will be blood return on aspiration along the catheter; if the obstruction has been passed with the help of a catheter, the guidewire is removed and contrast media injected through the catheter to define the run-off. A balloon catheter is positioned over the guidewire and the length and diameter of the balloon are chosen according to the arterial segment to be treated. To reduce the risk of complications (rupture of the wall, peripheral embolism a predilatation with a balloon catheter of small diameter can be performed.

Since the intraluminal PTA with bare balloon catheter is characterized by a high rate of restenosis [16], it was recently proposed to use drug-coated angioplasty balloons. These balloon catheters have shown a significant reduction in late lumen loss and target-lesion revascularization [17].

Subintimal technique

The most widely recognized angioplasty variation is the use of intentional subintimal angioplasty popularized by the Leicester group [18]. The goal of subintimal angioplasty is to intentionally maneuver the guidewire into the subintimal layer at the occlusion's origin. The inclusion morphological criteria for this technique are calcified and long occlusions (Fig. 6); when an occlusion is less than 3-month old, the procedure is not attempted. For the technique to be successful, the distal segment of the artery must be reasonably healthy; the presence of a disease-free segment distal to the arterial occlusion allows intraluminal return of the guidewire. Therefore extensively diseased distal segments beyond an occlusion are a relative contra-indication for the subintimal technique.

The technique as described above [18,19], includes a Van Andel 5 F catheter introduced antegradely up to the arterial occlusion. A curved

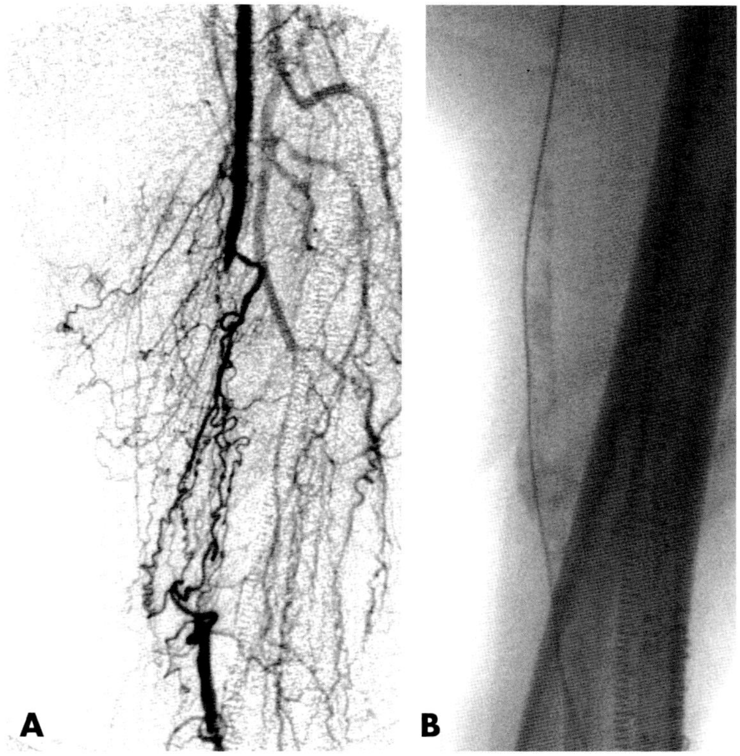

FIG. 6 Superficial femoral artery occlusion (A) with heavy calcification (B). Arterial recanalization through a subintimal approach (B).

tipped hydrophilic guidewire (floppy or stiff) introduced through the catheter is directed towards the wall of the artery at the level of the occlusion. Advancing this guidewire usually causes an arterial wall dissection; the guidewire is manipulated into a loop which is then used to dissect the entire length of the occlusion. The catheter is subsequently advanced in the arterial wall. Distal re-entry of the guidewire in the arterial lumen is the most critical and difficult part of the subintimal angioplasty. Once re-entry has been achieved (spontaneously, through angled catheters or through re-entry systems) the catheter is substituted for a balloon catheter of the appropriate size and the entire length of the dissection is dilated [20]. In many cases, the re-entry point of the guidewire is not at the end of the obstruction or at the beginning of the reconnection segment but more distally within the patent vessel.

Inflation of the balloon

When the balloon, by means of intraluminal or subintimal technique, is properly centered at the arterial lesion it is inflated. There is no absolute standard for inflation time or number of repetitions. Most operators inflate between 30 and 120 seconds and perform a total of 2 to 3 repetitions. During inflation the patient may experience pain which is caused by stretching of adventitial nerve fibres. Pain that persists after deflation is a warning of possible arterial rupture.

Post-procedural morphological result

To define the morphological post-procedure result, at the end of the PTA, intra-arterial angiography should be performed through the sheath with the balloon catheter well removed from the dilatation site and the guidewire left across the lesion.

Technical success is defined as achievement of a residual diameter stenosis < 30% on the procedural completion angiogram. If the residual stenosis is > 30% or if it appears a flow-limiting dissection it is necessary to repeat balloon inflation. In case of persistent residual stenosis > 30%, a flow-limiting dissection or an intraluminal thrombosis (suboptimal result) stent implantation should be performed (secondary stenting).

Stent implantation

At present primary stenting is only reserved for calcified lesions of the aorta and iliac axis whereas secondary stenting is indicated in suboptimal results. In the latter case, the stent can fixate the plaque, dissection or thrombosis against the arterial wall and can prevent elastic recoil and post-procedure arterial restenosis.

Stents can be divided into two basic categories: balloon-expandable (BES) and self-expanding stents (SES). BES have greater hoop strength, resulting in more resistance to elastic recoil after full expansion; they deploy more precisely than SES. SES have greater longitudinal flexibility to maximize ease of delivery into tortuous vessels, available in longer treatment lengths and recover from deformation secondary to flexion and extension. The stents most commonly used are constructed of stainless or thermomodulated nitinol.

In addition to the bare stent, the industries are proposing other types of stents: bioabsorbable, coated and drug-eluting stents. The rationale of the use of these stents is to remove or to mitigate the long-term stimulus for neointimal hyperplasia and to decrease in-stent restenosis.

Stents are also manufactured with either a Dacron or an expanded polytetrafluoroethylene (PTFE) covering. PTFE seems to be the better covering material as compared to Dacron. These so-called stent-grafts or covered-stents are now used with increasing frequency to treat long-segment occlusive disease (Fig. 7) aiming at decreased in-stent restenosis and improving vessel patency [21]. The rationale for using covered-stents is to exclude the plaque from the arterial lumen by creating a mechanical barrier that will isolate atheroma and smooth muscle cells from the circulating blood. Compared to conventional stents, stent-grafts may combine the radial resistence of the stent with a mechanical barrier to prevent restenosis.

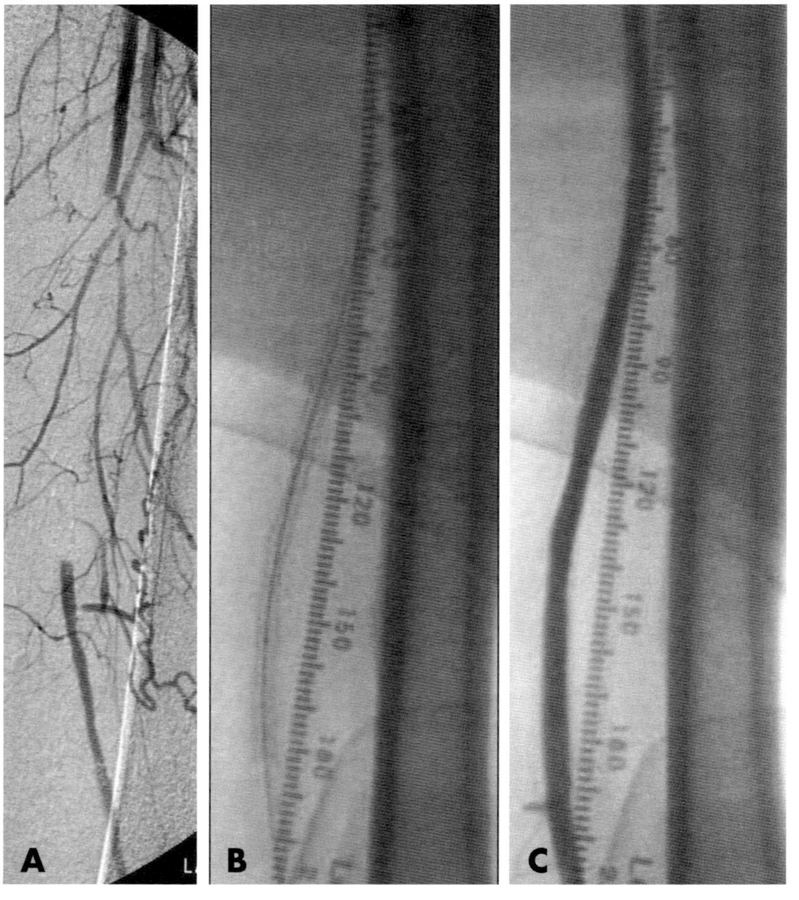

FIG. 7 Long chronic total occlusion of superficial femoral artery (A); release of the PTFE stent-graft (B); completion angiogram (C).

DEBULKING TECHNIQUES

A debulking strategy prior to balloon angioplasty is warranted in many cases. Removal of obstructive material can facilitate crossing of total occlusions, debulking and removal of the obstructive material to transform an occlusion into a more easily balloonable stenosis. Several techniques have been developed to remove the endoluminal occlusive material like laser and atherectomy devices.

The principle of laser-assisted angioplasty is debulking by means of laser light. The excimer laser facilitates successful treatment of the most severe PAOD by ablating and removing thrombus and other obstructive material [22]. The Rotablator is a high-speed rotating device for transluminal atherectomy with a central guidewire. The Rotablator works by means of the cutting action of the diamond fragments which are able to splinter and remove the plaque by reducing it to microparticles of a size inferior to that of the red globules. The removal action works efficiently on calcified plaques while leaving the arterial wall undamaged [23]. The SilverHawk plaque excision system consist of 2 components: a low profile catheter and a palm sized drive unit. A tiny blade on the tip of the catheter rotates when activated and removes the plaque from the arterial wall [24].

All devices designed for the debulking technique seem to work. However, the important question to be answered is whether these modalities have superior results as compared to PTA. Until now there is no answer to this question and it is difficult to justify the use of these devices considering costs, complex application and the frequent necessity of complementary techniques.

MEDICAL THERAPY

Antiplatelet and anticoagulant therapy play an important role before, during and after endovascular treatment of CLI. The majority of patients with CLI are on antiplatelet therapy (aspirin or clopidogrel) for primary or secondary prevention of any ischemic complication, such as myocardial infarction and stroke.

As soon as vascular access is obtained routine systemic heparinization (2 500 U-5 000 U) is performed before revascularization. Also, in order to prevent intra-arterial, peri-sheath or peri-catheter thrombosis, all devices introduced into the artery need to be frequently flushed with heparinized saline solution.

After endovascular treatment, patients are discharged with a combination of 100 mg/day acetylsalicylic acid or ticlopidine 500 mg/day and low molecular weight heparin for one month and long-lasting Aspirin 100 mg/day therapy or ticlopidine 500 mg/day afterwards. After a complex endovascular procedure with stent placement or tibial artery angioplasty with or without stent, before discharging patients, at least 48 hours heparin infusion is administered.

REFERENCES

1 Norgren L, Hiatt WR, Dormandy JA et al. Inter-Society Consensus for the Management of Peripheral Arterial Disease (TASC II). *Eur J Vasc Endovasc Surg* 2007; 33 (Suppl 1): S54-S64.

2 Faglia E, Clerici G, Caminiti M et al. Accuratezza della pressione arteriosa alla caviglia e della ossimetria transcutanea al dorso del piede per la diagnosi di ischemia critica nei pazienti diabetici. In: Stella A, Gargiulo M, editors. *Arteriopatia Diabetica Periferica*. Turin: Edizioni Minerva Medica; 2009. pp. 61-67.

3 Faglia E, Clerici G, Caminiti M et al. Predictive values of transcutaneous oxygen tension for above-the-ankle amputation in diabetic patients with critical limb ischemia. *Eur J Vasc Endovasc Surg* 2007; 33: 731-736.

4 Ascher E, Mazzariol F, Hingorani A et al. The use of duplex ultrasound arterial mapping as an alternative to conventional arteriography for primary and secondary infrapopliteal bypasses. *Am J Surg* 1999; 178: 162-165.

5 Lujan S, Criado E, Puras E et al. Duplex scanning or arteriography for preoperative planning of lower limb revascularisation. *Eur J Vasc Endovasc Surg* 2002; 24: 31-36.

6 Koelemay M, Legemate D, Reekers J et al. Duplex scanning and angiography of the lower leg and foot arteries. In: Brancherau A, Jacobs M, editors. *Critical limb ischemia*. Armonk NY: Futura Publishing Company; 1999. pp. 55-62.

7 Dotter CT, Judkins MP. Transluminal treatment of arteriosclerotic obstruction: description of a new technique and a preliminary report of its application. *Circulation* 1964; 30: 654-670.

8 Gruentzing A. Hopff H. Die perkutane rekanalisation chronisscer arterieller verschlusse mit einer neuen dilatationskatheter: modifikation der Dotter-technik. *Dtsch Med Wochenschr* 1974; 99: 2502-2505.

9 Seldinger SI. "Catheter replacement of the needle in percutaneous arteriography; a new technique". *Acta radiologica* 1953; 39: 368-376.

10 Noory E, Rastan A, Schwarzwälder U et al. Retrograde transpopliteal recanalization of chronic superficial femoral artery occlusion after failed re-entry during antegrade subintimal angioplasty. *J Endovasc Ther* 2009; 16: 619-623.

11 Fusaro M, Tashani A, Mollichelli N et al. Retrograde pedal artery access for below-the-knee percutaneous revascularisation. *J Cardiovasc Med* 2007; 8: 216-218.

12 Gandini R, Pipitone V, Stefanini M. The "Safari" technique to

perform difficult subintimal infragenicular vessels. *Cardiovasc Intervent Radiol* 2007; 30: 469-473.

13 Iyer SS, Dorros G, Zaitoun R et al. Retrograde recanalization of an occluded posterior tibial artery by using a posterior tibial cutdown : two cases report. *Cath Cardiovasc Diagn* 1990; 20: 251-253.

14 Montero-Baker M, Schmidt A, Bräunlich S et al. Retrograde approach for complex popliteal and tibioperoneal occlusions. *J Endovasc Ther* 2008; 15: 594-604.

15 Fusaro M, Agostani P, Biondi-Zoccai G. "Trans-collateral" angioplasty for a challenging chronic total occlusion of the tibial vessels: a novel approach to percutaneous revascularization in critical lower limb ischemia. *Catheter Cardiovasc Interv* 2008; 71: 268-272.

16 Anonymous. TASC TransAtalantic Inter-Society Consensus (TASC). Management of peripheral arterial disease (PAD). *Eur J Vasc Endovasc Surg* 2000; 19 (Suppl A): S88.

17 Tepe G, Zeller T, Albrecht T et al. Local delivery of paclitaxel to inhibit restenosis during angioplasty of the leg. *N Engl J Med* 2008; 358: 689-699.

18 Bolia A, Miles KA, Brennan J et al. Percutaneous transluminal angioplasty of occlusions of the femoral and popliteal arteries by subintimal dissection. *Cardiovasc Intervent Radiol* 1990; 13: 357-363.

19 Bolia A, Bell PR. Femoropopliteal and crural artery recanalization using subintimal angioplasty. *Semin Vasc Surg* 1995; 8: 253-264.

20 Hausegger KA, Georgieva B, Portugaller H et al. The outback catheter: a new device for true lumen re-entry after dissection during recanalization of arterial occlusions. *Cardiovasc Intervent Radiol* 2004; 27: 26-30.

21 McQuade K, Gable D, Hohman S et al. Randomized comparison of ePTFE/nitinol self-expanding setnt graft vs prosthetic femoro-popliteal bypass in the treatment of superfcial femoral artery occlusive disease. *J Vasc Surg* 2009; 49: 109-116.

22 Laird JR, Reiser C, Biamino G et al. Excimer laser assisted angioplasty for the treatment od critical limb ischemia. *J Cardiovasc Surg (Torino)* 2004; 45: 239-248.

23 Henry M, Amor M, Ethevenot G et al. Percutaneous peripheral rotational ablation using the Rotablator: immediate and mid-term results. Single center experience concerning 146 lesions treated. *Int Angiol* 1993; 12: 231-244.

24 Zeller T, Rastan A, Sixt S et al. Long-term results after directional atherectomy of femoro-popliteal lesions. *J Am Coll Cardiol* 2006; 48: 1573-1578.

7

BYPASS VERSUS ANGIOPLASTY IN SEVERE ISCHEMIA OF THE LEG (BASIL) TRIAL

ANDREW BRADBURY

Severe limb ischemia (SLI) manifests itself as rest (night) pain and/or tissue loss (ulceration/gangrene) and imposes a major health, social, and economic burden on all developed, and an increasing number of developing, countries. Our ageing populations, the increasing prevalence of diabetes and obesity and their vascular complications worldwide, together with the failure thus far to significantly reduce global tobacco consumption mean that, despite advances in medical therapies, the numbers of patients requiring lower limb revascularization for SLI are likely to increase significantly in the foreseeable future [1]). The two available interventions, bypass surgery (BSX) and balloon angioplasty (BAP), have been generally considered to have a number of relative advantages and disadvantages (Table I). Previous studies have attempted to compare BSX with BAP but all have had one or more serious methodological limitations [2-4]. The resulting absence of level 1 evidence has resulted in a lack of clarity as to whether BSX or BAP is associated with a better clinical outcome, and a more effective use of health care resources, in patients whose legs are threatened by SLI.

To address this problem the UK National Institute of Health Research (NIHR) Health Technology Assessment (HTA) program (http://www.hta.ac.uk/) funded the Bypass versus Angioplasty in Severe Ischemia of the Leg (BASIL) trial in 1998 [5-7]. The aim of BASIL trial was to compare, for the first time in a multi-center randomized controlled trial (RCT), the clinical and cost-effectiveness of a BSX and a BAP first revascularization strategy for SLI due to infra-inguinal disease.

Methods

Prior to the trial a Delphi consensus study of vascular surgeons' and interventional radiologists' views on the most appropriate treatment of SLI due to infra-inguinal disease was undertaken with the aim of identifying the "grey area of clinical equipoise" for the trial [8,9].

Between August 1999 and June 2004 452 patients presenting to 27 UK hospitals with SLI due to infra-inguinal disease, and who required immediate/early revascularization, were randomized to either a BSX first (n = 228) or a BAP first (n = 224) revascularization strategy [10]) (Fig. 1). The main outcomes were amputation-free survival (AFS), overall survival (OS), health related quality of life (HRQL), and use of hospital resources. All patients provided written informed consent and the study was approved by the Multi-center Research Ethics Committee (MREC) for Scotland. The BASIL trial was registered with the National Research Register (NRR) and the International Standard Randomised Controlled Trials Number (ISRCTN) Scheme (Number 45398889). Follow-up data were obtained from dedicated research nurses; the Information and Statistics Division (ISD) of the NHS in Scotland using record linkage to Scottish Morbidity Records (SMR01) and the General Registrar Office (Scotland); the Office of National Statistics (ONS) in England; paper and electronic hospital records; and General Practitioners. Pre-intervention angiograms were scored using the TASC II classification [1] and the Bollinger Scoring System [11].

Results

Delphi consensus studies

There was very substantial disagreement between and among vascular surgeons and interventional radiologists with regard to the appropriateness of BSX or BAP for SLI due to infra-inguinal disease across a wide range of different clinical and angiographic scenarios [8,9]. This disagreement

Table I The potential advantages and disadvantages of BSX and BAP as a first line treatment for SLI due to infra-inguinal disease (as often stated prior to the BASIL trial)

	BSX	*BAP*
Pros	Superior long-term anatomic patency and clinical durability	Low morbidity and mortality and requirement for urgent surgical intervention Low cost Quick to perform Shorter hospital stay Can be repeated Failed angioplasty has been said not to jeopardize subsequent surgery Preserves collaterals so that even if the angioplasty site occludes symptoms may not return and tissue loss may remain healed
Cons	Significant morbidity and mortality Significant resource utilization (theater time and personnel, prolonged hospital stay) Graft surveillance, often leading to repeated prophylactic re-intervention, required to optimize patency Vein as a conduit often unavailable, inadequate in length or poor quality Use of prosthetic material associated with poorer patency and risk of graft infection	Limited anatomic and hemodynamic patency and clinical durability Only a minority of patients may be suitable, especially with the trans-luminal technique The technique, particularly using the sub-intimal approach, is technically demanding and satisfactory results may not be widely achievable

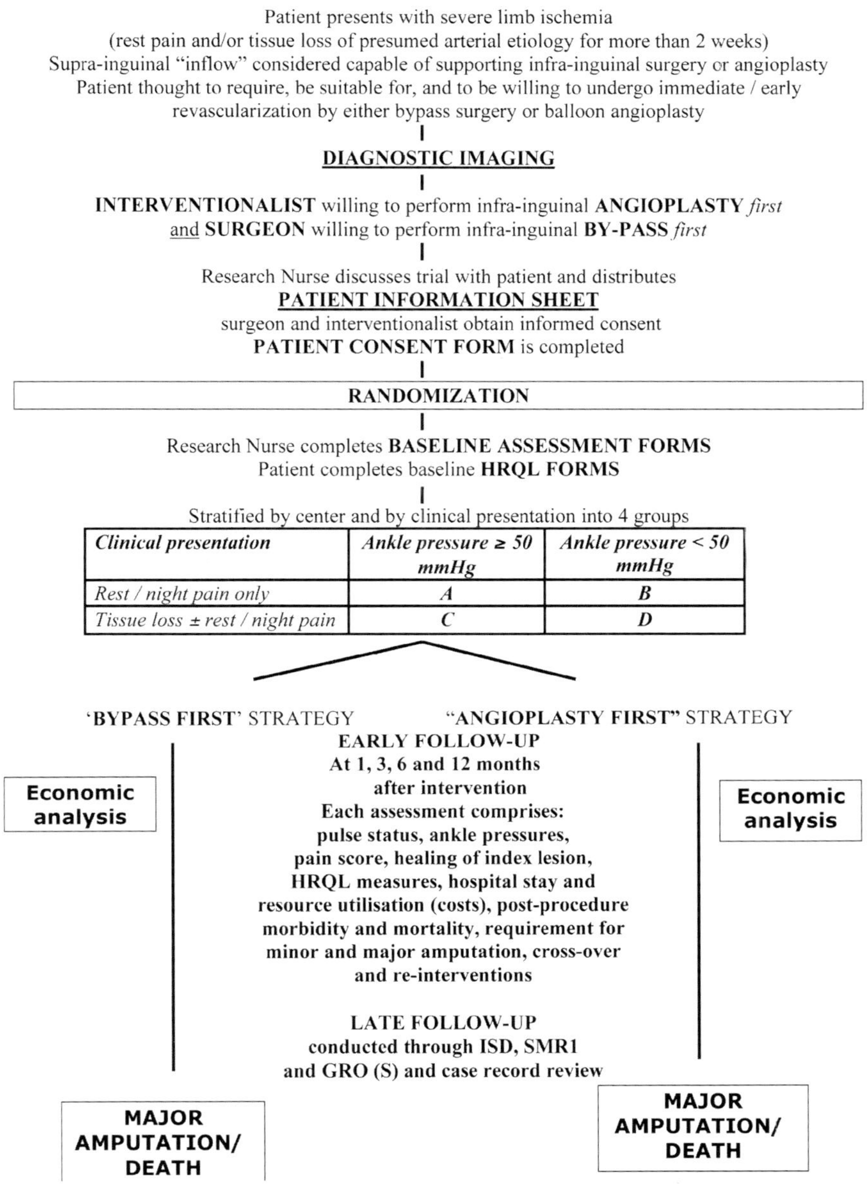

FIG. 1 Flow diagram of BASIL trial design.

was greater among surgeons. Surgeons and interventionalists viewed the risks and benefits of their own, and their counterpart's, treatment modality very differently.

BASIL trial audit

Approximately half of the patients presenting to the top six BASIL recruiting centers during the recruitment period with SLI due to infra-inguinal were judged to require, be suitable for, and gave their consent to, immediate/early revascularization by either BSX or BAP. Of these, approximately 30% were considered eligible for randomization in that they were judged by the responsible surgeon and interventionalist to be equally suitable for either a BSX first or a BAP first strategy; circa (c.) 70% of such patients were randomized (Fig. 2).

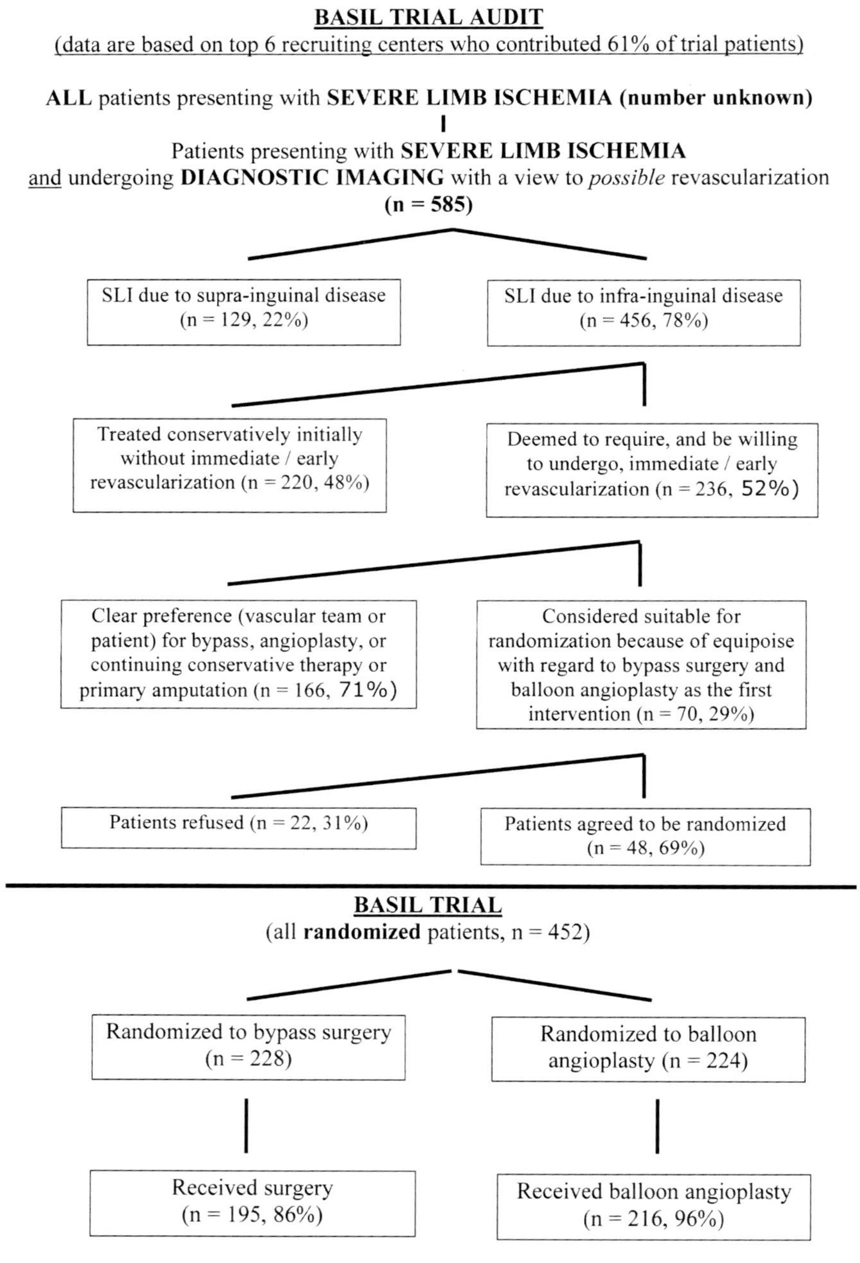

FIG. 2 BASIL trial audit: CONSORT diagram showing patients flow into trial.

Patient characteristics

Trial patients were well matched in terms of baseline clinical data and the angiographic severity and extent of disease. Over 40% patients had diabetes; over a third were still smoking; three-quarters had tissue loss; over a half had an ankle pressure < 50 mmHg; a quarter had bilateral SLI; and most were elderly with a significant cardiovascular past medical history. Despite this, a third of patients was not receiving an anti-platelet agent and only a third of patients was receiving a statin when referred to the vascular service for consideration of intervention. With regard the distribution and severity of infra-inguinal disease, over 40% of the cohort were TASC II group C or D and over 40% were TASC II B. The profunda femoris artery (PFA) was relatively spared with most disease being concentrated in the distal superficial femoral and proximal popliteal arteries where most patients had occlusion. Approximately one half of patients had occlusion in the proximal and/or distal half of the posterior tibial artery (PTA). The anterior tibial artery (ATA) was less affected with distal and/or proximal occlusions in approximately one third of patients. The peroneal artery (PerA) was relatively spared. Where forefoot views were available the plantar arch was considered occluded in almost 20% of cases.

Nature of the interventions received

A quarter of BSX involved prosthetic material; 90% of vein grafts were constructed using great saphenous vein; and the distal anastomoses were fashioned in approximately equal numbers at the above-knee popliteal, below-knee popliteal, and crural arteries. With regard to BAP, in c. 70% of patients, interventional radiologists attempted to treat a single length of disease; in the remainder attempts were made to treat several (up to 4) separate disease lengths. The numbers of trans-luminal and sub-intimal BAP were approximately equal with just over 10% being reported as mixed. Approximately 80% of the BAP patients underwent treatment of the superficial femoral artery either alone (c. 40%) or in combination with the popliteal artery (c. 40%) and crural arteries (c. 20%). Most of the remaining BAP patients underwent treatment of the popliteal segments either alone or more usually in combination with crural arteries; the number of isolated crural artery balloon BAP was small. Patients who had BAP first were significantly more likely to suffer an immediate technical or early clinical failure (c. 27%) than those who had BSX first (c. 7%). In over two-thirds of patients, a failed first attempt at BAP was followed by a further intervention and in over 90% of cases that was surgery.

Interim "intention to treat" analysis – 2005

Following randomization, 195/228 (86%) patients randomized to BSX and 216/224 (96%) to BAP underwent an attempt at their allocated treatment at a median (inter-quartile range) of 6 (3-16) and 6 (2-20) days respectively. BSX was associated with significantly lower immediate failure (3% vs. 20%), higher 30-day morbidity (57% vs. 41%) and lower 12 month re-intervention (18% vs. 26%) rates than BAP. The 30-day mortality was similar (BSX 5%, BAP 3%). By 2005, 99% of patients had been followed up for 1 year, 48% for 3 years, 248 (55%) patients were alive with their trial leg intact, 38 (8%) were alive with their trial leg amputated, 36 (8%) had died subsequent to having their trial leg amputated and 130 (29%) had died with their trial leg intact. AFS at 1 and 3 years was not significantly different; 68% and 57% for BSX and 71% and 52% for BAP. However, a post-hoc analysis found a significantly reduced hazard in terms of AFS (adjusted HR 0.37 [95% CI 0.17, 0.77], p = 0.008) and OS (adjusted HR 0.34 [95% CI, 0.17, 0.71], p = 0.004) for a BSX first strategy relative to a BAP first strategy beyond 2 years from randomization [10] (Figs. 3, 4). We therefore followed the patients for another 2½ years to gather further long term outcome data.

Final "intention to treat" analysis – 2008

Apart from 4 patients lost to follow up, by 2008 100% of patients were followed for 3 years and 54% for more than 5 years; the longest follow-up was over 7 years. At the end of follow-up, patients were either dead (n = 250, 56%), alive without amputation (n = 168, 38%), or alive with amputation (n = 30, 7%) (of the trial leg). Considering the follow-up period as a whole, AFS and OS did not differ between randomized strategies. However, for those patients surviving 2 years from randomization, a BSX first revascularization strategy was associated with a reduced hazard ratio (HR) for subsequent AFS (HR 0.85 [95% CI 0.5-1.07], p = 0.108) and for subsequent OS (HR 0.61 [95% CI 0.50-0.75], p = 0.009) in an adjusted, time-dependent Cox proportional hazards model. For those patients who survived for 2 years after randomization, initial randomization to a BSX first revascularization strategy was associated with an increase in subsequent restricted mean OS of 7.3 months (95% CI 1.2-13.4 months, p = 0.02), and an increase in restricted mean AFS of 5.9 months (95% CI 0.2-12.0 months, p = 0.06), during the subsequent mean (range) follow-up of 3.1 (1 to 5.7) years. A non-randomized "by treatment received" analysis showed that patients receiving vein BSX first fared better than those receiving prosthetic BSX first (p < 0.01 for AFS, p = 0.11 for OS, log-

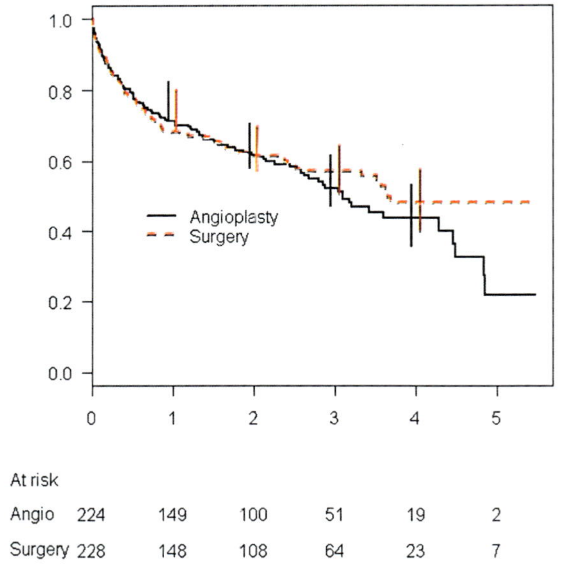

FIG. 3 Amputation free survival following BSX and BAP by intention to treat (2005 analysis).

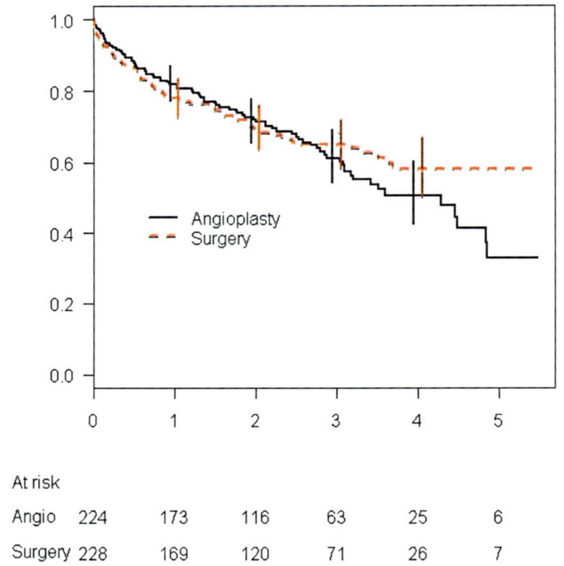

FIG. 4 All cause mortality following BSX and BAP by intention to treat (2005 analysis).

rank tests). There were no differences in outcome between transluminal and sub-intimal BAP. Overall, prosthetic BSX performed significantly worse than both transluminal and sub-intimal BAP. Patients who underwent BSX after failed BAP fared significantly worse in terms of OS and especially AFS than those who underwent BSX as their first treatment.

HRQL

HRQL response rates fell significantly over time (c. 70%-75% at 12 months and c. 40% at both 24 and 36 months) but were very similar for all HRQL instruments used (SF-36, VascuQol, and EuroQoL) and in the two arms. Amputation was associated with a significant reduction in HRQL. When compared to BAP, BSX was associated with (non-significantly) better HRQL before intervention and at all time intervals out to 3 years.

Use of hospital resources

Over the first year hospital costs in patients randomized to BSX (£ 22 002) were significantly higher than in those randomized to BAP (£ 16 582). This decreased to £ 3 533 (£ 29 006 BSX vs. £ 25 472 BAP, NS) by the end of year 3 and to £ 2 310 (£ 33 539 BSX vs. £ 31 228 BAP, NS) by the end of year 7. After three years, procedure costs accounted for 9% of the BAP group costs compared with 14% for the BSX group; most these were incurred in the first year following randomization. Over 7 years the average number of hospital stays for both groups was 4 and average total length of stay was just over 2 months (71 days). On average, BASIL patients spent 5-6 weeks of their first post-randomization year in hospital and then 2-3 weeks per year thereafter. Most of this was in the wards and not in high dependency (HDU) and intensive therapy units (ITU). Patients randomized to BSX used around a half day more of HDU and few more hours of ITU than those randomized to BAP. A 7-year (non-quality adjusted) perspective shows that patients randomized to BSX live, on average, 41 days longer with their trial leg intact at an additional average cost of £ 2 310 when compared to BAP. The additional cost per AFS year is, therefore, £ 20 579. The 7-year (non-quality adjusted) cost-effectiveness ratio for OS (additional 29 days) is £ 29 095. A 36-month quality-adjusted perspective generates a mean quality-adjusted life time of 442 days for BAP and 452 days for BAP (mean difference 10 days [95% CI -48, 68], NS). This extra 10 days is obtained at an estimated additional average hospital cost of £ 3 533 for BSX so giving point estimate of the cost-effectiveness of BSX compared with BAP over 3 years, the "cost per QALY", of £ 125 499.

Factors predicting survival to 2 years

The modelling of factors that might predict whether individual SLI patients might survive for two years after intervention is fraught with methodological and interpretational challenges. Any estimates of survival so produced must, therefore, be used with great care and in the context of the overall clinical situation for each individual patient. However, bearing those important caveats always in mind, we sought to examine whether easily obtainable baseline clinical and anatomic (angiographic) data might be used to make informed judgments about how long an individual "BASIL-like" patient is likely to live; and, specifically, how likely they are to survive beyond 2 years which appears to be the point where the relative merits of a BAP first and BSX first revascularization strategy change.

In a multivariate model factors including increasing age; presence of tissue loss (as opposed to ischemic pain only); diabetes; current smoking; a history of angina or myocardial infarction (MI), stroke or transient ischemic attack (TIA); increasing severity of below-knee disease (as measured by the Bollinger Angiogram Score [11]); abnormal Body Mass Index (BMI), low number of recordable ankle pressure measurements; and low ankle pressure were highly predictive of those patients likely (and unlikely) to survive 2 years after intervention (Table II).

Implications for practice going forward

Generalizability of the BASIL trial

One of the main criticisms levelled against all RCTs is their lack of generalizability; and BASIL is no exception. It is important to emphasize that BASIL was not a trial of all patients presenting with

Table II Predicted 6 month, 1 and 2-year survival for 5 hypothetical patients based on baseline data entered into the BASIL trial survival model

	A	*B*	*C*	*D*	*E*
Smoking status	Ex	Ex	Current	Current	Current
BMI	Desirable	Overweight	Desirable	Underweight	Overweight
Serum creatinine	Low	Low	Low	Low	Low
Tissue loss?	Yes	Yes	Yes	Yes	No
Number of ankle pressures detected	None	One	One	Two	All 3
Highest ankle pressure	0	60	30	56	136
Below knee Bollinger score	5 or more	Missing	Under 5	Under 5	Under 5
History MI / angina?	Yes	No	Yes	No	No
History stroke / TIA?	No	No	No	No	No
Age (years)	79	80	63	56	59
Predicted proportion (%) of such patients that will survive to:					
6 months	71	84	90	97	97
1 year	57	75	84	96	95
2 years	40	63	76	93	92

SLI any more than the landmark carotid or aortic aneurysm trial were studies of all patients presenting with those conditions. Patients were, of course, only eligible for BASIL if:

1) they required, were suitable (fit) for, and would give consent to immediate/early revascularization (about 50% of SLI patients presenting to the top BASIL recruiting centers);
2) in the joint opinion of the responsible surgeon and interventionalist they could reasonably be treated by either a BSX first or BAP first strategy (that was true of about a third of that 50% who had immediate/early intervention and c. 70% of those were randomized, a high proportion by RCT standards).

So BASIL was likely to have excluded those SLI patients with more:

1) limited (proximal) disease suitable for BAP where BSX was thought to be inappropriate;
2) extensive (distal) disease who were considered unsuitable for BAP and to be candidate for (often very) distal BSX.

All RCTs must driven by the "uncertainty principle" and operate in this "grey area of clinical equipoise" that characterizes patients who occupy the middle ground; not to do so would of course be ethically unacceptable and scientifically unsound.

BASIL trial patients had, for the most part, severe and extensive multi-level disease, and poor outcomes in terms of loss of life and limb almost regardless of what treatment was offered. However, as discussed above, this is despite the fact that likely to represent the "better" end of the SLI disease spectrum in that they were offered a revascularization procedure at all and, also, considered potentially suitable for BAP. Outcomes for the SLI (or critically ischemic) patient group as a whole are likely to be significantly worse still. By reporting the clinical and angiographic severity of disease of the BASIL trial cohort in great detail we believe we are allowing clinicians to assess for themselves with a high degree of accuracy and confidence whether and how the BASIL trial cohort (and its findings) relates to their own SLI patient population.

The greatest gains in SLI lie in early diagnosis, best medical therapy and prompt referral

Most BASIL patients had developed SLI slowly over months, often years. Despite this, and being at exceptionally high overall cardiovascular risk, many patients:

- had never received "best medical therapy" for their multi-system atherosclerotic disease;
- were referred (too) late to vascular services for (successful) revascularization;
- were far from medically optimized at the time of referral.
- It seems likely, therefore, that public health and primary and secondary care measures aimed at:
- detecting lower limb arterial disease at an earlier stage (before it becomes life and limb threatening);
- ensuring that all such patients are offered evidenced-based "best medical therapy";
- encouraging prompt referral to vascular services for specialist care;
- would significantly diminish the burden imposed by SLI on the health of the nation.

Thus, the humbling reality for vascular surgeons and interventionalists is that regardless of what form of revascularization we offer, most patients with SLI have an extremely poor prognosis. The answer to SLI as far as the "health of the nation" is concerned lies in better public health and primary medical care and not primarily in the operating room or interventional suite.

Cost-effectiveness

Although in the short term surgery was more expensive, overall, there was little difference in costs between the two trial arms. It is clear that in this highly morbid patient group of patients there was a wide range of medical and social factors (other than the status of the trial leg and its treatment) that determined admission, re-admission, length of stay in hospital and outcomes. Furthermore, the higher procedure costs and morbidity associated with BSX have to be weighed against the significantly higher immediate failure and re-intervention rates with BAP. Hospital costs were largely driven by the time spent in wards rather than in specialist HDU or ITU environments, or by procedure costs. In the context of the UK National Health Service discharging patients more promptly and effectively from expensive acute hospital beds to properly resourced, "step-down" convalescence and rehabilitation facilities would seem likely to both improve functional outcomes and reduce costs. There was no attempt in the BASIL trial to collect data on medical or social care resource utilization or costs from outside hospital. However, it is reasonable to assume that such costs will be considerable (perhaps as much as, or even more than, the direct hospital costs) and that they will be broadly similar in the two trial arms.

Although a 3-year quality adjusted perspective suggests BSX will be highly cost-ineffective when compared to BAP (£ 125 499 per QALY), a 7-year (non-quality adjusted) perspective suggests the additional cost per AFS year is £ 20 579 and per year of OS is £ 29 095. However, there remains a substantial possibility that surgery may in fact remain cost-ineffective at broadly accepted willingness to pay thresholds. Whether such economic analyses should affect clinical decision making when faced with a SLI patient who could reasonably be treated by either BSX or BAP is a matter for debate.

Clinical effectiveness

The BASIL data indicate that in SLI due to infra-inguinal disease requiring immediate/early revascularization, patients expected to live:

- less than 2 years should usually be offered BAP first, especially where there is no vein for bypass; this is because they are unlikely to reap the longer term benefits of BSX and BAP is significantly less expensive and less morbid in the short term;
- more than 2 years should usually be offered BSX first; especially where vein is available for bypass. Some might argue that these gains are not clinically meaningful. However, this survival advantage for BSX has to be viewed in the context of a condition that has an overall prognosis not dissimilar from many common malignancies. For such patients, an additional 6-7 months of quality life with leg(s) intact seems likely to be viewed as an important benefit.

Multi-disciplinary team working

BASIL strongly suggests that the best outcomes for SLI are achieved when vascular surgeons and interventional radiologists work closely together with other professionals as part of a multi-disciplinary team (MDT) in specialist, high volumes centres (http://www.vascularsociety.org.uk/).

Role of prosthetic bypass in the management of SLI

The BASIL trial confirms that prosthetic BSX usually performs poorly in this patient group; usually worse than BAP. Had only those patients able to undergo vein bypass been randomized in BASIL then the longer term advantages of BSX over BAP might have been substantially greater. However, the investigators believe that it was appropriate to include prosthetic grafts as it reflects real-world practice and because the trial was designed to be a comparison of "best" surgical option first versus "best" endovascular option first. However, a non-randomized "by treatment received" (as opposed to "intention to treat") analysis of the BASIL data suggests that many patients who could not undergo a vein BSX first would probably have been better served by a first attempt at BAP. The trial reaffirms once again that surgeons should make every effort to use vein and to view prosthetic material in such patients as a last resort.

Role of BAP in the management of SLI

The failure rate of BAP in SLI is high (c. 25%) and patients who underwent BSX after failed BAP fared significantly worse than those who underwent surgery as their first procedure. So, BAP does not appear to be a "free shot", as has often been claimed (without, it has to be said, much supporting evidence). It is not yet clear whether failed BAP merely selects out patients who were going to do badly whatever treatment they receive, or whether angioplasty per se reduces the chances of successful surgical revascularization. However, these BASIL data should be borne in mind when discussing the treatment options with patients.

An important question is whether BAP alone still represents "best" endovascular therapy for this patient group? Stenting, stent-grafting and various other adjuncts such as atherectomy may have reduced immediate technical and early clinical failure rate in the endovascular arm — but would they have improved longer term clinical and cost-effectiveness? At present there is little robust evidence that they would in this patient group. All we can be certain about at this stage is that such adjuncts would have significantly increased the costs of endovascular treatment.

There is clearly an urgent need for further research to:

- identify those patients and anatomies where BAP is unlikely to be successful;
- understand the mechanisms of failure;
- develop new procedures, techniques and devices that may increase the success of peripheral vascular endovascular interventions both initially and in the longer term in patients with SLI caused severe and extensive multi-level disease.

We respectfully suggest that it would be preferable if such research were not funded entirely by those with strong commercial interests.

The role of amputation in the management of SLI

Regrettably, despite the best efforts of vascular surgeons and interventionalists to revascularize the limb, many SLI patients soon go on to require major limb amputation and/or die, usually of their widespread cardiovascular disease. Clinical and resource utilization data from BASIL, taken together with the prediction model (discussed further below), suggest that the interests of a significant proportion of BASIL patients might have been best served by primary amputation, followed by high quality rehabilitation, rather than, often repeated, unsuccessful attempts at revascularization. Amputees tended to spend long periods on acute surgical wards where they consumed expensive acute resources while not receiving the rehabilitation they required. At least in the UK, there would seem to be a need to rethink amputation and services for vascular amputees so that the available resources can be used in a more clinically and cost-effective manner to patient and tax-payer benefit. Although controversial, many believe that the BASIL trial leaves the way open for a trial of (probably largely endovascular) revascularization versus primary amputation versus best medical and nursing care only in selected poor prognosis patients.

Will the BASIL trial lead to a convergence of views?

It would seem highly desirable to repeat the Delphi studies in due course to determine whether there has been any convergence of views as to the relative merits of BSX and BAP in SLI patients in the light of the BASIL trial data. If it hasn't then we need to know why. It is interesting that despite repeated calls for RCTs in all manner of areas of medicine, and vascular surgery is not exception, we have only limited data and so understanding on how the results of those trials impact real-life, everyday practice.

The BASIL trial prediction model

The BASIL trial suggests that chances of surviving for 2 years after intervention is the main factor that determines whether SLI patients with infra-inguinal disease suitable for both surgery and angioplasty are best served by a BSX or BAP first revascularization strategy. It seems entirely logical, therefore, to attempt to model those factors that might predict which patients will probably survive for 2 years and which will not. Many different groups of researchers have attempted to create models and scoring systems that will accurately predict patient outcomes following various vascular and endovascular interventions. Used across different health economies such tools may: allow important clinical decisions to be made in a more scientific manner, improve the process of obtaining informed consent from patients, mitigate against medico-legal activity, allow the performance different clinicians and hospitals to be fairly compared in the context of differing case-mix, and improve cost-effectiveness and value for money thus protecting patients, private health care providers and the tax payer.

However, for understandable reasons, many surgeons and interventionalists choose not to use such tools; preferring instead to rely on experience and intuition. While not wanting to devalue the all-important "art" of medicine, as was very clearly shown in the pre-BASIL Delphi consensus studies, the result is that same patient may be offered a wide variety of different treatments (associated with very different risk and benefits) depending which clinician and institution they attend. At least in the UK, this non-evidence based variability in practice and outcome is viewed as increasingly unacceptable. Routine submission of detailed "scoreable" prognostic patient data to the UK National Vascular Database for the purposes of comparative weighted outcomes analyses is now viewed by many as a sine qua non of reasonable, defensible practice.

Present data confirm that while all SLI patients are "high risk", in reality, they represent an extremely heterogeneous group with regard to the risks of death, limb loss, and other major cardiovascular events over different time horizons. This complicates clinical decision-making, especially when trying balance short term risks with longer term durability in individuals who could reasonably be treated by either standard surgical or endovascular techniques.

There is an almost limitless set of data that one could try to collect on every SLI patient due to undergo revascularization in an attempt to predict with perfect accuracy the likely outcomes for each possible treatment methodology. Such an approach is logistically and ethically impossible and very likely to nicely demonstrate the law of diminishing returns. What clinicians from around the world have told the BASIL investigators is that they want to see a survival model based on robust (objective) baseline variables that are easily and widely available in day-to-day clinical practice at the point of clinical decision making.

The modelling tool presented in brief here is the only one to be derived from an RCT comparing BSX and BAP. While it is possible that in certain health economies the other factors, such as race and socio-economic status, might be influential we think it unlikely that they would add much to what is already a highly predictive model. Notwithstanding important issues around generalizability, the specific intention here is to give clinicians an idea of how long an individual "BASIL-like" patient might live. The clinician can, if they so choose, use that information along with other data to counsel their patient, reach a decision about treatment, and take informed consent.

If the model suggests, say, that there is only a 10%-20% chance of that patient being alive at 2 years then BASIL suggests that a BSX first strategy is unjustified because of the associated increased morbidity and costs. Rather, the appropriate choice would seem to be BAP or perhaps even primary amputation or best medical and nursing treatment only. However, if the model suggests that the chances of a patient being alive at 2 years are predicted as 80%-90% then the BASIL trial data suggest that a BSX first strategy is preferable (especially if vein is available) as the patient will probably survive to enjoy the longer term benefits of BSX in terms of AFS and OS at no significant additional cost. In this case where the model predicts a c. 50/50 chance of 2-year survival the decision whether to attempt BSX or BAP first can reasonably decided on other factors; for example, institutional expertise, cost and importantly patient choice (based upon a full discussion of the likely medical journey the patient will take following each of the two strategies as described in the BASIL trial). Although not everyone will agree, used properly, we think our model will prove to be a useful addition to the clinician's armamentarium when facing these challenging patients. That said, it would seem important to validate the BASIL trial survival prediction model in a separate cohort of "BASIL-like" patients.

THE NEED FOR FURTHER PUBLICLY FUNDED TRIAL IN PERIPHERAL VASCULAR DISEASE

Given the huge socio-economic burden that SLI places upon developed and increasingly developing nations it seems quite extraordinary that, to our knowledge, BASIL remains the only RCT to compare the surgical and endovascular treatment of this condition. The BASIL investigators and participants would be delighted if others were to make the brave commitment to undertake further RCTs in this field and help validate (or not as the case may be) the BASIL trial findings. We respectfully but strongly suggest that it is not in the public interest that responsibility for such trials should be left entirely within the private sector where research is understandably driven by powerful commercial interests. The overwhelming and urgent need for further publicly funded trials in peripheral vascular disease, and SLI in particular, would seem all too clear.

Summary of research recommendations

We suggest that further research is required in order to:

1) develop treatment algorithms in primary and secondary care for the early detection and "best medical therapy" of patients with, and at risk of developing, peripheral arterial disease; some form of (targeted) population screening would seem an appropriate strategy;
2) repeat the Delphi studies to determine whether there has been a convergence of views as to the relative merits of BSX and BAP in SLI; and if not, why not;
3) confirm or refute the BASIL findings and recommendations in further publically-funded, non-commercial RCTs;
4) validate the BASIL trial survival prediction model in a separate cohort of SLI patients;
5) examine the clinical and cost-effectiveness of new endovascular techniques and devices (such as stents and stent-grafts) in the management of SLI; again such research should not be funded entirely by commercial interests;
6) compare, within the confines of a randomized controlled trial, revascularization versus primary amputation versus best medical and nursing care only in those SLI patients with the poorest overall survival prospects.

REFERENCES

1 Norgren L, Hiatt WR, Dormandy JA et al. Inter-Society Consensus for the Management of Peripheral Arterial Disease (TASC II). *Eur J Vasc Endovasc Surg* 2007; 33 Suppl 1: S1-75.

2 Bradbury AW. Angioplasty is the first line treatment for critical limb ischaemia: the case against. In: *Vascular and Endovascular Controversies.* London: WB Saunders; 2003. pp. 295-307.

3 Holm J, Arfridsson B. Chronic lower limb ischaemia. A prospective randomised controlled trial comparing the 1-year results of vascular surgery and percutaneous transluminal angioplasty (PTA). *Eur J Vasc Surg* 1991; 5; 517-522.

4 Wolf GL, Wilson SE, Cross AP. Percutaneous transluminal angioplasty versus operation for peripheral arteriosclerosis. *J Vasc Surg* 1989; 9: 1-9.

5 Bradbury AW, Ruckley CV. Angioplasty for lower limb ischaemia: time for randomised controlled trials. *Lancet* 1996; 347: 277-278.

6 Jackson MJ, Wolfe JH. Are infra-inguinal angioplasty and surgery comparable? *Acta Chir Belg* 2001; 101: 6-10.

7 Bell J, Papp L, Bradbury AW. Bypass or angioplasty for severe ischaemia of the leg: the BASIL trial. In: Greenhalgh RM, Powell JT, Mitchell AW, editors. *Vascular and Endovascular Opportunities.* London: WB Saunders; 2000. pp. 485-494.

8 Bradbury AW, Bell J, Lee AJ et al. Bypass or angioplasty for severe limb ischaemia? A Delphi consensus study. Eur J Vasc Endovasc Surg 2002; 24: 411-416.

9 Bradbury AW, Wilmink T, Lee AJ et al. Bypass versus angioplasty to treat severe limb ischemia: factors that affect treatment preferences of UK surgeons and interventional radiologists. J Vasc Surg 2004; 39: 1026-1032.

10 Adam DJ, Beard JD, Cleveland T et al. Bypass versus angioplasty in severe ischaemia of the leg (BASIL): multicentre, randomised controlled trial. *Lancet* 2005; 366: 1925-1934.

11 Bollinger A, Breddin K, Hess H et al. Semi-quantitative assessment of lower limb atherosclerosis from routine angiographic images. *Atherosclerosis* 1981; 38: 339-346.

8

DIABETIC FOOT DISEASE

MAYA HUIJBERTS

The development of diabetic foot ulcers is a well-known and important complication of diabetes. The pathophysiological mechanism is complex, and different clinical presentations are possible, depending on the specific underlying pathology. Diabetic foot ulcers are usually caused by several factors acting in concert, with polyneuropathy, altered biomechanics, inadequate shoes and peripheral arterial disease (PAD) as major factors. Neuropathy is present in most patients with diabetic foot ulcers, while PAD is present in 30%-50%; infection can be diagnosed in up to 50% of patients presenting with a foot ulcer. Foot ulcers often develop in elderly multi-complex diabetic patients. Careful examination of the patient and identification of these specific pathologies and co-morbidities is needed before the start of any treatment. Because most patients have lost the natural protective mechanism to relieve pressure from the wound, off-loading of these ulcers is extremely important.

Multifunctional influences

The presence of PAD is an important determinant of the outcome of diabetic foot ulcers. Therefore evaluation of the severity of PAD is indicated in many patients. Patients with critical limb ischemia should undergo revascularization as soon as possible, and both endovascular treatment and bypass surgery are suitable interventions to improve tissue perfusion. Advances in endovascular treatment of PAD have improved the outcome in diabetic foot disease and therefore interventional radiologists or angiologists play an important role in the multidisciplinary treatment of this condition. The recognition and treatment of infection is equally important. Diagnosing infection is a challenge in these patients because of the often relatively mild local and systemic signs and symptoms. The choice of the initial antimicrobial therapy is usually empiric and based on the severity of the infection, prior antibiotic use and local resistance to most common pathogens. Most other strategies to improve wound healing, such as local application of growth factors, have failed to show significant clinical benefits. Recently, negative pressure wound therapy was shown to improve wound healing in patients with a partial foot amputation in a large randomized trial. Many patients not only have foot problems but also other health problems such as cardiovascular and renal disease and self care problems. Therefore an integrated management program is needed, in which optimal regulation of diabetes and associated co-morbidity and regular communication and instruction of the patient and his or her caregivers are taken care of.

Diabetic foot disease

Diabetes mellitus is one of the important chronic diseases of our times. The World Health Organization predicts that the number of persons with diabetes worldwide will increase to 366 million by the year 2030. A large part of the burden of disease as well as health care costs are related to the development of chronic complications of diabetes. One of the most feared complications of diabetes is diabetic foot disease. Diabetic foot ulcers have a major impact on the patient as well as on the health care system. These ulcers tend to heal slowly, need intensive care and healing can be complicated by infection and gangrene, leading to long-term in-hospital treatment and/or amputation [1]. Every 30 seconds a leg is lost due to diabetes somewhere in the world. Moreover, foot ulcers have major negative effects on quality of life, due to loss of mobility, loss of work and reduction of social activities; one study has demonstrated that quality of life of diabetic foot ulcer patients was comparable to quality of life of patients with recurrent breast cancer. After an amputation prognosis is poor and quality of life is further reduced. In addition these ulcers and their consequences are associated with major health care consumption and high costs. Despite these poor outcomes, the feet of diabetic patients have traditionally received relatively little attention from health care workers and scientists. However, in recent decades our knowledge on diabetic foot ulcers has clearly increased, with a rise in the number of scientific publications and the production of guidelines on prevention and management [2].

Epidemiology and costs

On a population basis, diabetic foot ulcers are a relative rare disease: the prevalence in cross-sectional studies in the UK was 1%-2% of the diabetic patients screened, and the annual incidence of new ulcers in the Western world was approximately 2% in community based studies. This incidence rises to 5%-7% in patients with risk-factors, such as loss of sensation or foot deformities. Foot ulcers and their consequences are associated with major health care consumption and high costs. In view of the increasing number of diabetic patients and limited health care resources, data on cost-of-treatment are necessary to prioritize health care expenditures and, if possible, to determine which patients and aspects of treatment are the most important determinants of costs. Although only a minority of foot ulcers will result in a lower extremity amputation (LEA), such an amputation is one of the feared outcomes of a diabetic foot ulcer and a LEA is associated with the highest costs, as shown by several authors. Several retrospective, single center, studies, using different methodologies, indicate that costs for foot ulcer treatment in general are also high [3]. On the longer term, costs are probably much higher as diabetic foot ulcers are a recurrent disease, with recurrence rates up to 70% in centers of excellence, resulting in repeated interventions and progressive disability.

Pathways to ulceration and amputation

Diabetic foot ulcers are usually caused by several factors acting in concert, with polyneuropathy, altered biomechanics, peripheral vascular disease, and inadequate shoe wear as major factors. The course of the disease may be complicated by the occurrence of infection. Each of these components is usually not sufficient to cause ulceration, but it is the combination of two or more factors that typically results in a poorly healing foot ulcer [4].

Diabetic polyneuropathy and altered biomechanics

In daily life our feet are continuously threatened by multiple minor and major insults, and loss of protective sensation is a cardinal event in the pathway to foot ulceration in many patients. The sensory deficits include diminished perception of pain, temperature, light touch, and pressure [5]. Many patients do not have major symptoms and are not aware of the diminished protective sensation. The majority of neuropathic or neuro-ischemic ulcers are caused by chronic repetitive biomechanical stress with abnormal loading of the foot during standing and walking and/or ill-fitting shoes. This abnormal loading of the foot can be the consequence of loss of muscle function due to neuropathy, foot deformities (such as claw toes or bony prominences), changes in shock absorbing capacity and limited joint mobility of the joints of the foot. In the non-ischemic foot, the repetitive biomechanical stress induces the formation of callus at the sites of abnormal load. This callus further elevates pressures and is associated with a high risk of future ulceration in neuropathic patients. Finally the skin breaks down, with the formation of a painless neuropathic ulcer. According to current guidelines total contact cast treatment is the treatment of choice for these neuropathic ulcers. It is not known, however, to what extent this standard treatment is embedded in daily clinical practice. In patients with neuropathy and peripheral vascular disease this total contact casting should be carried out with caution, since (also in our hands) poor healing was observed in patients with both PAD and infection.

Peripheral vascular disease

The same pathways as described above are probably followed in neuro-ischemic ulcers. However, atherosclerotic, obstructive, PAD is a major determinant of poor outcome of a diabetic foot ulcer. PAD is a common finding in patients with type 2 diabetes mellitus, with a prevalence of approximately 20% to 40% [6]. In many patients the disease has no or few symptoms and runs a relatively benign course, but in others it leads to gangrene or impaired healing of foot ulcers. PAD in diabetes frequently has a specific anatomical pattern, which can be interpreted as a sign of premature ageing of the vascular tree. The proximal vessels are relatively spared, with less involvement of the aortic iliac arteries and more extensive disease in the arteries of the lower leg [7]. In diabetic patients, the atherosclerotic changes seem to be more extensive and also more aggressive, with a faster progression of disease compared to non-diabetic patients. McDaniel et al. [8] showed that patients with claudication and diabetes had a 35% risk of sudden ischemia and a 21% risk of major amputation, compared to 19% and 3%, respectively, in non-diabetic patients. Major risk factors for the development of PAD (other than diabetes) are older age, smoking, and possibly hypertension. Recently, several novel risk factors have been identified in the general population for the development of PAD), such as hyperhomocysteinemia, elevated markers of inflammation, and possibly insulin resistance.

DIAGNOSIS

Evaluation of the adequacy of tissue perfusion in the feet of diabetic patients can be a difficult clinical challenge, as almost all tests have a moderate accuracy in predicting outcome. Many patients do not have claudication or severe ischemic rest pain, probably due to sensory neuropathy. However, if claudication or rest pain are present, the probability of amputation is greatly enhanced. The pulses of the femoral, popliteal, dorsalis pedis, and posterior tibial artery should be palpated. The proximal vessels should be auscultated for bruits, particularly the iliofemoral segment. If both foot arteries are palpated, severe ischemia is unlikely. Additional signs of severe ischemia are skin necrosis, gangrene, and blanching of the feet on elevation with a red-purple discoloration on dependency (in the absence of infection). Other signs are probably of little value in diabetic patients. The color and temperature of the skin is usually not helpful as the feet of diabetic patients can be red and warm, despite (severe) ischemia, which is probably caused by the relative high (thermoregulatory) shunt blood in diabetic patients with peripheral ischemia [9].

Non-invasive vascular evaluation is indicated in case of nonpalpable pulses, or other signs of ischemia and in nonhealing ulcers. In nondiabetic patients measurement of the systolic arterial pressure at the ankle with a hand held Doppler is a reliable screening test for severe ischemia. Also, in diabetic patients an absolute ankle pressure less than 50 mmHg indicates critical limb ischemia. However, due to media calcification, these arteries can become less compressible in diabetic patients, resulting in falsely elevated ankle pressures. Ankle pressures above 50 mmHg, therefore, are of very limited predictive value. In contrast, measurement of systolic toe pressures is probably more reliable and can predict wound healing in diabetic patients. In particular, values below 30 mmHg are associated with a poor outcome, and values between 30 and 50 mmHg should alert the clinician of the possibility of severe PAD. Unfortunately, toe pressure measurements can also be affected by media calcification in a minority of patients. Measurement of the transcutaneous pressure of oxygen ($TcPO_2$) can give additional information on the probability of wound healing. Wound healing is very unlikely if $TcPO_2$ values are below 20 mmHg and healing is likely with a $TcPO_2$ value above 40 mmHg [10].

If clinical and noninvasive assessments suggest significant PAD with a low probability of wound healing, or if the patient has persistent rest pain, revascularization should be considered in all patients [2]. In these patients further investigations are necessary to localize arterial lesions, to grade their severity, and to assess the possibility of a revascularization procedure [10]. As stated in the International Consensus, in all cases the arterial tree of the lower extremity should be visualized. It is crucial to visualize the entire tibial and foot circulation, as the former is a common location of the most significant occlusive lesion and the latter is an important potential site for the anastomosis of a distal bypass. In most centers angiography will be performed, but this technique might be replaced progressively by magnetic resonance angiography.

Endovascular treatment

Endovascular treatment of PAD has a number of advantages over bypass surgery, including the low morbidity and mortality of the procedure, the short preparation time and the limited hospital stay. The main contra-indications are problems with hemostasis, severe heart failure or renal disease and specific anatomical characteristics of the lesions. The restenosis rate might be relatively high, especially in procedures below the knee in which restenosis over a 5 year period in 50% of cases has been reported [11]. However, in patients with a foot ulcer the main aim is to heal the ulcer and to save the limb. The temporary improvement of skin perfusion can be sufficient to promote healing of a chronic ulcer and to avoid amputation in a patient with a relatively short life expectancy. Moreover, once the ulcer is healed lower perfusion pressures are necessary to maintain skin integrity. Faglia et al. [12] reported on the results of peripheral angioplasty as first line revascularization therapy in 993 patients with diabetic foot ulcers. All patients with absent foot pulses and a $TcPO_2$ below 50 mmHg and stenoses > 50% of vessel diameter underwent angiography and if possible PTA. In 62% of patients obstructions both in the femoro-popliteal and infra-popliteal axis were present. With a mean follow-up of more than two years relatively good outcomes were reported: all but 6 ulcers healed, and major amputation was performed in only 17 patients (1.7%). The number of minor amputations was, however, high with almost 50% (478 patients). The estimate of clinical restenosis was 2.2% per year, but in most of these patients PTA could be repeated successfully; 12% of the patients died during follow-up. In a recent publication from the same group long-term follow-up of 554 diabetic patients with critical limb ischemia demonstrated that most of these patients (75%) could be treated with angioplasty. Overall major amputation rate was 13%, restenosis occurred in 17%, bypass failures in 6% and recurrent ulcers in 13%. In this cohort almost half of all patients died during follow-up. Factors independently associated with mortality were age, unfeasible revascularization, hemodialysis, history of cardiac disease and impaired ejection fraction [13]. In the multicenter randomized controlled BASIL trial, results of bypass surgery versus angioplasty in patients with severe limb ischemia with or without tissue loss have been evaluated; 42% of this cohort consisted of patients with known diabetes. The median results for the outcomes amputation-free survival, all cause mortality and Health Related Quality of Life (HR-QOL) were quite similar. In the first year bypass surgery resulted in increased morbidity, mortality and higher costs, but in the long term patients who underwent surgery seemed to have a reduced risk of future amputation and death [14]. Recently also promising results with laser ablation in total chronic obstructions (TASC II C and D) were reported by Serino et al. [15] with 94% limb salvage rates at 24 months. The results of these studies indicate that endovascular therapy should take a prominent place in the treatment of PAD, especially in patients with significant co-morbidity and a shorter life expectancy.

Peripheral bypass surgery

Peripheral bypass surgery remains an effective treatment in many diabetic patients with PAD and critical limb ischemia [16]. The basic principles of this type of surgery are that any artery can be used for the proximal anastomosis provided inflow is uncompromized. The graft should bypass the major obstructive lesions and for the distal anastomoses an artery relatively free of occlusive disease, providing the best outflow into the arteries of the foot, should be selected. The bypass graft should preferably be constructed with autogenous vein(s), although acceptable results have been obtained with prosthetic grafts that do not cross the knee. An adequate ipsilateral saphenous vein is preferred in a below-knee bypass, but other good quality veins can be used. If possible the contralateral saphenous vein should be spared, as a substantial number of patients will require a bypass on the contralateral leg in the future. The crural and pedal arteries are common outflow sites of the graft in diabetic patients, given the characteristic anatomic pattern of PAD. Long-term results of these distal procedures in diabetic patients are good, with 5-year secondary patency rates of ≥ 70% and limb salvage rates of 75%-85%. In addition, such distal procedures in diabetic patients are more cost-effective than primary amputation. Anti-platelet therapy should be started pre-operatively and continued after an endovascular or surgical procedure. In general diabetes does not seem to have an important negative effect on the long-term patency and limb salvage rates of bypass surgery.

Stimulation of neovascularization

Successful revascularization by means of endovascular intervention or peripheral bypass surgery is not always possible in patients with foot ulcers and ischemia. Failure to restore tissue perfusion is currently probably the most important determinant of lower extremity amputation in patients with diabetes. Stimulation of the formation of collateral arteries could form an attractive medical therapy to improve blood flow to the leg. Outward remodelling is an important process during the development of a collateral network. Animal studies suggest that in the legs these collaterals are preformed and in case of a severe reduction in blood flow, grow in diameter to restore peripheral blood flow in a process called arteriogenesis. However, as recently shown in the coronary circulation, the formation of these collateral vessels seems to be impaired in diabetic patients with ischemic heart disease. The same observation was made in diabetic animals with peripheral ischemia [17]. It is likely that in diabetic patients several mechanisms contribute to the impaired arteriogenesis during ischemia, such as endothelial dysfunction, diminished cellular responses to several growth factors or cytokines, and impaired degradation of the extracellular matrix. Also dysfunction of endothelial progenitor cells, that plays a role in neovascularization in response to tissue ischemia, has been demonstrated in patients with type 1 diabetes. Gene transfer using growth factors has been evaluated in a number of studies as a tool to enhance vascular growth. In the RAVE trial patients with intermittent claudication were treated with VEGF gene transfer (AdVEGF121) which did not result in improved exercise performance or quality of life [18]. However, in the TRAFFIC study repeated intra-arterial administration of FGF-2 slightly but significantly improved walking time in patients with intermittent claudication [19]. Currently there are however no studies that have demonstrated effects in patients with diabetes, critical limb ischemia and foot ulcers.

Hyperbaric oxygen therapy

For those patients with foot ulcers and severe ischemia in whom revascularization is not possible, improving oxygen delivery by hyperbaric oxygen (HBO) therapy might be a useful adjunctive therapy. Five randomized controlled trials (RCTs) in diabetic patients with chronic foot ulcers were recently analyzed in a systematic review [20]. HBO treatment was associated with a reduction in major amputations, but not in minor amputations nor was an effect on wound healing observed. The authors concluded that HBO may be regarded as a promising treatment option when other strategies have failed, but the small numbers of patients and methodological problems necessitate a cautious interpretation of the results and a large RCT is needed.

Infection

Infection in a diabetic foot ulcer is potentially a limb-threatening condition. It is generally assumed that poor metabolic control is associated with impaired immunity, but it is still a matter of debate whether patients with only moderately elevated blood glucose levels diabetes are more susceptible to infection. Neutrophil function is impaired in diabetic patients with poor metabolic control, resulting in defective chemotaxis, phagocytosis, and intra-cellular killing.

Infection is characterized by tissue damage due to multiplying micro-organisms and the host response. As open wounds tend to become colonized with micro-organisms and even virulent pathogens (e.g. Staphylococcus aureus) can sometimes be colonizers, isolating a micro-organism in a culture does not help to identify the patient with an infection and the diagnosis should be made on clinical grounds. Unfortunately, local signs of inflammation, such as erythema or pain, can be less apparent in diabetic patients with a foot infection, probably due to factors as ischemia and neuropathy. Also systemic signs of infection can be markedly absent. In one study of patients with a deep foot infection approximately 50% of the patients did not have systemic signs of inflammation, such as elevated body temperature or C-ractive protein (CRP) [21]. On the other hand when increased body temperature or laboratory parameters of inflammation are present, a severe infection is more likely. The specific anatomy of the foot can also affect the presentation and course of an infection. In case of a penetrating ulcer, infection of one of the muscle compartments of the foot can result in tissue oedema with a rise in compartmental pressure and subsequent microvascular occlusion. This foot compartment syndrome, with its vicious cycle of infection, edema and microvascular failure, can result in extensive tissue necrosis.

Superficial infections in patients not treated previously with antibiotics are usually caused by gram-positive micro-organisms, in particular Staphylococcus Aureus and bacteria such as β hemolytic streptococci. Deep foot infections, chronic infections and wounds that have previously been treated with antibiotics often have a mixed flora of gram-positive and gram-negative aerobes and anerobes. Multiresistant micro-organisms and methicillin-resistant S. Aureus (MRSA) are a growing problem and may be isolated in up to 20% of the cultures.

Diagnosis of infection

In patients in whom infection is considered the wound should be debrided aggressively to determine the extent of the infection. The depth of the wound should be determined, if necessary by probing the wound with a blunt instrument. If a deep foot infection is suspected, an X-ray of the foot should be obtained and in some cases a magnetic resonance imaging will be helpful to determine the extent of tissue involvement. Material for culture should be obtained, preferably pus or tissue of the base of the wound by scraping with a scalpel or a curette. If this is not possible, aseptically obtained aspirates of pus or tissue fluid can also provide good specimens for culture. Wound swabs are less preferable as they provide, in comparison to tissue specimens, less sensitive and specific results. The material obtained should be immediately processed for gram stain and culture, both aerobic and anaerobic.

Treatment of infected foot ulcers

Treatment of an infected diabetic foot ulcer should be based on the severity of the infection and the presence of ischemia. Superficial ulcers without severe ischemia, can usually be treated on an outpatient basis with repeated debridement, meticulous wound care, off-loading and oral antibiotics. Patients with deep foot infections, signs of systemic toxicity or severe ischemia should be admitted to the hospital; especially the combination of infection and ischemia should be considered as a medical emergency. Surgery should be considered in all patients, which may range from minor debridement or drainage to extensive resections or amputation. A surgical debridement in the operating theatre should therefore be considered in case of a deep soft tissue infection, with decompression of the infected compartment, removal of all necrotic tissue and the creation of adequate drainage. The choice of the initial antimicrobial therapy is usually empiric and based on the severity of the infection, prior antibiotic use and local resistance to most common pathogens. Unfortunately, there is currently little evidence in the literature to guide the clinician in the choice, the route (oral or parenteral) and the duration the antibiotic treatment. The number of RCT in which antibiotic regimens were compared are limited and interpretation is difficult as in these trials different classification systems and different end-points were used. Hopefully, the introduction of the PEDIS classification system by the International Consensus on the Diabetic Foot can help to standardize future clinical trials. As summarized in the guidelines of the Infectious Diseases Society of America guidelines, no single drug or combination of drugs seems superior to another. Superficial infections can usually be treated initially with oral antibiotics aimed at gram positive cocci, such as flucloxacillin or, in case of penicillin allergy, clindamycin. Deep soft tissue infections are initially treated with an i.v. broad spectrum regimen aimed at gram positive, gram negative aerobic and anaerobes, e.g. amoxicillin/clavulanate, piperacillin/tazobactam, or a combination of a third generation cephalosporin and clindamycin. After 2-3 days of empirical treatment, therapy should be modified on the basis of the clinical response of the patient and the results of the wound culture. The optimal duration of treatment for soft tissue infections is unknown, but mild infections can usually be treated for 7-10 days and more severe infections for 2-3 weeks. In our experience duration of treatment is especially difficult to determine in patients with infected ischemic wounds, in whom signs and symptoms of infection can be mitigated. Antibiotics may penetrate less effectively in bone and some (retrospective) studies suggest that the combination of a fluoroquinolon and clindamycin can be effective treatment in patients with (suspected) osteomyelitis. As these drugs have a high bioavailability they can be prescribed as oral agents and, in case of a (chronic) osteomyelitis, therapy can be continued until eradication of the infection is likely, which usually takes 2-3 months. However, some authors have argued that compared to antibiotic therapy conservative surgery could result in faster healing and shorter duration of antibiotic treatment. Future clinical trials, in which the cost-effectiveness of long term antibiotic treatment is compared with conservative surgery, are needed in order to guide the clinician in this difficult choice [22].

Tissue perfusion is a major determinant of the penetration of antibiotics and in one amputation study already moderate levels of ischemia resulted in poorer penetration of a third generation cephalosporin into skin, muscle and bone. Unfortunately, limb ischemia was an exclusion criterion in most RCTs on antibiotics and more insight is needed on the pharmacodynamics and efficacy of antibiotics in patients with infected ischemic wounds. Relatively high doses of antibiotics seem preferable in patients with ischemia to reach sufficient tissue concentrations. In patients with severe ischemia it is advisable to first treat the infection with broad-spectrum antibiotics and, if necessary, a drainage procedure or minor amputation. Once the infection is controlled a revascularisation procedure can be performed after 4-5 days; with this approach excellent long-term results have been obtained.

Diabetic foot disease in European perspective: The Eurodiale study

Several specialized diabetic foot centers in Europe joined forces some years ago in order to collect prospective data on patient characteristics, management, resource utilization and outcome of individuals with diabetes and a foot ulcer. This collaborative effort which was partly funded by an EC Fifth Framework program grant has resulted in the collection of prospective follow-up data on more than 1 000 patients with diabetes and a foot ulcer. The study has provided a clear insight into the impact of diabetic foot disease on a European scale. Baseline data show that throughout Europe diabetic foot ulcers occur most often in elderly male patients with longstanding diabetes. Many patients with diabetic foot ulcers are severely ill, as reflected by the severe underlying pathology and the presence of disabling co-morbidities in at least one third of these patients. PAD was present in half of all patients and infection at presentation in 58%. The combination of both PAD and infection was present in 31%. Overall clinical outcome was more favourable than reported previously: 77% of the patients healed, 5% underwent a major amputation, and 6% died. In patients with both PAD and infection outcomes were significantly worse; 64% overall healing, 10% major amputation and 13% mortality. Multivariate analysis showed that age, male sex, heart failure, end stage renal disease, the inability to stand or walk without help, ulcer size, the presence of PAD and the presence of peripheral neuropathy were independent predictors of healing [23]. In the Eurodiale study, prospective data on resource utilization were collected on a large scale. These unique data indicated that average total direct and indirect cost for the treatment of a diabetic foot ulcer was more than € 10 000, based on the costing data of 821 patients from seven of the 10 participating countries and corrected for Purchasing Power Standards. Costs for patients with PAD (especially in combination with infection) were almost twice as high [24]. Data on management strategies demonstrated that there is a substantial gap between recommendations in multidisciplinary guidelines and every day clinical practice. Recommendations on referral, the use of total contact casting and vascular work-up and revascularization were often not followed. In the Eurodiale cohort only 43% of patients with critical limb ischemia were revascularized. Factors related to this underuse of resources included reimbursement policies, personal beliefs of professionals, lack of patient acceptance, spontaneous healing of the ulcer and very poor health status of the patient. Nevertheless these data suggest that the management of diabetic foot ulcers in Europe can be improved substantially.

Conclusion

Diabetic foot disease is an important complication of longstanding diabetes, with substantial impact on the patient and the health care system. Foot ulcers occur typically in elderly patients with significant co-morbidities such as heart failure and end stage renal disease. PAD is an important factor in the pathogenesis of diabetic foot ulcers and (especially in combination with infection) is associated with poor prognosis. Adequate treatment of these patients requires a multidisciplinary approach in which issues such as treatment of PAD, treatment of infection, and treatment of diabetes and associated co-morbidities are addressed. In view of the underlying peripheral neuropathy and loss of protective sensation adequate pressure relief of the ulcer is also a mainstay of foot ulcer treatment. Diabetologists, vascular surgeons, radiologists or angiologists, specialized nurses, and shoemakers should therefore collaborate closely and should be able to consult infectious disease specialists, plastic surgeons, rehabilitation specialists and dermatologists. Recent data have shown that aggressive revascularization is associated with favourable outcomes in diabetic foot ulcer patients but is so far no standard policy in the treatment of these patients. Increasing awareness of the importance of diagnosing and restoring impaired tissue perfusion in diabetic foot disease, is therefore still an important task for vascular disease specialists in Europe.

REFERENCES

1 Boulton AJ, Vileikyte L, Ragnarson-Tennvall G et al. The global burden of diabetic foot disease. *Lancet* 2005; 366: 1719-1724.

2 Apelqvist J, Bakker K, van Houtum WH et al. *International Consensus on the Diabetic Foot.* Maastricht: Schaper NC (Ed); 1999.

3 Matricali GA, Dereymaeker G, Muls E et al. Economic aspects of diabetic foot care in a multidisciplinary setting: a review. *Diabetes Metab Res Rev* 2007; 23: 339-347.

4 Reiber, GE, Vileikyte L, Boyko EJ et al. Causal pathways for incident lower-extremity ulcers in patients with diabetes from two settings. *Diabetes Care* 1999; 22: 157-162.

5 Boulton AJ, Vinik AI, Arezzo JC et al. Diabetic neuropathiesy: A statement of the American Diabetes Association. *Diabetes Care* 2005; 28: 956-962.

6 Beks PJ, Mackaay AJ, de Neeling JN et al. Peripheral arterial disease in relation to glycaemic level in an elderly Caucasian population: the Hoorn study. *Diabetologia* 1995; 38: 86-96.

7 Jude EB, Oyibo SO, Chalmers N et al. Peripheral arterial disease in diabetic and nondiabetic patients: a comparison of severity and outcome. *Diabetes Care* 2001; 24: 1433-1437.

8 McDaniel MD, Cronenwett JL. Basic data related to the natural history of intermittent claudication. *Ann Vasc Surg* 1989; 3: 273-277.

9 McGee SR, Boyko EJ. Physical examination and chronic lower-extremity ischemia: a critical review. *Arch Intern Med* 1998; 158: 1357-1364.

10 Norgren L, Hiatt WR, Dormandy JA et al. Inter-Society Consensus for the Management of Peripheral Arterial Disease (TASC II). *J Vasc Surg* 2007; 45 Suppl S: S5-S67.

11 Balmer H, Mahler F, Do DD et al. Balloon angioplasty in chronic critical limb ischemia: factors affecting clinical and angiographic outcome. *J Endovasc Ther* 2002; 9: 403-410.

12 Faglia E, Dalla Paola L, Clerici G et al. Peripheral angioplasty as the first-choice revascularization procedure in diabetic patients with critical limb ischemia: prospective study of 993 consecutive patients hospitalized and followed between 1999 and 2003. *Eur J Vasc Endovasc Surg* 2005; 29: 620-627.

13 Faglia E, Clerici G, Clerissi J et al. Long-term prognosis of diabetic patients with critical limb ischemia: a population-based cohort study. *Diabetes Care* 2009; 32: 822-827.

14 Adam DJ, Beard JD, Cleveland T et al. BASIL trial participants. Bypass versus angioplasty in severe ischaemia of the leg (BASIL): multicentre, randomised controlled trial. *Lancet* 2005; 366: 1925-1934.

15 Serino F, Cao Y, Renzi C et al. Excimer laser ablation in the treatment of total chronic obstructions in critical limb ischaemia in diabetic patients. Sustained efficacy of plaque recanalisation in mid-term results. *Eur J Vasc Endovasc Surg* 2009; [Epub ahead of print].

16 Beard JD. Which is the best revascularization for critical limb ischemia: Endovascular or open surgery? *J Vasc Surg* 2008; 48 (Suppl 6): 11S-16S.

17 van Golde JM, Ruiter MS, Schaper NC et al. Impaired collateral recruitment and outward remodeling in experimental diabetes. *Diabetes* 2008; 57: 2818-2823.

18 Rajagopalan S, Mohler ER 3rd, Lederman RJ et al. Regional angiogenesis with vascular endothelial growth factor in peripheral arterial disease: a phase II randomized, double-blind, controlled study of adenoviral delivery of vascular endothelial growth factor 121 in patients with disabling intermittent claudication. *Circulation* 2003; 108: 1933-1938.

19 Lederman, RJ, Mendelsohn FO, Anderson RD et al. Therapeutic angiogenesis with recombinant fibroblast growth factor-2 for intermittent claudication (the TRAFFIC study): a randomised trial. *Lancet* 2002; 359; 2053-2058.

20 Roeckl-Wiedmann, I, Bennett M, Kranke P. Systematic review of hyperbaric oxygen in the management of chronic wounds. *Br J Surg* 2005; 92: 24-32.

21 Eneroth, M., Apelqvist J, Stenstrom M. Clinical characteristics and outcome in 223 diabetic patients with deep foot infections. *Foot Ankle Int* 1997; 18: 716-722.

22 Prompers L, Schaper N, Apelqvist J et al. Prediction of outcome in individuals with diabetic foot ulcers: focus on the differences between individuals with and without peripheral arterial disease. The EURODIALE Study. *Diabetologia* 2008; 51:747-755.

23 Prompers L, Huijberts M, Schaper N et al. Resource utilisation and costs associated with the treatment of diabetic foot ulcers. Prospective data from the Eurodiale Study. *Diabetologia* 2008; 51: 1826-1834.

24 Lipsky BA. New developments in diagnosing and treating diabetic foot infections. *Diabetes Metab Res Rev* 2008; 24 (Suppl 1): S66-S71.

9

OPEN AND ENDOVASCULAR TREATMENT OF TYPE A DISSECTION

CHRISTOPH NIENABER, STEPHAN KISCHE

Type A aortic dissection and other pathologies confined to or involving the ascending aorta are traditionally repaired with open surgery on cardio-pulmonary bypass and cooling or selective perfusion of the head. Despite well-established procedures and standardized operations mortality and morbidity of open approaches are not trivial, especially considering the emerging need to care for an ageing population with multiple co-morbidities. Besides explaining those traditional approaches, this chapter will also introduce new emerging interventional techniques to tackle proximal aortic pathologies under certain conditions of elevated surgical risk and anatomic suitability.

Surgical repair

Classic repair of pathologies involving the ascending or proximal aorta affords an open surgical approach with thoracotomy, cardio-pulmonary bypass and usually selective head perfusion. Even though such surgical approaches have been standardized, 30-day mortality and collateral changes are considerable. Nevertheless, open surgery has demonstrated to improve survival and outcomes when offered in timely fashion to patients with aortic dissection [1] (Fig. 1). The surgical techniques applied vary from simple supracoronary interposition graft to more complex procedures such as hemi- or complete arch replacement with or without aortic root replacement or reconstruction by either the David procedure (that exists in various styles from I-IV with Stanford modification) or the Yacoub reconstruction. On aggregate, open surgical repair has proven survival benefits in proximal pathologies of the aorta. With our current demographic changes, however, we are facing an increasing number of elderly patients who will not necessarily benefit from open aortic surgery, but who may become candidates for less traumatic interventions for proximal disease. Some anatomic features are being addressed.

Type A aortic dissection

Even today proximal aortic dissection is a life-threatening condition with a mortality up to 50%

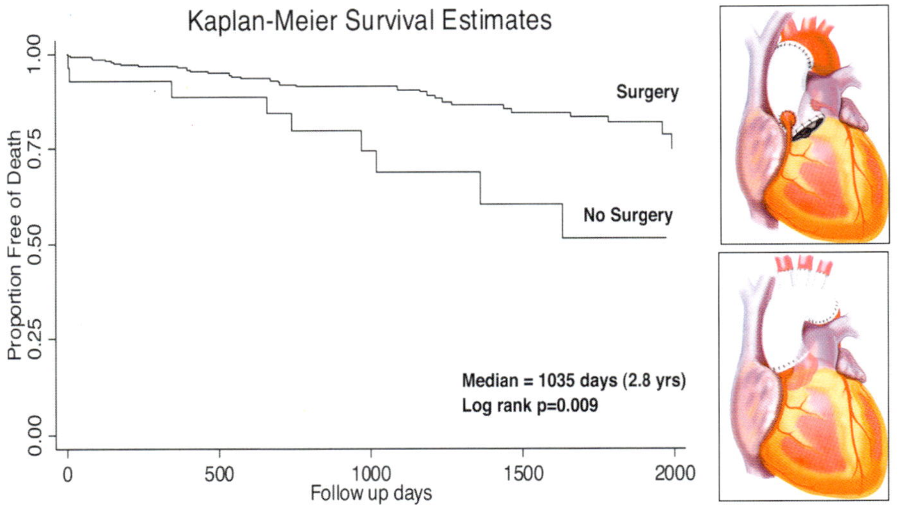

FIG. 1 Surgical repair of type A aortic dissection improves long-term survival as documented in IRAD [1]. The surgical options may vary from simple supracoronary interposition to complex solutions such as conduits or total arch replacement.

in the initial 2 days if left untreated. Therefore, the dissected ascending aorta needs to be repaired without any delay, in the attempt to limit mortality to approximately 23% in patients ≤ 70 years of age [1]. Conversely, elderly patients experience up to 37% mortality with surgical repair [2] as documented in IRAD. Moreover, up to 20% of patients with type A dissection are not accepted for surgery because of advanced age and co-morbidities [3]. These patients have been targeted recently for endovascular and minimally invasive interventions.

As a typical example a 89-year-old woman was the first case subjected to proximal endovascular stent-grafting as she refused open surgery; she received a stent-graft to cover the entry to the dissection in the ascending aorta and a chimney bare stent via the right carotid artery in the brachiocephalic trunk (Fig. 2). Similarly, a 84-year-old patient with acute type A dissection was successfully subjected to customized stent-graft placement in the ascending aorta (Fig. 3). In such desperate setting we have so far successfully treated 5 cases of proximal dissection with one fatality only; in all cases cerebral perfusion and function of the aortic valve were preserved while the proximal entry was successfully sealed. Chronic situations appear to be more difficult to manage because of both progressive aneurysmal expansion and aggravating valvular insufficiency [4]. Nevertheless, reasonable follow-up data are not available yet in such elderly patients, who are expected to live only a few years. Conversely, younger patients with proximal dissection are mostly suffering from hereditary fibrillinopathies with a need for open surgical repair at all costs [5].

Pseudoaneurysm of the ascending aorta

Different from a true aneurysm a pseudoaneurysm combines perforation of parts of the aortic wall layers often with surrounding hematoma, a finding that may occur in up to 13% after previous aortic surgery for dissection [6]. Most frequently pseudoaneurysm develops along an anastomotic suture line, expands steadily before rupture, or compresses adjacent structures with typical symptoms. They may develop even after routine cardiac operations at the site of aortotomy or after mediastinal infection, along with intra-operative use of gelatine-resorchine glue or after trauma. It may take days to years for a pseudoaneurysm to form after an initiating event. Open surgical repair is often a complex endeavour and can be associated with 12%-41% mortality [7,8] due to the nature of redo-operation, and the chance of traumatizing the situs, although surgical standards have markedly been improved.

Considering the associated high mortality with

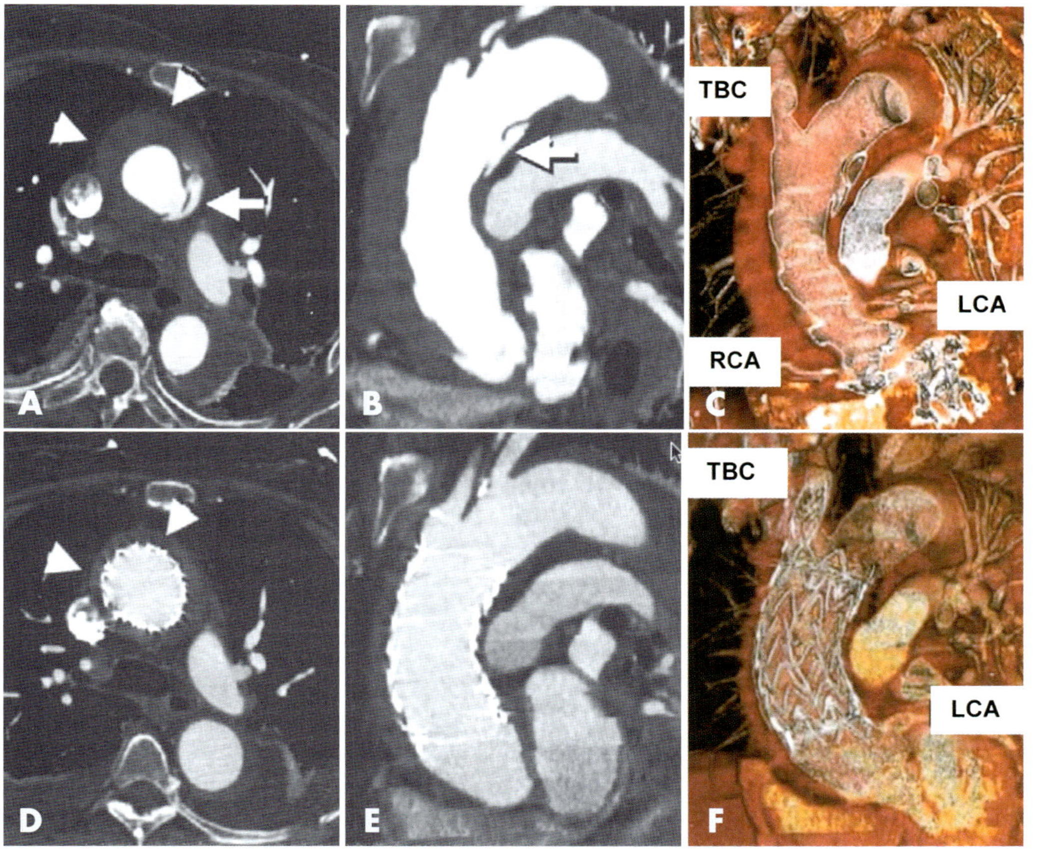

FIG. 2 A-C) Acute type A aortic dissection with proximal entry (white arrow) and intramural hematoma (arrowhead); D-F) Results after stent-graft and chimney for repair of proximal dissection.

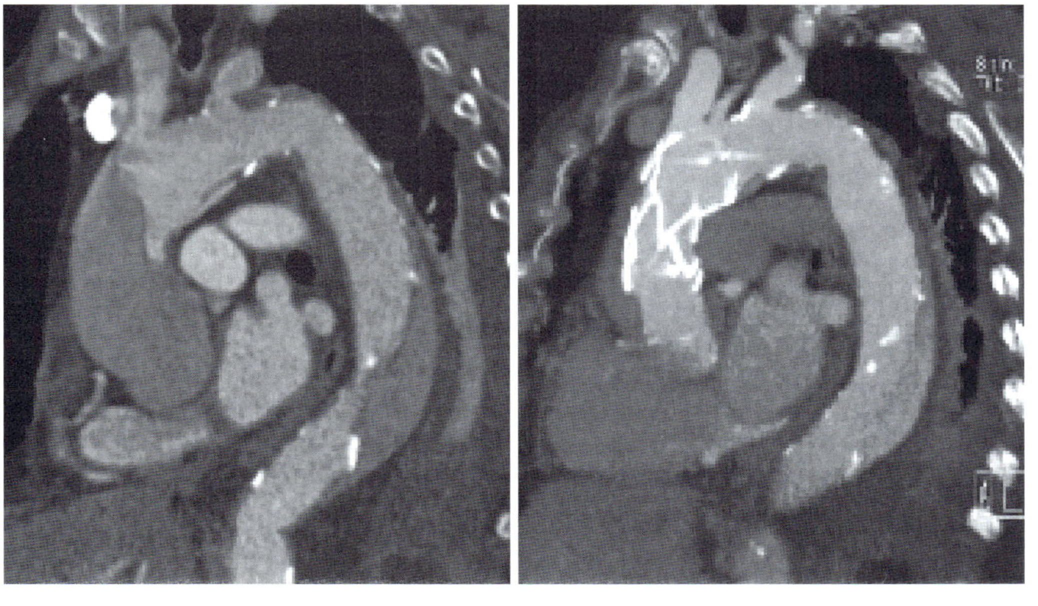

FIG. 3 Acute type A dissection before and after proximal stent-graft placement for entry sealing.

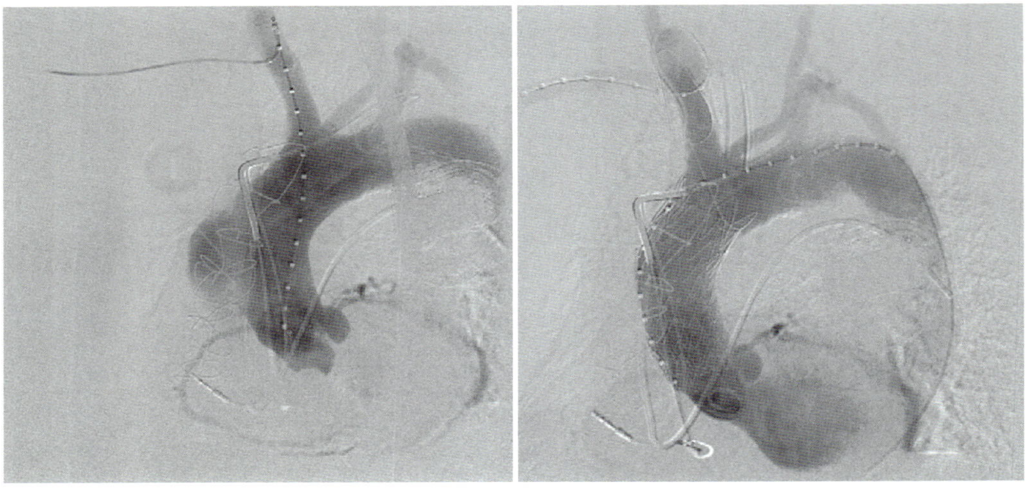

FIG. 4 Pseudoaneurysm after surgical repair of iatrogenic dissection (type A); complete reconstruction with total exclusion of the aneurysm.

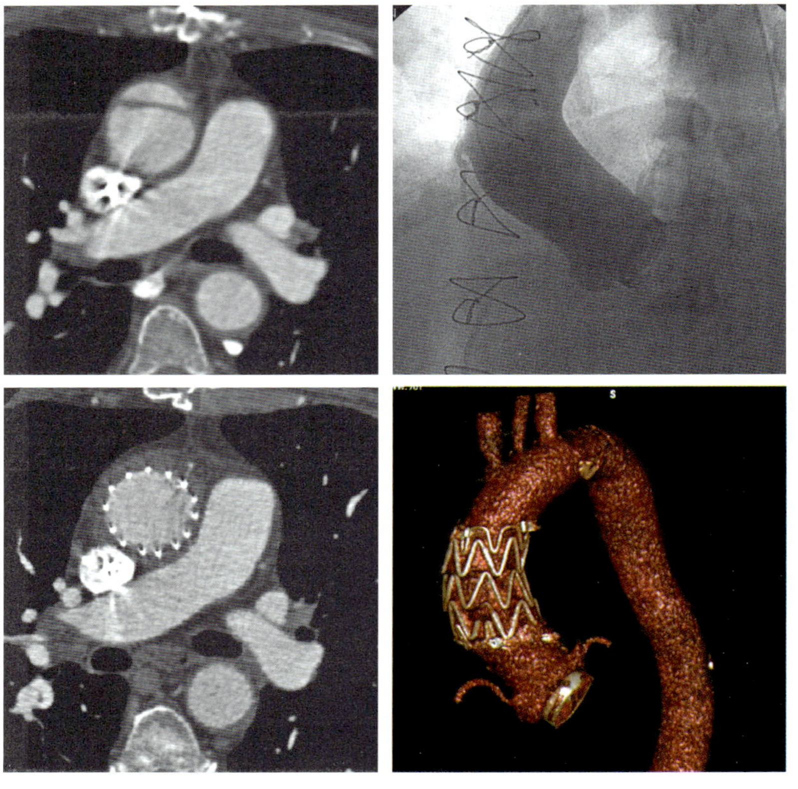

FIG. 5 Dissected ascending aorta after previous bypass- and valve replacement surgery treated by customized stent-graft to seal entry.

open surgery, however, minimally invasive endovascular strategies are desperately needed. A limited number of reports surfaced so far describe interventional approaches to such highly fragile patients. A 78-year-old man who had developed a pseudoaneurysm 4 years after coronary bypass grafting was successfully treated by exclusion of his growing pseudoaneurysm by use of Zenithe endografts introduced over the left common carotid artery in retrograde fashion [9]. Another case is a 82-year-old woman developing a pseudoaneurysm after surgical repair of iatrogenic dissection; this pseudoaneurysm was eventually covered with a Tag endograft (Fig. 4). We were able to collect 3 cases referred for similar interventions; one of 3 women with an aortic ulceration or localized dissection after previous aortic valve replacement is displayed in Fig. 5. All such cases show the feasibility of endovascular approaches for chronic pathologies of the ascending aorta in selected patients as an alternative to a redo open surgical procedure, but hint also to a multitude of current limitations.

Mycotic aneurysm of the ascending aorta

Mycotic aneurysms are rare and often associated with high mortality due to the acuity from hematogenic dissemination; infected pseudoaneurysms are found after conventional cardiac surgery or after heart transplantation. In general immuno-compromized patients are more likely to be affected accounting for an occurrence of 4% to 8% after orthotopic cardiac transplantation [10-14].

The standard procedure of course is open resection of the affected aortic segment and extensive debridement of infected and surrounding tissues. Despite refined surgical techniques open surgical repair carries a burden of 40% mortality. Although many details are still nebulous, endovascular techniques may even find a place in the treatment of mycotic aneurysm. To date there are some data on the endovascular use in the descending aorta with reasonable success [15,16] while the ascending aorta was only tackled in a few instances [17,18]. Again, for critically ill patients the less aggressive endovascular approach may be advantageous especially since re-thoracotomy is avoided. More experience, however, is needed before valid conclusions can be drawn. In cases of contained rupture of pseudoaneurysm, regardless of location, a specialized "aortic team" may be able to safe lives offering endovascular technology as a bridging maneuver for definitive surgical repair.

Rapid, but comprehensive imaging is important for any therapeutic approach to aortic diseases. With modern computed tomography (CT) angiography complex 3-dimensional image information is collected within 20 to 30 seconds. With refined post-processing routines including volume-rendering techniques "virtual angioscopy" becomes feasible. Both CT and magnetic resonance imaging technologies allow relatively simple post-processing and enable intuitive reading of diagnostic and follow-up image information.

On aggregate, previously established and accepted application of endografts to the descending aorta cannot be simply applied to the ascending aorta in similar fashion. Hemodynamic forces in the ascending aorta are markedly higher than elsewhere in the aorta and ankering as well as potential migration may become important issues. Pulsatile changes in the proximal aortic diameter are significantly higher here than more distally, and the application and launching of a stent-graft in the proximal aorta requires the delivery system to cross the aortic valve and enter the left ventricle. For wider and more general use important refinements are necessary.

Summary and therapeutic applications

With recently emerging fenestrated and branched endografts and particularly with the acceptance of hybrid procedures in the aortic arch, the use of endovascular interventions with stents or stent-grafts has been expanded to the ascending aorta. The technology is constantly adapting to the needs of higher flexibility, individual custom-design, miniaturization and endurance in order to be potentially used in the ascending aorta [19]. Procedural results, with emphasis on safety, are currently being collected and monitored in participating specialized centers; the field is emerging although still confronted with a number of obstacles and short-comings. Flexibility and apposition beyond current standards, adaptation to the pulsative aorta and non-traumatic launching in type A dissection are important characteristics to be developed. New endografts with interjacent bare stent (open) segments and proximal valvular ankering are being discussed. The technology and its miniaturization is a moving target; clinical centers of excellence need to cooperate closely in a multi-disciplinary fashion and with industry to further advance endovascular strategies to the ascending aorta.

REFERENCES

1 Tsai TT, Evangelista A, Nienaber CA et al. Long-term survival in patients presenting with type A acute aortic dissection: insights from the International Registry of Acute Aortic Dissection (IRAD). *Circulation* 2006; 114: 350-356.

2 Mehta RH, O'Gara PT, Bossone E et al. Acute type A aortic dissection in the elderly: clinical characteristics, management and outcomes in the current era. *J Am Coll Cardiol* 2002; 40: 685-692.

3 Mehta RH, Suzuki T, Hagan PG et al. International Registry of Acute Aortic Dissection (IRAD) Investigators. Predicting death in patients with acute type a aortic dissection. *Circulation* 2002; 105: 200-206.

4 Palma JH, Gaia DF, Guilhen JS et al. Endovascular treatment of chronic type A dissection. *Interact Cardiovasc Thorac Surg* 2008; 7: 164-166.

5 Ince H, Rehders TC, Petzsch M et al. Stent-grafts in patients with marfan syndrome. *J Endovasc Ther* 2005; 12: 82-88.

6 Mesana TG, Caus T, Gaubert J et al. Late complications after prosthetic replacement of the ascending aorta: what did we learn from routine magnetic resonance imaging follow-up? *Eur J Cardiothorac Surg* 2000; 18: 313-320.

7 Dumont E, Carrier M, Cartier R et al. Repair of aortic false aneurysm using deep hypothermia and circulatory arrest. *Ann Thorac Surg* 2004; 78: 117-121.

8 Mohammadi S, Bonnet N, Leprince P et al. Reoperation for false aneurysm of the ascending aorta after its prosthetic replacemtn surgical strategy. *Ann Thorac Surg* 2005; 79: 147-152.

9 Lin PH, Kougias P, Huynh TT et al. Endovascular repair of ascending aortic pseudonaeurysm: technical considerations of a common carotid artery approach using the Zenith aortic cuff endograft. *J Endovasc Ther* 2007; 14: 794-798.

10 Macedo TA, Stanson AW, Oderich GS et al. Infected aortic aneurysms: imaging findings. *Radiology* 2004; 231: 250-257.

11 Katsumata T, Moorjani N, Vaccari G et al. Mediastinal false aneurysm after thoracic aortic surgery. *Ann Thorac Surg* 2000; 70: 547-552.

12 Knosalla C, Weng Y, Warnecke H et al. Mycotic aortic aneurysms after orthotopic heart transplantation: a three-case report and review of the literature. *J Heart Lung Transplant* 1996; 15: 827-839.

13 Follis FM, Paone RF, Wernly JA. Mycotic aneurysm of the ascending aorta after coronary revascularization. *Ann Throac Surg* 1994; 58: 236-238.

14 Palanichamy N, Gregoric ID, La Francesca S et al. Myocotic pseudo-aneurysm of the ascending thoracic aorta after cardiac transplantation. *J Heart Lung Transplant* 2006; 25: 730-733.

15 Razavi MK, Razavi MD. Stent-graft treatment of myocotic aneurysms: a review of the current literature. *J Vasc Interv Radiol* 2008; 19: 51-56.

16 Kan CD, Lee HL, Yang YL. Outcome after endovascular stent graft treatment for mycotic aortic aneurysm: a systematic review. *J Vasc Surg* 2007; 46: 906-912.

17 Rayan SS, Vega JD, Shanewise JS et al. Repair of mycotic aortic pseudoaneurysm with a stent graft using transesophageal echocardiography. *J Vasc Surg* 2004; 40: 567-570.

18 Heye S, Daenens K, Maleux G et al. Stent-graft repair of a mycotic ascending aortic pseudoaneurysm. *J Vasc Interv Radiol* 2006; 17: 1821-1825.

19 van Prehn J, Vincken KL, Muhs BE et al. Toward endografting of the ascending aorta: Insight into dynamics using dynamic cine-CTA. *J Endovasc Ther* 2007; 14: 551-560.

10

INNOVATIVE TREATMENT OF ARCH ANEURYSMS

PETER HOLT, ROB HINCHLIFFE, IAN LOFTUS

Endovascular therapy is now a treatment of choice for thoracic aortic pathology including degenerative thoracic aneurysms, acute complicated and chronic dissections, acute aortic syndromes and for aortic trauma. It has been suggested that both mortality and morbidity are significantly reduced with endovascular interventions when compared with open surgery [1-3].

Lesions that affect the aortic arch are the most technically challenging endovascular procedures, but also those for which the benefits of minimally invasive surgery might be the most easily demonstrated. The challenges for this technique revolve around aortic arch morphology. The three-dimensional angulations of the aortic arch and large hemodynamic forces coupled with manipulating an endograft through tortuous, calcified access vessels make accurate endograft placement a significant challenge. The supra-aortic trunks add to the complexity of managing these lesions endovascularly, as they can impinge on the potential proximal landing zone. A range of hybrid techniques have developed in tandem with arch endografting that have allowed for an expansion in the indications for surgical intervention.

This chapter discusses the major options and evidence for the management of aortic arch aneurysms, ways in which complications might be minimized and the potential future directions for intervention.

Open or endovascular repair

Conventional surgical repair of aortic arch pathologies requires median sternotomy and cardio-pulmonary bypass with circulatory arrest. This has quoted mortality rates of between 5% to 20%, even in series of highly selected patients. Aside from operative mortality, the devastating complications of disabling stroke and spinal cord ischemia (SCI) occur in up to 20% and 30% of patients, respectively. Even with significant advances in pre-operative assessment and optimization, advanced anesthetic techniques and intensive care, aortic arch repairs remain amongst the highest risk of across all surgical specialties. The advent of endovascular technologies for infra-renal aneurysm repair with well-documented reductions in mortality and morbidity from these procedures has inevitably led to the application of these techniques to pathology within the thoracic aorta. Interest is now firmly focused on the aortic arch, but this region of the aorta provides special challenges. Dedicated devices for the management of thoracic aneurysms have made endografting of the aortic arch a more realistic option but the outcomes remain poorly defined as a limited number of surgeons have embraced the procedures. Despite this, early experience would suggest that endovascular arch repair can be carried out at an acceptable mortality and morbidity.

Indications for thoracic endovascular repair

The indications for intervention in the repair of aortic arch pathologies are poorly defined. However, until a larger body of evidence is available the indications should be a threshold of 5.5 cm for elective repair of non-symptomatic thoracic aneurysms and chronic dissections. Acute type B thoracic dissections should be treated when complicated by rupture, impending rupture (i.e. rapid expansion, intra-mural hematoma, left-sided pleural effusion) or malperfusion as described [4].

In order to land a stent-graft in the thoracic aorta a proximal landing zone of 20 mm is required. For pathologies in the arch this mandates the creation of a landing zone, measured on the lesser curve, through extra-anatomic bypass procedures followed by stent-graft placement. A similar endovascular-open hybrid approach has been usefully utilized in the repair of thoraco-abdominal aneurysm repair for those patients unfit to undergo extensive open surgical repair.

Pre-operative assessment

As with any major surgical procedure, an appropriate pre-operative assessment of patients with aortic arch pathology is of paramount importance. Aside from the standard work-up such as an assessment of cardio-respiratory function and reserve and of renal function, accurate pre-operative imaging is crucial.

This would include computed tomography (CT) visualization of the access vessels and of the carotid arteries with a thorough assessment of aorto-iliac morphology being necessary prior to endovascular repair. Heavily diseased carotid arteries would preclude carotid bypass procedures in the absence of concomitant carotid endarterectomy.

There are three key components: endovascular access, the state of aortic side branches including cerebral circulation and the site and suitability of stent-graft landing zones. The aortic arch should be accurately visualized with multi-slice CT images suitable for 3D-reconstruction with a view to examining not only aneurysm morphology, but also the degree of arch atheroma that might lead to embolic stroke secondary to manipulation within the arch. In cases where the left subclavian artery ostium will be covered some authors have suggested the routine CT angiographic, or magnetic resonance (MR) angiographic, assessment of the circle of Willis in addition to the patency and dominance of the vertebral circulations although this might be debated in view of more recent results discussed below. It is important to recognize congenital abnormalities of the left vertebral artery and vertebra-basilar system. The left vertebral artery is usually the dominant artery in 60% of individuals and arises from an anomalous location in up to 5%. Anomalous left vertebral arteries most frequently arise from the aortic arch between the left common carotid artery and the left subclavian artery and are visible on CT. A study by Tsuchida et al. [5] found that 13% of patients had inadequate vertebra-basilar communications on pre-operative cerebral angiography. In 7% the left vertebral artery supplied a large area of the posterior fossa and a hypoplastic vertebral artery was observed in 10%-40% of normal angiograms. In addition to the posterior cerebral circulation, the vertebro-basilar system makes important contributions to the spinal cord and the anterior spinal artery arises from one vertebral artery in 21% of cases, with approximately equal incidence from each side.

Arch endovascular-open hybrid approaches

Ishimaru's [6] anatomical landing zone map was devised to assist in operative planning and reporting of arch endografting (Fig. 1). Zones 0-3 relate

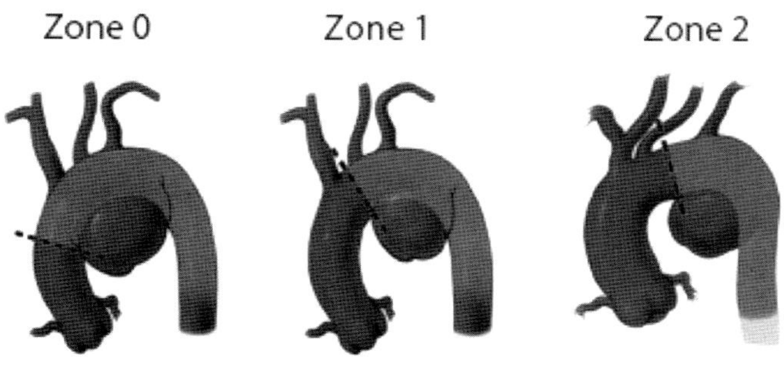

FIG. 1 The landing zones of the aortic arch. From Ishimaru [7].

to the arch and zones 4 and above to the relatively straight segment of the descending thoracic aorta. Aneurysms with proximal deployment in zones 0 to 2 encompass the coverage of one or more supra-aortic trunk ostia to create a satisfactory proximal seal. Zone 0 lesions require coverage and revascularization of the brachiocephalic trunk and the left common carotid artery. Coverage of the left common carotid artery origin and revascularization by carotid-carotid bypass is mandated for pathology with a zone 1 landing zone. Management of the left subclavian artery (LSA) is through carotid-subclavian bypass or transposition. The outcomes of hybrid approaches when compared with open surgery are summarized in Table I.

An endovascular procedure might also be use-

Table I THIRTY-DAY OUTCOMES OF OPEN ARCH REPAIR AND ENDOVASCULAR-OPEN HYBRID ARCH REPAIR. THESE REPORTS OF OPEN REPAIRS ARE LIMITED TO THOSE REPORTING ARCH REPAIRS SEPARATELY FROM ASCENDING AND THORACO-ABDOMINAL ANEURYSMS AS SUCH, PARAPLEGIA RATES ARE NOT REPORTED

First author (ref.)	*Method of repair*	*Mortality (%)*	*Stroke (%)*	*SCI (%)*
Hayashi [8]	Open	25	10	Not reported
Okita [9]	Open	10	4	Not reported
Yamashiro [10]	Open	20		Not reported
Czerny [11]	Open	11.6	5	Not reported
Holt [12]	Hybrid	6	7.7	3.8
Funovics [13]	Hybrid	4.5	0	0
Melissano [14]	Hybrid	6.3	3.1	3.1
Weigang [15]	Hybrid	15	0	0
Czerny [16]	Hybrid	7.4	0	0
Bergeron [17]	Hybrid	8	8	4
Saleh [18]	Hybrid	0	0	0
Schumacher [19]	Hybrid	20	4	0

fully employed where a previous elephant trunk repair has been performed. In this situation endovascular completion of the elephant trunk via a retrograde approach avoids a further thoracotomy, although the longer-term outcomes are unknown. It has also been suggested that an elephant trunk might be completed via an antegrade approach through the graft fabric to avoid thoracotomy.

Thoracic debranching procedure details

Zone 0

Zone 0 lesions are treated by debranching the innominate and left common carotid arteries, followed by deployment of the thoracic endografts. This can be achieved through median sternotomy, application of a side-biting clamp to the ascending aorta and end-to-end anastomoses of individual Dacron grafts, or a bifurcated graft, to transected innominate and left common carotid arteries. The use of a trifurcated graft has been described to revascularize all supra-aortic trunk ostia, but access to the LSA is often difficult and this approach may be best avoided and a carotid-subclavian by-pass undertaken instead.

Zone 1

Pathologies with a zone 1 proximal landing zone are treated through carotid-carotid cross-over bypass using a Dacron conduit tunnelled either pre-pharyngeally or retro-pharyngeally (Fig. 2). A decision must be made as to which route to use based on the degree of respiratory co-morbidity and the likely clinical requirement for post-operative tracheostomy. LSA revascularization can be performed synchronously with a bypass from the cross-over graft to the LSA.

Zone 2 and indications for LSA revascularization

LSA revascularization can be performed by a left carotid-subclavian bypass using a Dacron conduit or LSA transposition. However, there remains disagreement regarding the operative management of the LSA for pathology in any of zones 0 to 2. Early reports on the use of stent-grafts in the aortic arch suggested that the LSA need not be revascularized in the majority of cases, and that this might avoid the operative morbidity of a hybrid procedure [16,19-24]. A number of studies defined the absolute indications for LSA revascularization, which were long thoracic aortic segment coverage (more than 20 cm), prior abdominal aortic aneurysm re-

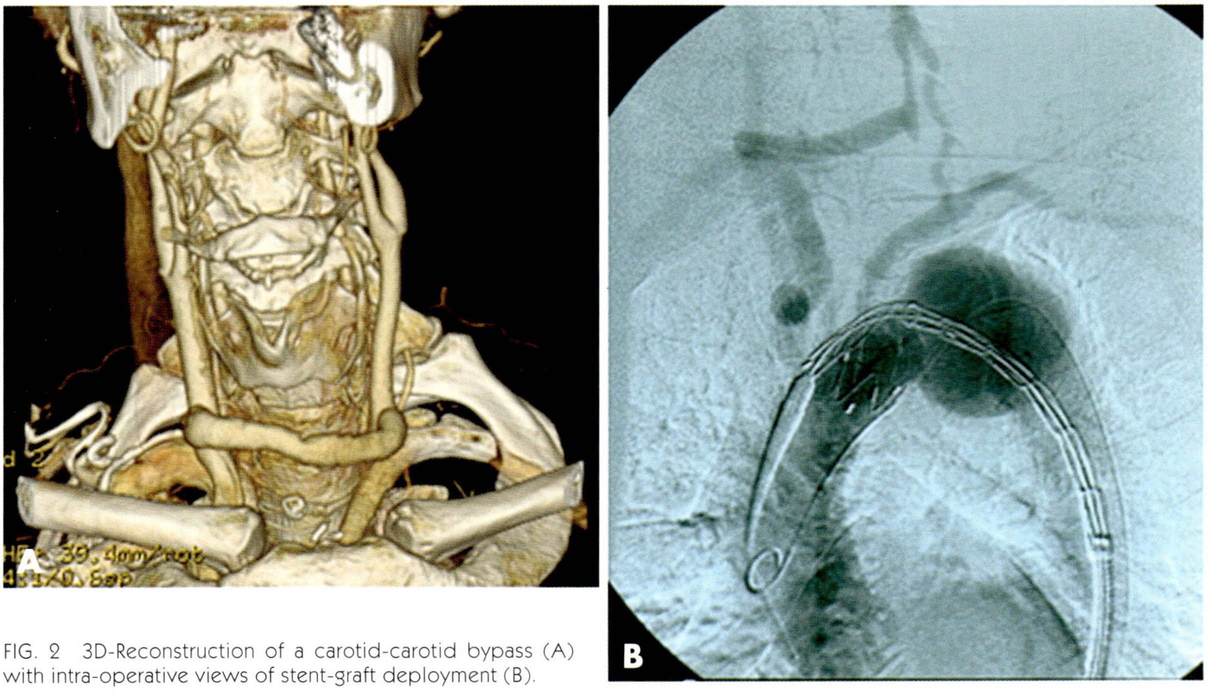

FIG. 2 3D-Reconstruction of a carotid-carotid bypass (A) with intra-operative views of stent-graft deployment (B).

Table II THE EFFECT OF LEFT SUBCLAVIAN ARTERY (LSA) REVASCULARIZATION ON THE OUTCOMES OF ARCH REPAIR FROM ONE LARGE SERIES DEMONSTRATING A PROTECTIVE EFFECT OF REVASCULARIZATION ON THE KEY OUTCOMES OF DEATH SPINAL CORD ISCHEMIA (SCI) AND STROKE, AND A COMBINED OUTCOME MEASURE (HOLT ET AL.) [12]

	LSA revascularized (n = 35)	*LSA not revascularized (n = 43)*	*p-value*
Stroke (%)	0	11.6	0.046
SCI (%)	0	6.98	NS
Death (%)	0	14.0	0.024
Combined Outcome (%)	0	27.9	< 0.0001

pair, upper limb ischemic symptoms post endografting [25], coronary artery bypassing with the left internal mammary artery and current hemodialysis access in the left upper limb or a hypoplastic/absent right vertebral artery [26-28].

More recent data, however, have been contradictory with the majority supporting LSA revascularization [29-32] to prevent neurologic sequelae during thoracic endovascular repair (TEVR) [32-33]. The largest reported case series of arch aneurysm to date suggested that there was a significant reduction in morbidity and mortality in arch aneurysm repair with LSA revascularization (Table II). Following revascularization an endovascular plug should be placed to occlude the LSA ostium as back bleeding in to the aneurysm sac in this situation may be considered to be a high-pressure endoleak.

TIMING OF TEVR

The repair of aortic arch pathology can be performed as staged or single-stage procedures although the evidence is limited for the adoption of a single protocol over another. In one large series, all patients underwent endografting with no interval ruptures, or failures to complete treatment due to unfit patients, which is in contrast to reports of endovascular-surgical hybrid procedures with visceral revascularization for thoraco-abdominal aneurysms [11]. This would suggest that this might be the best strategy for treating elective cases, whereas a single-stage procedure might be best adopted for emergency cases.

ENDOVASCULAR PROCEDURE

A number of thoracic endografts are available from each of the major stent-graft manufacturers and considerable resources are being placed into their continued development. The endovascular procedure can be performed under general or local anesthesia and in general a retrograde femoral approach is utilized, via iliac conduits when indicated. Other approaches have been described, including the subclavian and carotid arteries. A critical stage in the management of aortic arch pathology is in the accurate placement of the proximal stent. A number of factors combine to make this a challenging process and these include difficulties with access to the aortic arch leading to losses in pushability and torque of the delivery device and the high hemodynamic forces within the arch. In order to increase the accuracy of stent-graft placement a variety of hemodynamic manipulations are used. These include a temporary reduction of the systolic pressure to below 80 mmHg for deployment of the most proximal endograft, ventricular over-pacing or pharmacologically induced systole.

MANAGEMENT OF THE SPINAL CORD

One of the major complications of TEVR is SCI. This presents a higher-risk in patients who have had previous aortic surgery, including internal iliac artery embolization, in whom a long distance of the thoracic aorta is likely to be covered (> 20 cm) and in emergency cases [26]. The use of lumbar spinal drains causes a degree of debate with different authorities suggesting the routine use for all thoracic aortic cases, selective use or insertion only when patients are symptomatic. One further indication is the insertion of a prophylactic lumbar drains pre-operatively in patients who might require prolonged ventilation that might prevent recognition of neurological deficit. Protocols for the management of lumbar spinal drain differ along with their indications for use. One suggestion would be to set the drain to a fixed pressure of 10 cm H_2O and leave it on free drainage, up to a maximum of 30 mL cerebrospinal fluid per hour. Irrespective of spinal drain placement the mean arterial pressure should be maintained above 90 mmHg in the peri-operative period, with the use of inotropes if required to reduce the incidence of SCI through maintenance of the spinal perfusion pressure.

Complications of aortic arch repair

Revascularization

Reports from the literature suggest that the surgical procedures in open/endovascular hybrid procedures can be delivered with a very low morbidity. From a series of 88 cases there were only two complications as a result of the revascularization procedures themselves: one chronic sinus to an infected graft and one post-operative hematoma requiring re-intervention [11]. All patients were medically fit to go on to have the TEVR procedure with no interval ruptures. These findings are in contrast to open arch repair and hybrid repairs for thoracoabdominal aortic aneurysms, both of which carry significant morbidity and mortality.

Thoracic endovascular repair

Peri-operative death

Mortality rates for arch repair have been reported to be between 0% and 20%, with most series in the region of 8% for all landing zones. There are conflicting results as to the outcomes of arch repair with respect to the proximal landing zone. One series found that endografting the proximal arch was achievable at a lower risk [12], which was in contrast to the findings of Melissano et al. [14] (Table III). These conflicting results, not only for mortality, need clarification through the ongoing critical assessment of outcomes.

Stroke

Stroke has been reported in up to 10 % of arch aneurysm repairs. Previous studies have reported a variable effect for LSA revascularization and stroke, with the EUROSTAR experience suggesting that revascularization was not protective [19,20,28-32]. However, the latter authors routinely documented vertebral artery dominance and patency pre-operatively [19,20]. Conversely, not revascularizing the LSA has been suggested as a risk factor for stroke in a number of studies [23,33-35]. Recent data have suggested that LSA might be protective against all strokes post arch aneurysm repair with rates of

Table III Contrasting outcomes of aortic arch endografting by Ishimaru zone from two large series

	Holt [12]				*Mellisano [14]*			
Ishimaru Zone	0	1	2	All	0	1	2	All
Number of cases	9	17	52	78	14	12	38	64
30-day mortality (%)	0	0	9.4	6	14	0	5.3	6.3
SCI (%)	0	0	5.7	3.8	0	0	5.3	3.1
Stroke (%)	11	0	9.6	7.7	14.3	0	0	3.1
Type I / III endoleak (%)	11	11.7	7.7	8.9	7.1	33	7.9	12.5

SCI: spinal cord ischemia

11% in non-revascularized patients against 0% in revascularized patients. In these series emergency presentations were also at higher risk of post-operative stroke when compared to elective cases (14% against 2%).

Strokes have been reported to occur in both posterior and carotid circulation territories suggesting a multi-factorial etiology. In particular emboli from arch instrumentation and wire manipulation must be considered in addition to the hemodynamic risks of over-stenting the LSA and this embolic risk must be assessed preoperatively.

SCI

Whilst the proposed mechanisms underlying SCI in endografting differ from those in open repair, the risks remain significant and units must have robust policies in place for lumbar spinal drainage and post-operative blood pressure manipulation. The reported paraplegia rates following thoracic endovascular procedures are significantly lower (1%-6%) than those from open surgery which can be as high as 21% [1,27,36-38]. It is likely that LSA revascularization plays an important role in reducing the risk of SCI, with recent data demonstrating SCI rates of 0% in a cohort of patients in whom the LSA was revascularized group and nearly 7% in the non-revascularized group.

Endoleak

Proximal (Ia) endoleak rates have been reported at between 0% and 20%. Although the management of these leaks follows standard lines, there are intrinsic difficulties due to the short landing zone. Consequently the options are balloon dilation or the placement of an extension cuff or a Palmaz stent, but if these fail then further debranching might be necessary, where possible, to extend the proximal landing zone. To manage this problem, some authors have suggested when median sternotomy is to take place then endografting should be performed with open access. In this situation, an aortic tie can be placed to abolish a proximal endoleak at the primary sitting.

The high endoleak rates associated with thoracic stent-grafts are due to poor alignment of the stent-grafts in the region of the aortic arch. Conventional stent-grafts do not conform easily to the angles in the arch and in-vitro analysis suggests most stent-grafts permit peri-graft flow (endoleak) at angles of less than 30 degrees. The size of the endoleak increases with the degree of vessel angulation. One way to address this problem is to create a more proximal landing zone, pushing the stent-graft further around the arch, thus improving alignment. However, there is no guarantee that extending the proximal landing zone and improving alignment will ensure adequate seal.

Endograft non-conformation and collapse

In tandem with endoleak, it is important to recognize that the potential non-conformability of the currently available endografts can lead to "fishmouthing" of the graft with subsequent graft fracture or collapse. In the thoracic aorta, graft fracture has been associated with subsequent aortic rupture. Stent-graft collapse, often associated with multiple stent fractures, leads to pseudo-coarctation and can be fatal if not recognized and treated emergently. The true incidence of stent-graft collapse is unknown, but it might be more prevalent in cases where there is a poor apposition of the graft to the lesser curve at the completion of the procedure and where there is a protrusion of the stent into the aortic lumen by more than 50%. Management includes relining the stent-graft and the placement of large balloon expandable stents.

Retrograde type A dissection

Although rare, there is a possibility of a retrograde type A dissection (propogation of a dissection into the ascending aorta) secondary to stent-graft placement in the arch. This complication is unique to thoracic endografting and is a higher risk in the management of aortic dissection then atherosclerotic aneurysms. The etiology is through either a progression of the pre-existing disease, or more usually, intimal trauma from wire manipulation or from the device itself. Presentation may be acute or delayed. It has been suggested that devices with a proximal bare stent or those with proximal hooks or barbs are more likely to be associated with this complication, or when then endograft is oversized by more than 20%. These factors should be taken into consideration when planning arch endograft placement.

Consensus statement

One factor of importance for these cases is a current variability in reporting standards. It would be of use to gain a consensus statement from the vascular community not only for the management of the LSA, but also for the use of spinal drains and in the reporting of adverse neurological outcomes. The routine use of the Tarlov score for paraplegia and post-operative assessment by a specialist neurologist where SCI or stroke are suspected would seem to be a minimum requirement.

Future direction

The future of treatment of aortic arch aneurysms has been usefully debated by a number of authorities. It remains unclear whether the direction lies with a total endovascular solution through fenestrated or branched grafts or through endovascular-surgical hybrid procedures. Certainly current solutions involving in-situ fenestrations and chimney grafts (double barreled-techniques) represent a compromise in management at best and must be currently considered purely experimental. In-situ fenestration does not require a pre-loaded customized stent-graft but there are a number of drawbacks. First, it is possible that the orientation of the stents in the main graft may preclude satisfactory fenestration and second, there are concerns regarding the consequences of an uncontrolled graft fabric tear created in-situ with the cutting balloons.

Conclusion

Arch aneurysm repair can be carried out at a low mortality and acceptable morbidity using a staged endovascular-open hybrid approach with minimal morbidity from the surgical stage. The endovascular stage continues to carry a significant risk, although this is lower than traditional surgical repair. As well as assiduous endovascular planning for stenting the aortic arch should be undertaken with high quality imaging and 3D-reconstructions. It would appear that LSA revascularization is mandated in these procedures whether elective or emergency to reduce the incidence of death, SCI and stroke.

References

1 Stone DH, Brewster DC, Kwolek CJ et al. Stent-graft versus open-surgical repair of the thoracic aorta: mid-term results. *J Vasc Surg* 2006; 44: 1188-1197.

2 Dake MD, Miller DC, Semba CP et al. Transluminal placement of endovascular stent-grafts for the treatment of descending thoracic aortic aneurysms. *N Engl J Med* 1994; 331: 1729-1734.

3 Greenberg RK, Lu Q, Roselli EE et al. Contemporary analysis of descending thoracic and thoracoabdominal aneurysm repair: a comparison of endovascular and open techniques. *Circulation* 2008; 118: 808-817.

4 Sayer D, Bratby M, Brooks M et al. Aortic morphology following endovascular repair of acute and chronic type B aortic dissection: implications for management. *Eur J Vasc Endovasc Surg* 2008; 36: 522-529.

5 Tsuchida K, Hashimoto A, Aomi S et al. Prevention of cerebral complications during thoracic aortic aneurysms operation: study of preoperative selective cerebral arteriography. *Kyobu Geka* 1991; 44: 380-383.

6 Mitchell RS, Ishimaru S, Ehrlich MP et al. First International Summit on Thoracic Aortic Endografting: roundtable on thoracic aortic dissection as an indication for endografting. *J Endovasc Ther* 2002; 9 (Suppl 2): II98-1105.

7 Ishimaru S. Endovascular stent-graft repair for thoracic aortic aneurysm. *Kyobu Geka* 2006; 59(8 Suppl): 666-673.

8 Hayashi J, Eguchi S, Yasuda K et al. Aortic arch operation using selective cerebral perfusion for nondissecting thoracic aneurysm. *Ann Thorac Surg* 1997; 63: 88-92.

9 Okita Y, Takamoto S, Ando M et al. Mortality and cerebral outcome in patients who underwent aortic arch operations using deep hypothermic circulatory arrest with retrograde cerebral perfusion: no relation of early death, stroke, and delirium to the duration of circulatory arrest. *J Thorac Cardiovasc Surg* 1998; 115: 129-138.

10 Yamashiro S, Sakata R, Nakayama Y et al. One-stage thoracic aortic aneurysm treatment and coronary artery bypass grafting. *Jpn J Thorac Cardiovasc Surg* 2001; 49: 236-243.

11 Czerny M, Fleck T, Zimpfer D et al. Risk factors of mortality and permanent neurologic injury in patients undergoing ascending aortic and arch repair. *J Thorac Cardiovasc Surg* 2003; 126: 1296-1301.

12 Holt PJE, Johnstone CJ, Hinchliffe RJ et al. Outcomes of the endovascular management of aortic arch aneurysm and the implications for management of the left subclavian artery. *J Vasc Surg* 2009; In Press.

13 Funovics M, Blum M, Langenberger H et al. Endovascular repair of the descending aorta and the aortic arch with the Relay stent graft. *Ann Thorac Surg* 2009; 88: 637-640.

14 Melissano G, Civilini E, Bertoglio L et al. Results of endografting of the aortic arch in different landing zones. *Eur J Vasc Endovasc Surg* 2007; 33: 561-566.

15 Weigang E, Parker J, Czerny M et al. Endovascular aortic arch repair after aortic arch de-branching. *Ann Thorac Surg* 2009; 87: 603-607.

16 Czerny M, Gottardi R, Zimpfer D et al. Mid-term results of supraaortic transpositions for extended endovascular repair of aortic arch pathologies. *Eur J Cardiothorac Surg* 2007; 31: 623-627.

17 Bergeron P, Mangialardi N, Costa P et al. Great vessel management for endovascular exclusion of aortic arch aneurysms and dissections. *Eur J Vasc Endovasc Surg* 2006; 32: 38-45.

18 Saleh HM, Inglese L. Combined surgical and endovascular treatment of aortic arch aneurysms. *J Vasc Surg* 2006; 44: 460-466.

19 Schumacher H, Von Tengg-Kobligk H, Ostovic M et al. Hybrid aortic procedures for endoluminal arch replacement in thoracic aneurysms and type B dissections. *J Cardiovasc Surg* (Torino) 2006; 47: 509-517.

20 Gorich J, Asquan Y, Seifarth H et al. Initial experience with intentional stent-graft coverage of the subclavian artery during endovascular thoracic aortic repairs. *J Endovasc Ther* 2002; 9(Suppl 2): II39-1143.

21 Rehders TC, Petzsch M, Ince H et al. Intentional occlusion of the left subclavian artery during stent-graft implantation in the thoracic aorta: risk and relevance. *J Endovasc Ther* 2004; 11: 659-666.

22 Cina CS, Safar HA, Lagana A et al. Subclavian carotid transposition and bypass grafting: consecutive cohort study and systematic review. *J Vasc Surg* 2002; 35: 422-429.

23 Ozsvath KJ, Roddy SP, Darling RC et al. Carotid-carotid crossover bypass: is it a durable procedure? *J Vasc Surg* 2003; 37: 582-585.

24 Peterson BG, Eskandari MK, Gleason TG et al. Utility of left subclavian artery revascularization in association with endoluminal repair of acute and chronic thoracic aortic pathology. *J Vasc Surg* 2006; 43: 433-439.

25 Greenberg RK, O'Neill S, Walker E et al. Endovascular repair of thoracic aortic lesions with the Zenith TX1 and TX2 thoracic grafts: intermediate-term results. *J Vasc Surg* 2005; 41: 589-596.

26 Tiesenhausen K, Hausegger KA, Oberwalder P et al. Left subclavian artery management in endovascular repair of thoracic aortic aneurysms and aortic dissections. *J Card Surg* 2003; 18: 429-435.

27 Greenberg R, Resch T, Nyman U et al. Endovascular repair of descending thoracic aortic aneurysms: an early experience with intermediate-term follow-up. *J Vasc Surg* 2000; 31: 147-156.

28 Chiesa R, Melissano G, Marrocco-Trischitta MM et al. Spinal cord ischemia after elective stent-graft repair of the thoracic aorta. *J Vasc Surg* 2005; 42: 11-17.

29 Leurs LJ, Bell R, Degrieck Y et al. Endovascular treatment of thoracic aortic diseases: combined experience from the EUROSTAR and United Kingdom Thoracic Endograft registries. *J Vasc Surg* 2004; 40: 670-680.

30 Orend KH, Zarbis N, Schelzig H et al. Endovascular treatment (EVT) of acute traumatic lesions of the descending thoracic aorta–7 years' experience. *Eur J Vasc Endovasc Surg* 2007; 34: 666-672.

31 Rodriguez JA, Olsen DM, Shtutman A et al. Application of endograft to treat thoracic aortic pathologies: a single center experience. *J Vasc Surg* 2007; 46: 413-420.

32 Melissano G, Civilini E, Bertoglio L et al. Endovascular treatment of aortic arch aneurysms. *Eur J Vasc Endovasc Surg* 2005; 29: 131-138.

33 Buth J, Harris PL, Hobo R et al. Neurologic complications associated with endovascular repair of thoracic aortic pathology: Incidence and risk factors. a study from the European Collaborators on Stent/Graft Techniques for Aortic Aneurysm Repair (EUROSTAR) registry. *J Vasc Surg* 2007; 46: 1103-1111.

34 Fattori R, Nienaber CA, Rousseau H et al. Results of endovascular repair of the thoracic aorta with the Talent Thoracic stent graft: the Talent Thoracic Retrospective Registry. *J Thorac Cardiovasc Surg* 2006; 132: 332-339.

35 Woo EY, Bavaria JE, Pochettino A et al. Techniques for preserving vertebral artery perfusion during thoracic aortic stent grafting requiring aortic arch landing. *Vasc Endovascular Surg* 2006; 40: 367-373.

36 Criado FJ, Clark NS, Barnatan MF. Stent graft repair in the aortic arch and descending thoracic aorta: a 4-year experience. *J Vasc Surg* 2002; 36: 1121-1128.

37 Chaikof EL, Mutrie C, Kasirajan K et al. Endovascular repair for diverse pathologies of the thoracic aorta: an initial decade of experience. *J Am Coll Surg* 2009; 208: 802-816.

37 Cambria RP, Brewster DC, Lauterbach SR et al. Evolving experience with thoracic aortic stent graft repair. *J Vasc Surg* 2002; 35: 1129-1136.

11

OPEN AND ENDOVASCULAR TREATMENT OF DESCENDING THORACIC ANEURYSMS

ROBERTO CHIESA, EFREM CIVILINI, YAMUME TSHOMBA,
ENRICO MARIA MARONE, LUCA BERTOGLIO, GIOVANNI COPPI,
DAVIDE LOGALDO, FABIO CALLIARI, GERMANO MELISSANO

Aortic aneurysm is a potentially serious condition and if it affects the descending thoracic segment it can cause life threatening situations. Luckily, in many cases thoracic aortic disease can be diagnosed and treated before it becomes dangerous. The most appropriate management is related to the severity, extension and site of disease and to the specific patient's clinical characteristics and risk factors. This chapter summarizes etiology and indications for treatment, imaging modalities of open and endovascular techniques as well as personal and worldwide results.

Degenerative aneurysms

The incidence of degenerative aneurysms involving the descending thoracic aorta (DTA) is considered approximately 10 in 10 000 adults, with 30%-40% of these aneurysms limited to the intrathoracic segment of the descending aorta [1]. The pathogenesis of DTA is in most ways similar to the more frequent infra-renal aneurysms and is due to progressive destruction of the lamina media. Considering the inherent risk of complications, an aortic diameter of 5.5 cm is widely recognized as the threshold for interventions, while no benefit from treatment exists in case of aneurysms smaller than 5.5 cm [2]. These criteria apply only to asymptomatic patients; symptomatic aneurysms should be treated regardless of size if there are no other contra-indications, because symptoms often portend rupture. No level A or B scientific evidence from prospective, randomized studies exists related to the timing of operative intervention according to aneurysm size, as in the case for abdominal aortic aneurysms (AAAs).

The surgical open repair is currently considered the first therapeutic choice, and the thoracic endovascular aortic repair (TEVAR) should be chosen in selected patients with a suitable anatomy allowing a safe and effective endograft deployment, on a predicted operative risk that is clearly lower than the risk of either conventional open repair or optimal medical management.

Dissecting aneurysm

In the acute setting, uncomplicated type B dissection is best managed with medical therapy, however, almost half of all patients develop or present with complications requiring intervention and therefore have a marked increase in mortality. There are at present four indications for acute intervention: unrelenting pain, progressive aortic dilatation, malperfusion syndromes, or imminent rupture [3]. The role of primary open procedures for visceral, renal, and limb ischemia is nowadays unclear given the rapid advancement of percutaneous endovascular techniques. The goal of TEVAR in a complicated acute dissection is to occlude the primary tear(s) and relieve malperfusion syndromes.

Once a patient survives 14 days after initial onset of an acute aortic dissection, it is defined as chronic. Data suggest that TEVAR in patients with chronic aortic dissection can be performed with satisfying technical success. Indications are a maximal thoracic aorta diameter greater than 5.5 cm, documented increase of aortic diameter of more than 1.0 cm within one year, resistant hypertension despite antihypertensive combination therapy associated with a small true lumen or renal malperfusion, or recurrent episodes of chest/back pain that cannot be attributed to other causes [2].

Connective tissue disorders

One contra-indication to endovascular approaches seems to be defined by connective tissue disorders. Although endografts have been used in Marfan cases in the setting of aneurismal disease, there is too high a risk for creating retrograde dissection or acute or delayed perforation [4]. This concept is particularly relevant when considering that centers with extensive experience have excellent results with open repair. Endovascular approach may play a role in the treatment of recurrences when a previously implanted surgical graft can be used as a landing zone.

Imaging modalities

In order to plan the best possible treatment modality for each individual patient, accurate imaging must be obtained pre-operatively. There are many different modalities that allow to image the thoracic aorta, each one having its own advantages and drawbacks:

- chest XR (a valuable basic screening exam);
- ultrasonography (in particular trans thoracic and trans-esophageal echography);
- digital subtraction angiography (implies arterial catheterization, contrast media injection and exposure to ionizing radiation);
- magnetic resonance (MR)-angiography (no radiation involved but an intravenous contrast agent may still be necessary);
- computed tomography (CT)-angiography (exposure to ionizing radiation, intravenous contrast agent injection).

Thoracic aorta CT-angiography and OsiriX

There are several reasons why most surgeons who treat thoracic aortic disease choose CT-Angio as their preferred imaging modality, provided that there are no specific contra-indications. State-of-the-art multi-detector CT scanners produce excellent imaging. Typically, a complete exam to study the thoraco-abdominal aorta consists of at least 1 000-2 000 scans. To obtain optimal information from the CT dataset one must be able to navigate through the images and manipulate them (reformatting techniques) in order to extract the most appropriate images that are needed. Until recently, reformatting the CT dataset in order to obtain for planning the procedure was only possible on dedicated imaging workstations which are expensive and usually located in the radiology department, making practical access to them rather difficult. Since 2004 and especially in the last years the situation has changed considerably. We owe to the ingenuity of Dr. Ratib and his co-workers from the University of Genève for the creation of the OsiriX software. OsiriX is dedicated to "DICOM" images (Digital Imaging and Communications in Medicine) produced by current medical equipment, and runs on regular Mac OS X computers. It has been specifically designed for navigation and visualization of multi-modality and multidimensional images, including CT. It is world widely available to be freely downloaded on the Internet, and is released under GNU free software license, which grants recipients rights to use, modify and

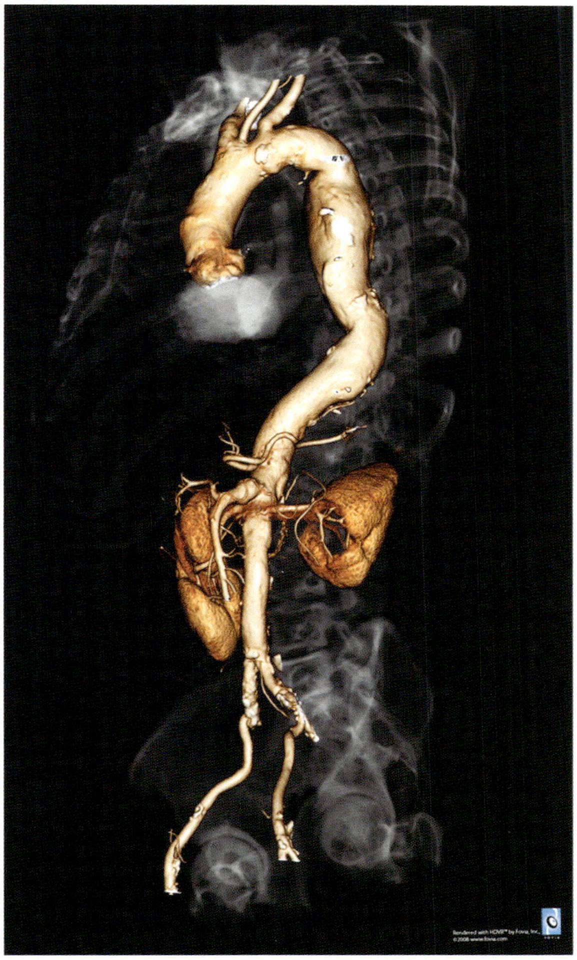

FIG. 1 This image depicts a three-dimensional rendering of the entire aorta in a patient with a descending thoracic aortic aneurysm obtained with the OsiriX and the Fovia high definition volume rendering software.

redistribute copyrighted work. It is possible to create personalized plug-ins which perform desired actions.

With the help of the OsiriX software we started working on our CT dataset to obtain the necessary images of the aorta (Fig. 1).

The classical way to show a CT dataset is by means of axial (transverse) scans. However, the dataset contains the entire volume of the body, and we are allowed to view the structure we are studying in a very realistic three-dimensional way using 3D rendering tools.

Furthermore, the slices of our dataset can be cut not only in a transverse (axial) plane but also in a frontal (coronal) or in a lateral (sagittal) plane. Scrolling these three sets of scans, adjusting the window level and width, zooming and modifying the slice thickness will allow us to gain a lot of information, however, the important structures in our body do not follow orthogonal planes and the aorta in particular has a tortuous path that curves in all directions of space. An oblique multi-planar reconstruction (MPR) may therefore help us producing a scan, the angulation of which matches that of the aorta, or the vessel we need to study (Fig. 2).

If the vessel (for example an iliac axis for peripheral access of a device) we are studying is too tortuous to be followed even in an appropriate oblique MPR we can use a more sophisticated tool: a curved MPR where the plane we are going to extract from the dataset is hand-drawn on the scan offering the precise course of the anatomical structure we need to follow (Fig. 3).

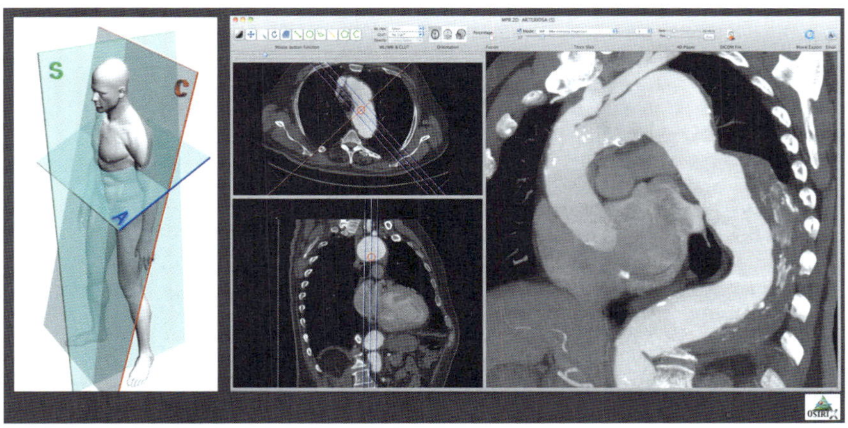

FIG. 2 Customized angulated (non orthogonal) cutting planes are extremely useful when studying a particularly angulated descending thoracic aneurysm. (Osirix screen capture – right).

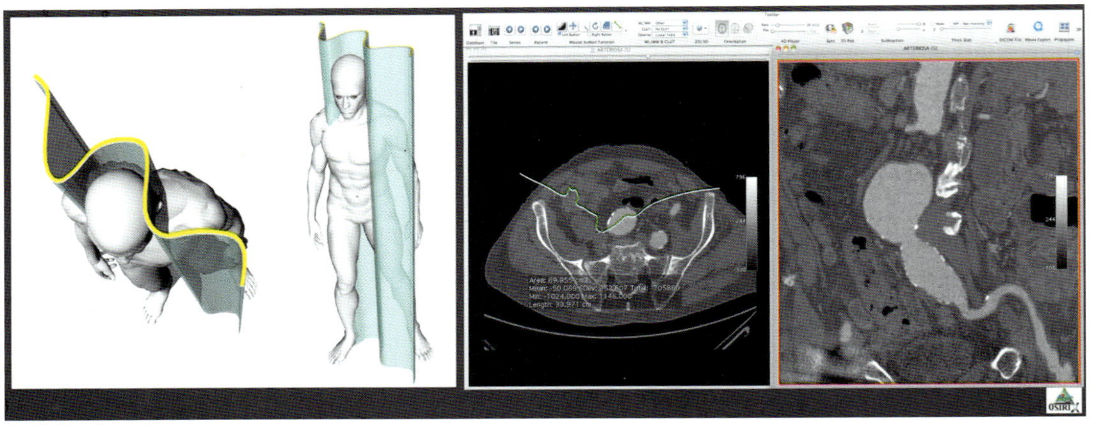

FIG. 3 A very tortuous structure may not be represented by a straight cut. A curved cut, opportunely hand-drawn on the axial scan (green line) can depict the course of this iliac access in a single reformatting plane. (Osirix screen-capture - right).

Curved MPR for critical intercostal artery study

The mechanism underlying the occurrence of spinal cord ischemia after open and endovascular thoracic aortic repair is still not completely understood.

Several authors believe that the presence of one or more critical intercostal arteries providing spinal cord blood flow play a crucial role in the development of postoperative spinal cord ischemia. Kieffer et al. [5] recently published a remarkable large single-center study of open and endovascular repair of descending thoracic aortic aneurysms in which endovascular repair was carried out exclusively in high-surgical risk patients in whom pre-operative spinal cord arteriography demonstrated the origin of the critical intercostal arteries outside the zone to be covered by the endograft.

A curved MPR may provide pre-operative imaging not only of intercostal arteries, but of all the vascular collateral network providing flow to spinal cord (Fig. 4) including vertebral, hypogastric and mammary arteries. Although this method to study spinal cord blood supply is extremely interesting from an academic perspective, it is probably still

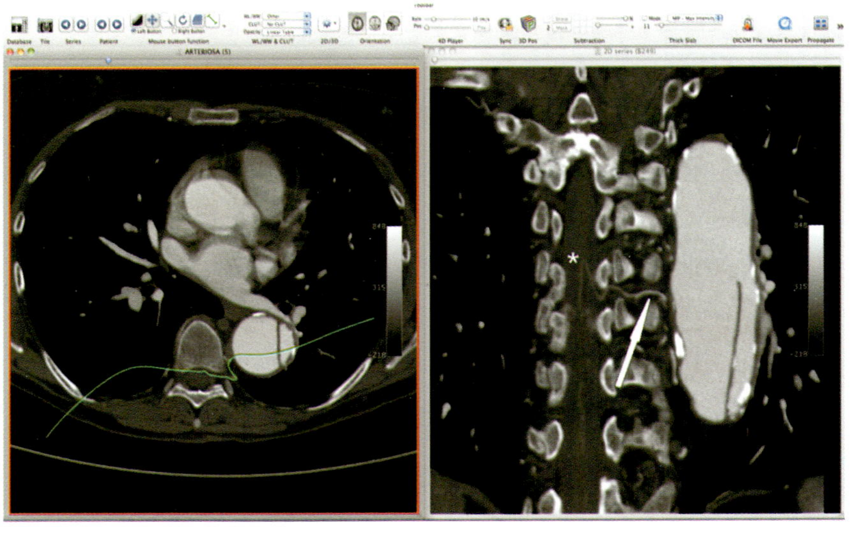

FIG. 4 Curved plane (green line) depicts the path of the Adamkiewicz artery(*) in this patient, clearly showing its continuity with the false lumen of the dissected aorta (arrow). (OsiriX screen capture).

not accurate enough to act as a base for operative strategies. Furthermore it only depicts the vascular anatomy without providing any functional information.

Once validation and improved understanding of the information acquired with CT-based angiography (or alternatively MR-angiography) of the spinal cord vasculature are realized, several important clinical benefits are possible:

1) pre-operative stratification of the risk of spinal cord ischemia;
2) selective intercostal/lumbar artery re-implantation (open surgery);
3) avoidance of unnecessary coverage of intercostal feeders of the artery of Adamkiewicz (TEVAR);
4) selective revascularization of left subclavian artery or hypogastric artery;
5) selective use of adjuncts that have an intrinsic risk of complications, such as cerebrospinal fluid drainage (CSFD).

Open repair

Open surgery for DTA is a major vascular procedure with substantial mortality and morbidity rates. However, thanks to the multimodality approaches of organ protection, the outcomes have considerably improved in the last decades, especially in "high-volume" centers as shown in Table I.

Pre-operative evaluation

Imaging

In addition to assess the aorta and spinal cord arteries, a pre-operative angio-CT with 3D volume rendering tools may play a role in understanding the conformation of the patient and locating the most appropriate intercostal space to perform thoracotomy (Fig. 5). Also, the most safe site of proximal and/or distal aortic cannulation can be visualized with regard to intraluminal thrombus and thereby reduce the risk of potential embolization.

Physiologic reserve

An adequate pre-operative assessment of physiologic reserve of cardiac, pulmonary, and renal function and an accurate knowledge of cerebral and spinal cord vascular anatomy are mandatory in evaluating operative risk, planning the best operative strategy and take early additional peri-operative precautions.

Cardiac evaluation

Pre-operative transthoracic echocardiography is a satisfactory noninvasive screening method which

Table I Results of open descending aortic repair. Updated personal series (*)

First author (ref.)	*Patients*	*Operative mortality (%)*	*Paraplegia/paraparesis (%)*	*Stroke (%)*	*Renal failure (%)*
Estrera [6]	300	24 (8.0)	7 (2.3)	6 (2.1)	12 (4.2)
Coselli [7]	387	11 (2.8)	10 (2.6)	/	29 (7.5)
Borst [8]	132	4 (3)	12 (9.1)	/	2 (1.3)
Svensson [9]	832	63 (8)	90 (10.8)	29 (3.5)	58 (6.9)
Verdant [10]	267	39 (15)	0 (0)	/	1 (0.4)
Kouchoukos [11]	65	2 (3)	2 (3)	1 (1.5)	0 (0)
Fehrenbacher [12]	63	2 (3)	0 (0)	/	0 (0)
Chiesa (2009)*	194	8 (4.1)	9 (4.6)	4 (2.0)	14 (7.2)

* Endoleaks were not consistently reported among the published series. Some authors reported only type I or type III leaks or none at all, and consequently, endoleak reporting is incomplete.

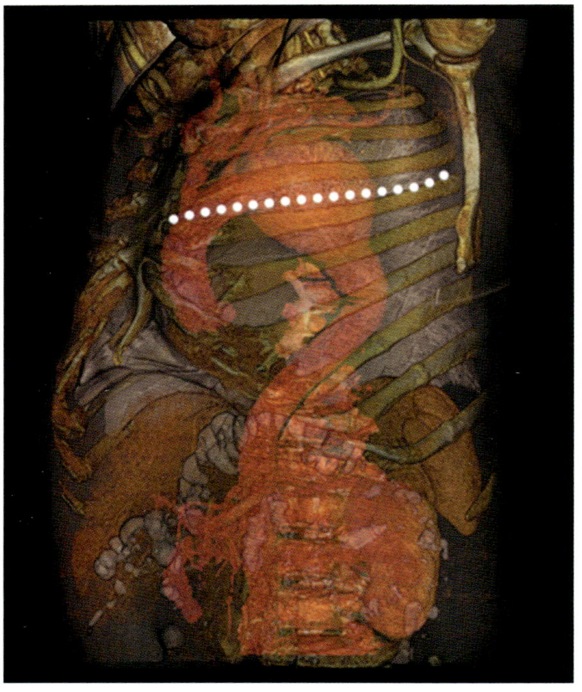

FIG. 5 This image obtained with the OsiriX software and the Fovia high definition volume rendering software allows a pseudo-realistic three-dimensional depiction of the human body highlighting different structures. This kind of images can be useful to plan the surgical access to the thoracic aorta and the ideal intercostal space for thoracotomy.

evaluates both valvular and biventricular function. Exercise testing or dipyridamole-thallium myocardial scanning identifies regions of myocardium which are reversibly ischemic and, in patients with a significant history of angina or reduced ejection fraction, cardiac catheterization with coronary arteriography should be performed. CT coronary angiography has recently emerged as a less-invasive, alternative method to visualize the coronary arteries anatomy. Interestingly, new multi-row (256) scanners, allow to obtain images of the coronary arteries and thoracic aorta in a single scan, thus improving spatial resolution with reduced radiation dose [13].

In patients with an asymptomatic thoracic aneurysm, severe coronary artery occlusive disease should be treated with percutaneous transluminal angioplasty prior to aneurysm repair, preferably avoiding use of drug-eluting stents requiring prolonged double anti-platelet therapy. The surgical myocardial revascularization should be limited to very selected patients with severe high-risk coronary lesions inadequate for percutaneous transluminal angioplasty.

Renal evaluation

Renal function is an established predictor of postoperative outcome. The National Kidney Foundation currently recommends the use of estimated glomerular filtration rate to assess renal function in order to avoid the misclassification of patients on the basis of serum creatinine levels alone [14]. Based on this indicator, chronic kidney disease has been shown to be a strong predictor of death after open and endovascular repair thoracic aneurysm, even in patients without clinical evidence of preoperative renal disease [15].

Respiratory evaluation

Pulmonary function assessment with arterial blood gases and spirometry is mandatory in all patients undergoing open surgery of the descending aorta. In patients with a forced expiratory volume lower than 1.0 and a PCO_2 more than 45, pulmonary function should be improved by stopping smoking, active treatment of bronchitis, losing weight, and following a general exercise program for a period of 1 to 6 months before operation. However, in patients with symptomatic aortic aneurysms, despite a poor pulmonary function, the operation can not be delayed.

Intra-operative monitoring

A right radial and right femoral arterial pressure line are always inserted in order to guarantee continuous intra-operative arterial blood pressure monitoring. Temperature monitoring is essential to guide hypothermia especially in time-consuming operations and if a period of circulatory arrest is required. Nasopharyngeal and bladder temperature sensors are inserted to monitor brain and core temperature, respectively.

Single lung ventilation by means of a double-lumen endobronchial tube is required in order to obtain adequate surgical exposure and to limit compression of the heart by retractors. Fiberoptic bronchoscopy is recommended to check correct positioning of the endotracheal tube, especially in large aneurysms of the descending aorta that may lead to distortion of the trachea or the left main bronchus.

Trans-esophageal echocardiography

Intra-operative trans-esophageal echocardiography (TEE) performed either by the operating room anesthesiologist or by the cardiologist (the presence of the cardiologist is strongly suggested

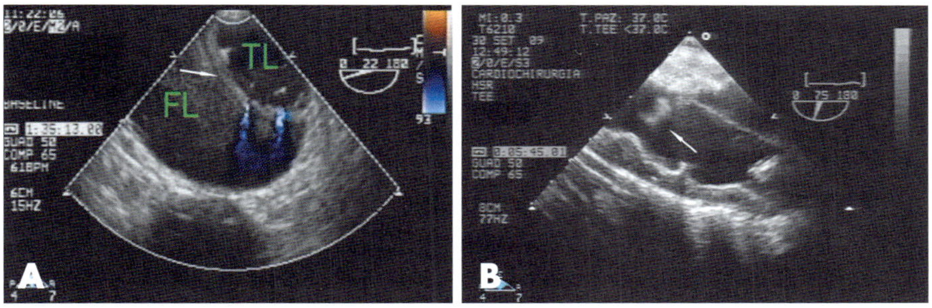

FIG. 6 The TEE examination may provide the most effective means of intra-operative assessment of aortic dissection, intramural hematoma, intraluminal thrombus, etc. A. Intra-operative TEE showing a large dissecting aneurysm involving the DTA. Of note the dissecting membrane (arrow) with 2 large tears with flow from the true lumen (TL) to the false lumen (FL). B. Intra-operative TEE showing a "shaggy aorta" with large thrombus (arrow) floating in the proximal DTA, detected before aortic clamping during a DTA aneurysm open repair.

in patients with concomitant severe heart disease) is a very helpful tool during thoracic aortic surgery (Fig. 6).

TEE enables dynamic monitoring of hemodynamics and modification of therapeutic management. Furthermore, the central venous pressure, right atrial pressure, and pulmonary capillary wedge pressure may be significantly influenced by the patient's right lateral decubitus position during surgery and may provide unreliable cardiac volume and function. Both systolic and diastolic changes which may occur during the different stages of the surgical procedure can be real time assessed and patients at risk for peri-operative hemodynamic deterioration may be identified. To assess the systolic function, ejection fraction is commonly used. Transmitral flow and pulmonary vein flow patterns are often measured to assess the diastolic function. Myocardial performance index can be used to assess both systolic and diastolic functions and is also useful to interpret right ventricular function. Recently developed real time 3-dimensional systems may provide adjunctive accurate cardiac informations, such as left ventricle volumetry, wall motion, dyssyncrony and valvular pathology.

CSFD

In order to reduce the incidence of spinal cord ischemic complications, we routinely utilize CSFD except in cases of planned hypothermic arrest [16]. Cerebrospinal fluid is freely drained during aortic clamping, and in the first 72 post-operative hours we drain fluid to maintain a target pressure of less than 10 cm H_20.

SURGICAL PROCEDURE

Access

The patient is positioned in a right lateral decubitus position on a beanbag with the shoulders at 60° and the hips flexed back to 30° to access the entire left thorax, the abdomen and the left groin. A circulating water mattress with heat exchanger is placed between the beanbag and the patient, in order to assist body temperature management.

An adequate exposure is mandatory for a safe surgical control at the distal and proximal neck. The thoracotomy incision varies in length and level, depending on the aneurysm extent.

It is our standard practice to deliberately cut the rib of the incised intercostal space posteriorly for a better mobilization. When required, rib resection or a double thoracotomy can be performed in order to improve proximal exposure (Fig. 7).

Surgical dissection of the deflated lung is kept to a minimum. Large aneurysms that extend proximally require an aortic clamping between the left common carotid and left subclavian artery and repair of the entire DTA.

In these cases, the distal aortic arch is mobilized gently and dissected by dividing the arterial ligament and the left subclavian artery is circumferentially mobilized. Mean aortic pressure should not be above 60 mmHg during arch manipulation. Preservation of the vagus and left recurrent laryngeal nerves is strived for. If a prior left internal mammary arterial bypass graft is present, either a left common carotid to subclavian bypass or a left subclavian to carotid transposition is required to

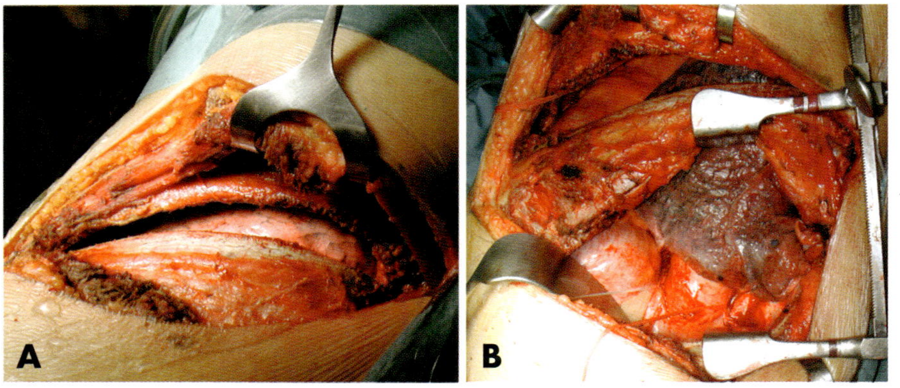

FIG.7 The picture shows a left thoracotomy in the fifth intercostal space. The left lung has not been excluded yet (A). In rare cases the we perform a double left thoracotomy (B) in order to have a better access to the distal and proximal descending aorta.

avoid cardiac ischemia when the cross-clamp is applied proximal to the left subclavian artery.

Distal aortic perfusion

Distal aortic perfusion has been shown to be an effective adjunct in reducing incidence of paraplegia in patients undergoing surgical repair of extensive thoraco-abdominal aortic aneurysms (TAAAs) [17]. The utility of distal aortic perfusion during less invasive repairs such as for DTA is still controversial. Although the "clamp-and-sew" technique has been shown to be a suitable approach to descending thoracic aneurysms repair if performed by experienced surgeons, we try to limit it's use to emergency cases with hemodynamic instability. We used hypothermic circulatory arrest selectively in cases of challenging proximal aortic clamping like huge aneurysms or proximal dissections, or as a bail out procedure in case of intraoperative distal arch rupture.

Methods of distal aortic perfusion may include passive aortic shunts, partial femoral-femoral cardiopulmonary bypass with or without hypothermia, complete cardiopulmonary bypass, and, as in our series, left heart bypass (LHBP). Our choice for distal aortic perfusion is the use of a LHBP composed by two cannulas (in and out) connected to a Bio-pump (Biomedicus, Medtronic, Inc., Eden-Prairie, MN). The Bio-Pump is an extracorporeal, cell-preserving centrifugal device that can provide support for circulation during open DTA repair. The transparent pump housing is shaped like a cone. The pump consists of an acrylic pump head with inlet and outlet ports placed at right angles to each other. The impeller, which is a stack of parallel cones, is driven by an external motor and power console. Rotation of this impeller at high speeds creates a vortex, which drives blood flow in relation to rotational speed. Blood enters through an inlet at the top of the cone and exits via an outlet at the base. The pump can rotate up to 5 000 rpm and can provide flow rates of up to 10 liters per minute. The heparin-coated inner surface of the circuit allows to lower systemic heparin administration and to minimize the inflammatory response. Besides, the Bio-Pump allows better platelet preservation and reduced haemolysis.

The aim of the LHBP is:

- support the heart function, particularly in case of underlying heart disease;
- prevent proximal hypertension;
- minimize visceral and spinal cord hypoperfusion;
- reduce the need for pharmacologic intervention to maintain hemodynamic stability during the different steps of surgical procedure;
- keep the cerebrospinal fluid pressure low by enhancing the collateral perfusion.

LHBP is usually achieved from the left superior pulmonary vein to either the left femoral artery or distal DTA. Alternatively to the left superior pulmonary vein, the left atrium or distal arch or descending aorta proximally to the aneurysm can be cannulated (Fig. 8).

Before cannulation for LHBP, 50 IU/Kg of heparin are administered, distal aortic perfusion is instituted and the thoracic aorta is clamped. The bypass flows are targeted towards a value between

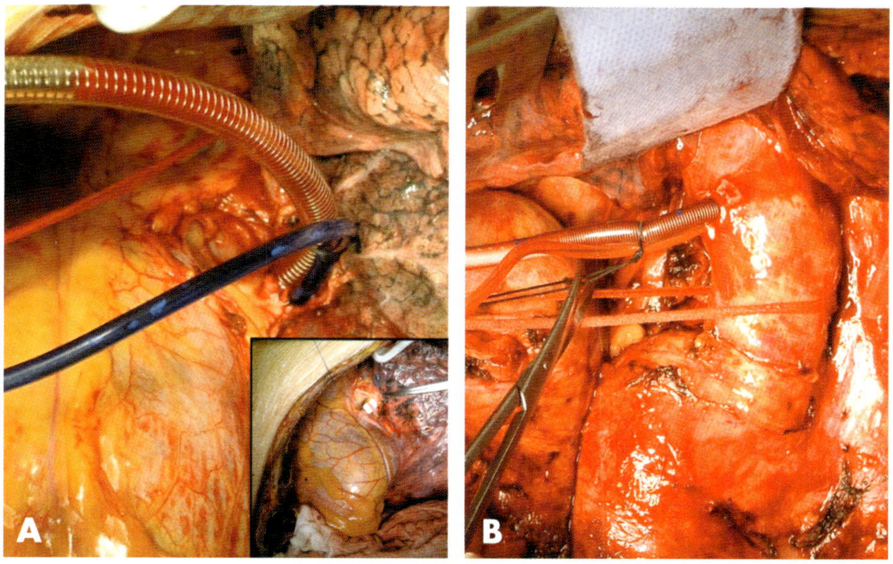

FIG. 8 Intra-operative pictures showing two alternative inflow sites for left heart bypass. A: cannulation of the left superior pulmonary vein; B) Cannulation of the proximal descending thoracic aorta. A single purse string suture reinforced with pledgets is generally used on the vein and a double one on the aorta.

1 500 and 2 500 mL/min in order to maintain a mean distal arterial pressure of 70 mmHg.

Since the flow of the LHBP is not as high as in cardiopulmonary bypass, pediatric cannulas can be used (14 F). This is especially advantageous when distal aortic perfusion must be instituted through small common femoral arteries and/or stenotic iliac vessels. In these cases, smaller cannulas do not occlude the vessels, allowing ipsilateral lower limb perfusion during LHBP, reducing the risk of femoral and iliac arteries injury and thrombosis. For the proximal cannulation we usually prefer a 20 F mouldable cannula when we cannulate the left superior pulmonary vein, and a 16-18 F standard cannula for the proximal aortic cannulation.

Normally the priming of the circuit is 400 mL. In particular clinical condition (anemia, dialysis) the priming can be replaced with the patient's autologous blood. Technically, this maneuvre can cause hemodynamic instability which can be resolved pharmacologically or by homologous blood transfusion.

Aortic clamping

During aortic clamping, the importance of cardiovascular stability cannot be overstated and the mean aortic pressure should not be lower than 70 mmHg in order to reduce the risk of spinal cord ischemia [18]. The use of TEE to monitor cardiac changes and to guide hemodynamic management in this critical surgical phase is now widely accepted as a routine monitoring and diagnostic tool in our protocol. The patient's temperature is allowed to drift down to a rectal temperature of 32 °C to 33 °C. Sequential clamping technique is our preferred technique although it is often not feasible due to aneurysm size, quality of aortic wall, and reduced intrathoracic space. In these cases proximal and distal necks are clamped, and the entire aneurysm is longitudinally opened. In case of dissections, rubber-shod Fogarty aortic clamps are preferred, especially in acute situations, in order to reduce the clamping-related aortic damage. Possible critical intercostal arteries are always temporarily occluded with 3 or 4 French occlusion-perfusion balloon catheters (Pruitt, Lemaitre Vascular, Inc. Burlington-MA-USA), suturing the other ones with 2-0 pledgeted polypropylene. The proximal aortic neck is transsected and circumferentially isolated to reduce the risk of injuring the esophagus through the aortic wall during proximal aortic anastomosis.

Aortic repair

Routinely, a collagen- or a gelatin-impregnated woven Dacron graft was used for aortic repair (Fig. 9).

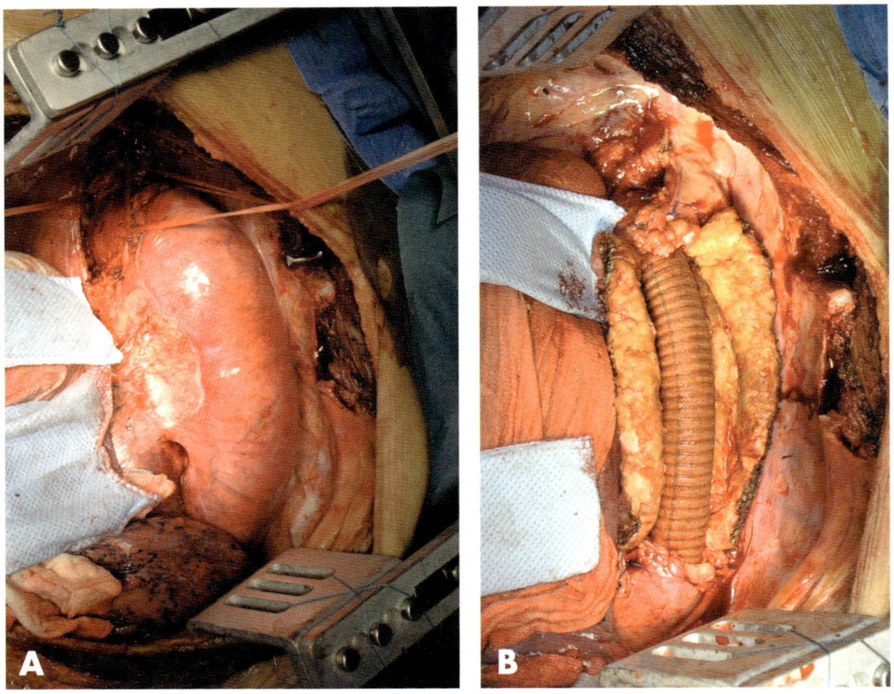

FIG. 9 A: depicts complete surgical dissection of a large aneurysm involving the entire descending aorta just before cross-clamping of the proximal neck between left common carotid and subclavian arteries. B: shows final aortic reconstruction with a conventional Dacron graft.

At present our current preferred graft material is Triplex prosthetic conduit (Vascutek Terumo, Renfrewshire, Scotland) consisting of an inner layer of standard uncoated woven dacron and an outer layer of a standard expanded polytetrafluoroethylene graft fused together by a central layer of self-sealing elastomeric membrane. In our experience, this prosthetic graft combines good handling and tailoring with a remarkable reduction of blood oozing from suture lines, even at full heparinization (Fig. 10).

The proximal anastomosis is usually made with a running suture with 2-0 polypropylene suture; in dissecting lesions 3-0 or 4-0 sutures are preferred. In aneurysms involving the distal arch, in which

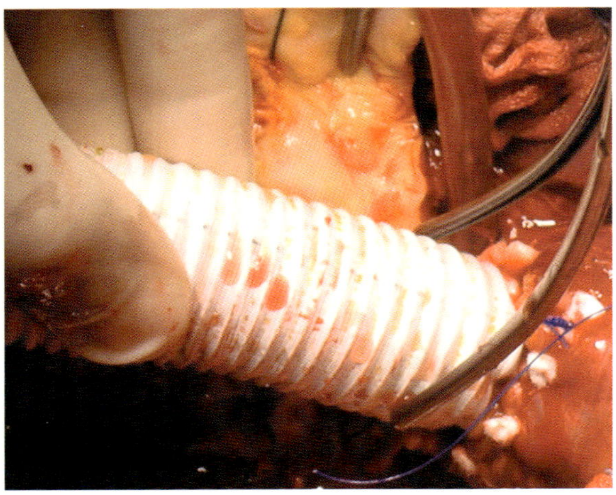

FIG. 10 Intra-operative picture showing the minimal bleeding at declamping of Triplex prosthetic conduit.

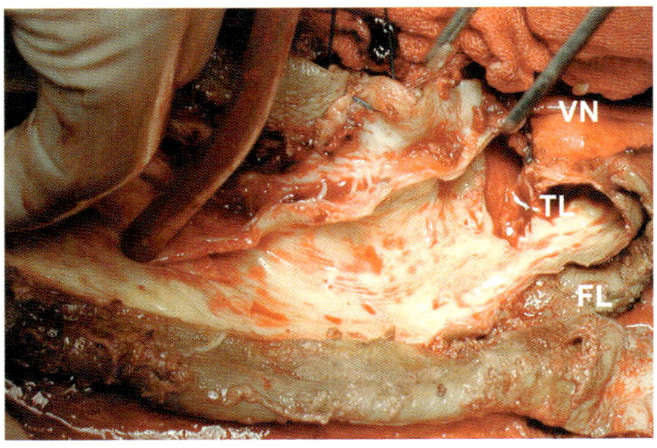

FIG. 11 Surgical treatment of a chronic dissection using deep hypothermic circulatory arrest (note the absence of aortic cross-clamping). The true (TL) and the false lumen (FL) are clearly recognizable. The origin of the left subclavian artery (LSA) and the vagus nerve (VN) are also visible.

the left subclavian artery can not be included in a bevelled proximal anastomosis a selective bypass is required. In case of chronic dissecting aneurysms (Fig. 11) the distal clamp is temporarily opened and a distal fenestration performed before performing the distal anastomosis, both containing the true and false distal aortic lumen.

In acute dissection the distal anastomosis is only performed with the true lumen, thereby obliterating the false lumen. After performing the distal anastomosis, the thoracic aorta is unclamped and the possible critical intercostal arteries temporarily occluded with balloon catheters. These arteries are subsequently reimplanted or revascularized by means of a bypass (Fig. 12).

Usually, intercostal artery reimplantation in acute dissection is avoided because of the friable aortic wall and risk of rupture and bleeding from the reimplanted tissues.

Completion of procedure

LHBP is subsequently used to rewarm the patient, discontinued and proximal and distal cannulae are removed. Especially in patients with dissecting aneurysms, detection of visceral organ ischemia immediately after aortic declamping is important. Femoral pulses and arterial lines are carefully assessed, and renal perfusion is checked by monitoring diuresis after distal clamp removal. When a good peripheral perfusion is confirmed, protamine sulphate is administered based on the activated clotting time values. After left heart bypass and especially after long periods of deep hypothermia, achieving hemostasis usually requires prompt administration of agents improving coagulation such as protamine, fresh-frozen plasma, thrombocytes, and, when deficient, concentrates of several coagulation factors. The aneurismal wall is then wapped around the aortic graft with a running suture. Two posterior thoracic drainage tubes are placed prior to closure at the apex and at the base of left pleural cavity.

Early post-operative management

The main focus of the immediate post-operative management of these patients in the intensive care unit is early detection of any possible neurological and cardiovascular complication, allowing selective prophylactic or therapeutic intervention. As soon as normal pressure and body temperature are achieved, the patient is allowed to wake up even if controlled ventilation is still necessary for pulmonary reasons. In case of clinical evidence of neurological damage, immediate CT scanning or nuclear magnetic resonance imaging is performed to exclude intracerebral bleeding or spinal cord

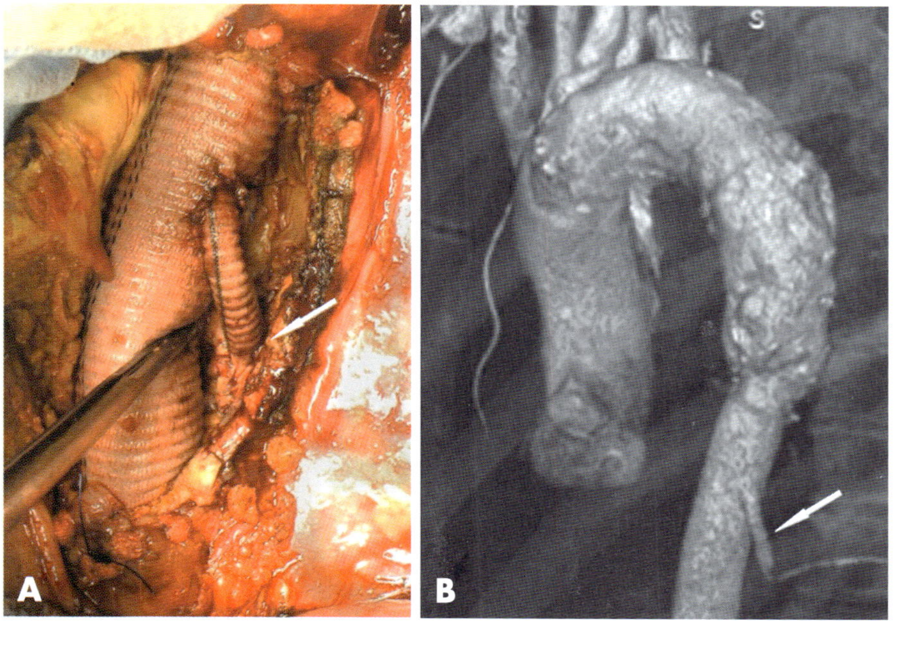

FIG. 12 Surgical picture (A) and postoperative CT (B) showing critical intercostal artery revascularization (arrow) by means of single Dacron bypass.

compression by an intradural hematoma. When spinal cord ischemia is detected, mean arterial pressure is maintained above 80 mmHg, spinal fluid is freely drained, and methylprednisolone (1 g in bolus, than 4 g in 24 hours in continuous perfusion) and 18% mannitol (5 mg/kg 4 times/die) are administered.

If signs of lower limb, renal or visceral malperfusion develop in the post-operative period, immediate diagnostic measures should be taken to assess organ blood supply and to appropriately plan surgical revascularization procedures. For a precise visualization of visceral organ perfusion, emergency arteriography or angio CT scanning is recommended.

In uncomplicated cases, drainage tubes are removed 36 to 48 hours post-operatively, while the intrathecal catheter for CSFD is usually removed after 72 hours if coagulation parameters and platelets counts are normal.

Personal results

Our experience with descending aortic open repair started in 1993. Since then we have performed a total of 194 surgical procedures for several patterns of disease: 54% of procedures was conducted for degenerative aneurysms, 34% for dissections and 12% for other acute and chronic conditions. We used LHBP in 82% of cases, clamp-and-sew technique in 16% and hypothermic arrest in 2%. Overall peri-operative mortality in open surgery of DTA was 4.1%. The rate of pulmonary complications, i.e. the need for more than 24 hours of mechanical ventilation was 8.8%. The rate of cardiac complications, i.e. new onset myocardial infarction demonstrated by positive blood tests was 6.2%. The rate of renal complications, i.e. the need for temporary or permanent hemodialysis, has been 7.2%. Cerebrovascular accident, defined as a new neurologic deficit lasting more than 24 hours confirmed by CT/MRI, has occurred in 2.0% of patients. Spinal cord ischemia, manifesting either as paraplegia or paraparesis was encountered in 4.6%.

Endovascular repair

A number of publications on TEVAR demonstrate a clear reduction in peri-operative mortality and morbidity, particularly for pulmonary, cardiac and renal complications as compared to open repair (Table II). However, we must consider the fact that these data report on devices which in the coming years will not be marketed anymore.

Pre-operative planning and sizing

Accurate planning is mandatory when a TEVAR is considered because precise quantitative measurements are needed for optimal device selection. Diameters, lengths and angles need to be measured very accurately including the presence of thrombus, calcifications, anomalies, etc. (Fig. 13).

Endovascular procedure

We perform all procedures in the operating room, using a portable digital C-arm image intensifier with road-mapping capabilities (series 9600, OEC Medical System or Moonray, Simad Medical Technology). As described before CSFD has a protective role in open surgical repair of DTAs and TAAAs, however its role in TEVAR is less defined.

Our current indications for CFSD in TEVAR includes:

1. long coverage (predicted use of more than one endograft);
2. coverage of high risk area including T10-T12;
3. previous abdominal or thoracic aortic surgery;

In our experience we installed CSFD in 48% of patients.

Intra-operative TEE monitoring was routinely used during all thoracic endovascular procedures. In our experience TEE allows assessment of the most appropriate landing zone of the endograft (in particular when the LSA origin has to be spared). At a later moment TEE is capable of documenting thrombosis or the presence of low flow inside the aneurysm sack after deployment of the endograft, thus avoiding repeated angiography and the use of high doses of contrast media. In the treatment of type B dissection, TEE can show whether the guide wire is correctly positioned inside the true lumen or whether it has moved inside a patent false lumen. TEE can also easily depict the presence and position of the proximal entry tear, the presence of additional distal tears (eventually not detected by angiography) and thrombosis or reperfusion of the false lumen.

Our preferred strategy is to perform the endovascular procedure under general anesthesia. In selective cases, depending of the patient general condition and comorbidity, access and endograft insertion can be performed under local or spinal anesthesia.

Table II Compiled data from published series of thoracic aortic endografting for predominantly aneurysmal disease: postoperative data. Updated personal series of descending thoracic aortic endovascular repair*

First author [ref.]	*Number of patients*	*Operative mortality (%)*	*Cerebrovascular events (%)*	*Paraplegia (%)*	*Early endoleak %*	*Late endoleak %*
Bavaria [19]	140	3 (2.1)	5 (3.6)	4 (2.9)	10	0
Wheatley [20]	156	6 (3.8)	7 (4.5)	1 (0.6)	11.5	NA
Ricco [21]	166	17 (10.2)	2 (1.2)	6 (3.6)	16.2	NA
Glade [22]	42	2 (5)	0 (0)	1 (2)	NA	NA
Greenberg [23]	100	7 (7)	3 (3)	2 (1)	10.3	6
Riesenman [24]	50	4 (8)	2 (4)	0 (0)	10	10
Bortone [25]	110	4 (3.6)	1 (1)	0 (0)	NA	NA
Czerny [26]	54	2 (3.7)	0 (0)	0 (0)	5.6	8.9
Neuhauser [27]	31	6 (19)	1 (3.2)	2 (6)	29	28
Bell [28]	67	1 (2)	3 (4)	3 (4)	NA	4.8
Bergeron [29]	33	3 (9)	1 (3.1)	0 (0)	0	0
Chabbert [30]	47	3 (6.4)	3 (6)	0 (0)	25.5	NA
Marin [31]	94	NA	6 (0.7)	NA	25	NA
Orend [32]	74	7 (9.5)	0 (0)	0 (0)	20.3	NA
Schoder [33]	28	0 (0)	0 (0)	0 (0)	21.4	NA
Criado [34]	47	1 (2.1)	0 (0)	0 (0)	8.7	NA
Mitchell [35]	103	9 (9)	7 (6.8)	3 (2)	24	2
Chiesa *	172	5 (2.9)	2 (1.2)	9 (5.2)	1 (0.6)	0

NA: not available

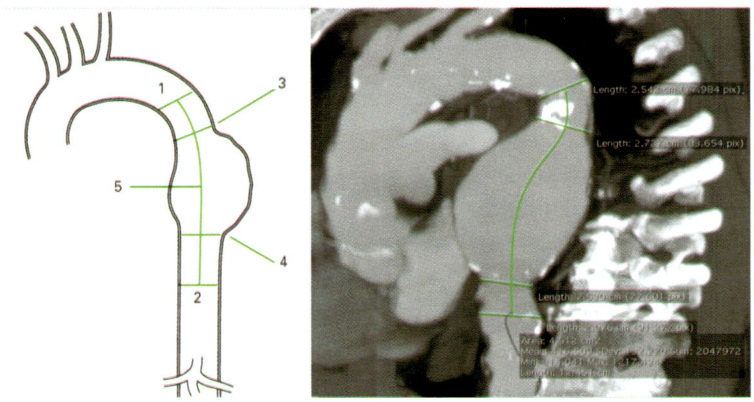

FIG. 13 An example of sizing in the work-up of an endovascular procedure for a thoracic aortic aneurysm.

Patients are placed in the dorsal decubitus position and the operative field is prepared in such a way that it allows access of the abdominal aorta and/or iliac arteries. In most cases the common femoral artery is exposed through an inguinal transverse incision. A bolus of heparin (70 IU/Kg) is administered. The contralateral femoral artery is percutaneously punctured for diagnostic guidance. In case of extremely calcified external iliac arteries we routinely use the common iliac through a paramedian extraperitoneal approach for access site. In rare cases the abdominal aorta has been used for access with direct puncture and subsequent closure with a purse string suture. A 260-cm long, 0.035-inch precurved super stiff guidewire (Lunderquist, Cook Medical Inc.) is advanced up to the aortic arch under fluoroscopic guidance.

The endograft is then passed over the guide wire into the appropriate position within the DTA or aortic arch under fluoroscopic guidance. During deployment, a mild systemic hypotension is induced pharmacologically by the anesthesiologist with a bolus of fast-acting venous or arterial vasodilators such as nitrates or urapidil. Nitroprusside or adenosine-induced asystole is never used. After deployment of the endograft on the selected location a completion angiogram is performed.

Endograft

The objective of a device for treatment of an aortic aneurysm is clear: it must prevent aneurysm rupture. This is achieved by excluding blood flow and pressure within the sac. Thrombus will form and with time the sac itself may regress or disappear altogether. In acute uncomplicated aortic dissection without dilatation of the aortic wall, closure of the proximal intimal tear may initiate healing of the aorta. However, the device itself may produce additional tears at both the proximal and distal level of the fragile diseased aorta. Most available endografts are not primarily intended for the treatment of this condition, especially if they contain proximal or distal uncovered stents, hooks or barbs. For chronic cases, closure of the intimal tear may produce thrombosis of the false lumen. Stabilization of the flap and enlargement of the true lumen are also desirable. It must be remembered that effective obliteration of the false lumen may compromise the circulation to arteries that arise from the false lumen itself (i.e. left renal artery). Flow to all important vessels must therefore be verified and additional procedures (i.e. stenting) may be necessary to restore flow to these vessels.

Follow-up

Once an endograft has been successfully implanted, the patients need to undergo follow-up imaging to confirm proper and stable position of the graft.

The presence of metal parts (which are very radio-opaque) in the endovascular prostheses allow postoperative assessment of graft position and side branch patency (Figs. 14,15).

Personal results

Our experience with thoracic endovascular aortic repair started in 1998. Since then we have performed 322 procedures. Of these, 116 involved the aortic arch with partial/total rerouting of the supra-aortic vessels; 172 involved the DTA, and 34 were hybrid procedures for pathology of the thoracoabdominal segment. A total of 126 procedures were conducted for degenerative aneurysms of the DTA.

When specifically considering the DTA, our technical success rate, indicating deployment of the endograft with complete exclusion of the lesion/minimal endoleak, has been 99.4% (with one case requiring emergent open conversion). Perioperative mortality has been 2.9% (5 patients).

The rate of pulmonary complication, i.e. the need for more than 24 hours of mechanical ventilation, has been 1.2%. The rate of cardiac complication, i.e. new onset of myocardial infarction demonstrated by positive blood tests, has been 0.6%. The rate of renal complication, i.e. the need for temporary or permanent hemodialysis, has been 1.9%. Cerebrovascular accident, defined as a new neurologic deficit lasting more than 24 hours confirmed by CT/MRI, has occurred in 1.2% of patients.

The rate of spinal cord ischemia, manifesting either as paraplegia or paraparesis, has been 5.2%. We have experienced an even distribution between early and delayed onset paraplegia/paraparesis. Delayed onset spinal cord ischemia has had a tendency towards amelioration with adequate arterial pressure support and CSFD.

Complications

In spite of the great enthusiasm that endovascular techniques provoked, it must be remembered that particularly at the level of the thoracic aorta these techniques are by no means completely safe.

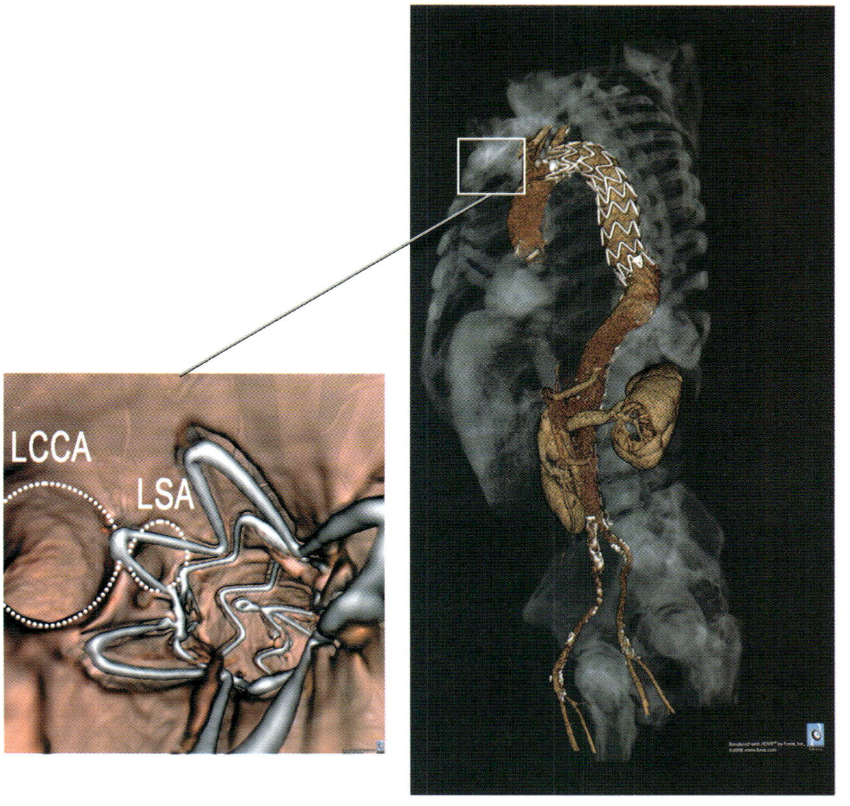

FIG. 14 This image obtained with the OsiriX and the Fovia high definition volume rendering software shows the post-operative angio-CT follow-up of a patient who underwent thoracic endovascular exclusion of a DTA. In the box a virtual endoluminal aortic view shows the proximal free-flow overstenting the left subclavian artery (LSA) and reaching the origin of the left common carotid artery (LCCA).

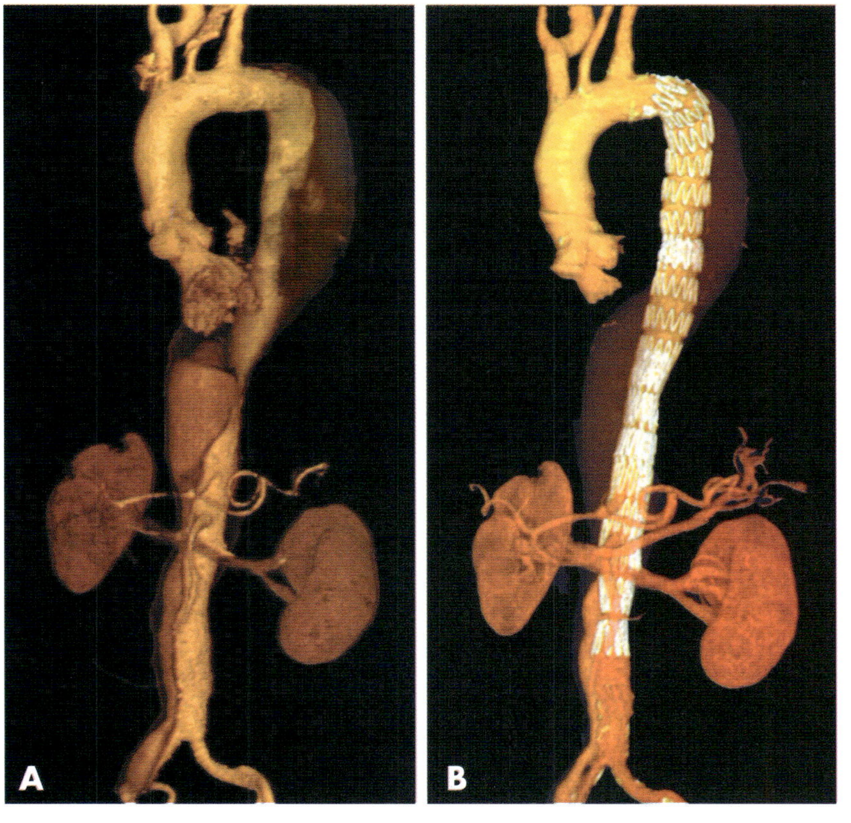

FIG. 15 A Pre-operative angio CT 3D reconstruction obtained with the OsiriX software of a type B chronic aortic dissection complicated by an aneurismal evolution. B: final result of TEVAR using the Cook TX2 and the specific device designed for dissection TXD. Note that patency of the visceral vessels is maintained.

A significant mortality and morbidity is described in all published series. A French report from Ricco et al. [36] analyzed a countrywide experience over two years and showed even more complications than in papers coming from single centers.

Damage to access vessels

Several literature reports have pointed out that serious and even fatal problems may arise from introduction of the device via the femoral artery. In particular rupture or avulsion of the external iliac artery have been reported. This usually becomes evident at the time the large introducer sheath used for endograft delivery is withdrawn. We therefore liberally switch to extraperitoneal surgical exposure of the common iliac artery or even the distal aorta if it is difficult to advance the device through the femoral artery.

Stroke

Cerebrovascular accidents are the most common and dreaded complications of endovascular therapy of thoracic aortic disease. They are mainly linked to atheromatous embolization into the cerebral arteries caused by guide wires, catheters, introducer sheath manipulation or the endograft itself [37]. It should be remembered that angiography for diagnostic purposes alone carries a 1%-2% risk of complications [38]. Second generation commercial grafts are definitely less prone to this complication as compared to the home made devices used initially. This is due to the better flexibility and smaller diameters of the grafts and sheaths. Minimal manipulation of the wires and catheters and a meticulous technique do play a significant role in the prevention of peri-operative stroke.

Paraplegia

Endoluminal repair avoids aortic cross clamping and its related sequelae, however, the intercostal arteries covered by the endograft cannot be reimplanted. The reported incidence of both immediate and delayed paraplegia in patients undergoing endovascular procedures of TAAA can be as high as 12% [28,34,39]. The coverage of a long thoracic aortic segment has been reported to be a significant risk factor for spinal cord ischemia [40]. Patients who had open AAA repair also appear to be prone to such a risk because of the marginal spinal cord collateral blood supply secondary to the ligation of lumbar arteries performed during the surgical procedure. Also, proximal collateral circulation of the spinal cord may be at risk by the occlusion of the left subclavian artery (landing zone 2) that abolishes the contribution to the blood supply provided by the anterior spinal artery, a branch of the ipsilateral vertebral artery. In a recent study [41], we analyzed our recent 5-year experience with repair of thoracic aortic pathology to evaluate the incidence and determinants of spinal cord ischemia in endovascular procedures. Our data showed that the lack of collateral spinal cord blood supply through the lumbar arteries in patients with previous aortic repair appear was a relevant risk factor even though it did not reach statistical significance. The intentional occlusion of the left subclavian was not a predictor of paraplegia and neither was the exclusion of an extensive thoracic aortic segment. Among the peri-operative variables, only a lowest mean arterial pressure (MAP) of < 70 mm Hg was a statistically significant determinant of delayed neurologic deficit ($p < 0.0001$). A delayed neurologic deficit developed in four patients and completely resolved after the institution of CSFD, steroids administration, and pharmacologically increased arterial pressure pharmacologic adjustment.

Our experience addresses the importance of hemodynamic control to prevent postoperative neurologic deficits and encourages aggressive, post-operative care of these patients. In our practice, we now try to maintain a peri-operative MAP of >90 mmHg and use of CSFD in patients deemed at high risk, including those who underwent AAA repair. In this respect, patients with synchronous thoracic and AAA, who we treated simultaneously before for both aneurysms, currently undergo staged procedures to allow development of collaterals for spinal cord blood supply. In the case of delayed paraplegia, prompt CSFD, if not previously instituted, is also used to keep the CSF pressure < 10 mmH_2O and possibly reverse the deficit.

Aorto-esophageal fistula

As follow-up is becoming longer and the reported series larger, new serious complications are emerging. One of the most dreaded is endograft infection (Fig. 16), especially if sustained by an aorto-esophageal fistula (Fig. 17). There are at this time several reports in the literature. It may be caused by erosion of the endograft through the aortic wall into the esophagus and we may speculate that excessive over-sizing may contribute. This complication does not seem to be specific to a sin-

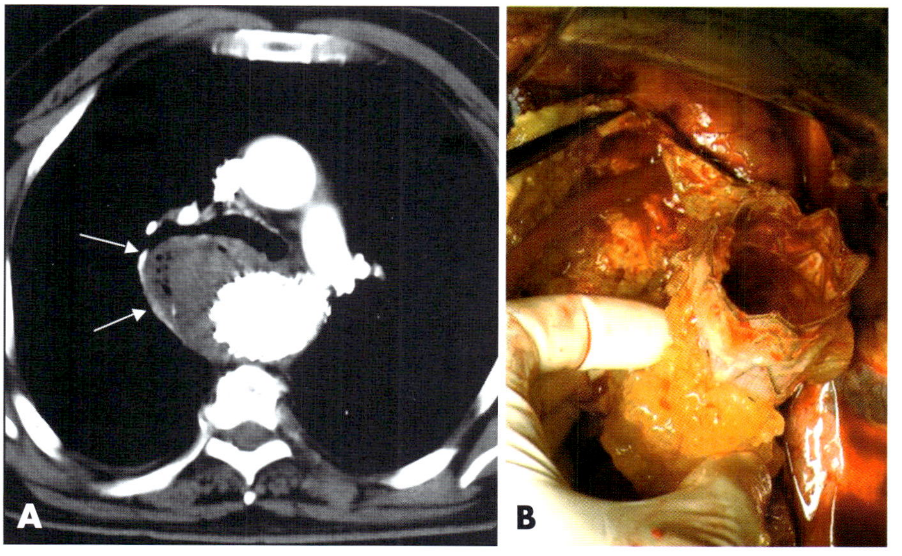

FIG. 16 A) Post-operative axial CT scan showing an endograft infection in a patient who underwent endograft exclusion of an aneurysm for DTA in another center. Note the presence of air bubbles (arrows) clearly indicating the presence of bacterial flora. B) Intra-operative image of our operation through a left thoracotomy of thoracic fluid collection evacuation and endograft removal.

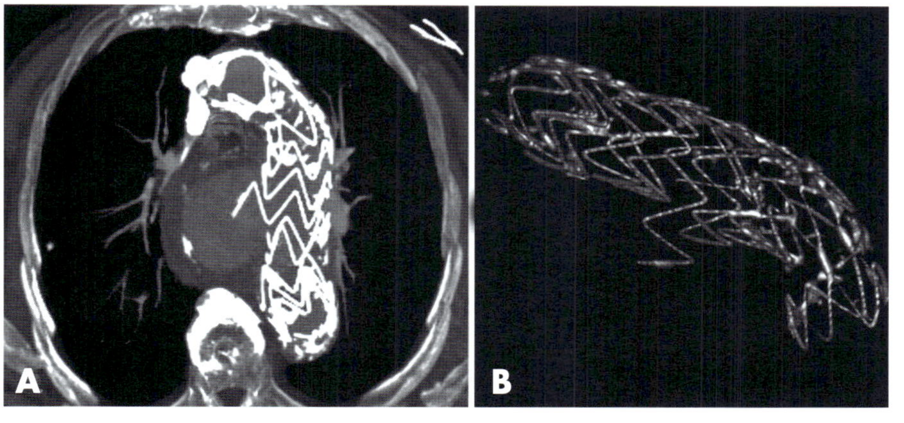

FIG.17 A) Post-operative CT showing endograft stent rupture leading to a large pseudoaneurysm complicated by an aorto-esophageal fistula. B) 3D volume rendered reconstruction of the stent structure of the same case obtained with the OsiriX software.

gle device. Sometimes it presents as a fatal hemorrhage, however, presentation can be less dramatic with pain, dysphagia, hematemesis, and septic symptoms. Treatment is very problematic, however, outcome without treatment is fatal.

Migration

Successful long-term aneurysm exclusion requires durability of the proximal and distal fixation sites against the bloodstream forces, the fatigue of the material and the morphological behavior of the aneurysm. The Society for Vascular Surgery/American Association for Vascular Surgery (SVS/AAVS) standards [42] defined endograft migration as any movement relative to the initial position (Fig. 14). To address this problem, a variety of fixation methods such as hooks, barbs, free-flows and longitudinal support devices have been developed [43], and each present peculiar advantages and drawbacks.

Conclusion

The DTA is the ideal morphological site for application of endograft technology since it constitutes the largest straight tubular arterial segment of the human body. It has been the first site of aortic aneurysm endograft exclusion as published by Volodos et al. [44], 3 years before Parodi et al. [45] reported the first series of AAA stent-graft repair. Since the pioneering experience of Volodos and the first renowned short series of TEVAR published by Dake et al. (46), many series, registries and trials have confirmed its feasibility and reduced invasivity, leading to a worldwide revolution in the therapeutic approach of descending aortic diseases.

This new development has limited the number of open repair in most European vascular centers dealing with thoracic aneurysms. Even in our center, we have experienced a progressive shift towards TEVAR for descending thoracic aortic aneurysms. At the beginning of our experience (the first 4-5 years) TEVAR was limited to those patients presenting with one or more serious co-morbitidies, while open surgery remained the choice for those in fair clinical conditions. In particular TEVAR was the treatment of choice in the elderly (> 77 years), in patients with a depressed ejection fraction (< 40%), in patients with severe pulmonary disease (home oxygen therapy, sever obstruction) and with a life expectancy of less than 5 years.

Since three years, mainly within investigational protocols and trials, we have gradually increased the rate of patients undergoing TEVAR. We have experienced really appealing results with TEVAR, also in good surgical patients, especially with critical intercostal arteries left uncovered. However, studies clearly addressing the respective roles of open and endovascular repair are still not available. It should be emphasized that endografts have been designed to have a durability of 10 years based on ISO (International Standardization Organization) stress testing and that the series with the greatest number of patients reach a maximum of 5-year follow-up, showing significant rates of reinterventions [47].

This all indicates that open surgery remains the best choice for patients with a long life expectancy, patients with connective tissue diseases and those not amenable for TEVAR.

Open repair should be part of the therapeutic armamentarium of all centers dealing with thoracic aortic diseases.

Open surgery is presently the gold standard against which endovascular techniques need to be compared. Patient age, comorbidity, symptoms, expected life expectancy, quality of life (if asymptomatic), aortic diameter, aneurysm morphology, aneurysm extent, suitability of landing zones, and operator experience are all distinctly relevant parameters to consider.

REFERENCES

1 Clouse WD, Hallett JW Jr, Schaff HV et al. Improved prognosis of thoracic aortic aneurysms: a population-based study. *JAMA* 1998; 280: 1926-1929.

2 Svensson LG, Kouchoukos NT, Miller CD et al. Expert consensus document on the treatment of descending thoracic aortic disease using endovascular stent-grafts. *Ann Thorac Surg* 2008; 85: S1-41.

3 Erbel R, Alfonso F, Boileau C et al. Diagnosis and management of aortic dissection. *Eur Heart J* 2001; 22: 1642-1681.

4 Coselli JS. Panel discussion: session III-natural history and dissection. *Ann Thorac Surg* 2007; 83: S846-50.

5 Kieffer E, Chiche L, Cluzel P et al. Open surgical repair of descending thoracic aortic aneurysms in the endovascular era: a 9-year single-center study. *Ann Vasc Surg* 2009; 23: 60-66.

6 Estrera AL, Miller CC III, Chen EP et al. Descending thoracic aortic aneurysm repair: 12-year experience using distal aortic perfusion and cerebrospinal fluid drainage. *Ann Thorac Surg* 2005; 80: 1290-296.

7 Coselli JS, LeMaire SA, Conklin LD et al. Left heart bypass during descending thoracic aortic aneurysm repair does not reduce the incidence of paraplegia. *Ann Thorac Surg* 2004; 77: 1298-1303.

8 Borst HG, Jurmann M, Buhner B et al. Risk of replacement of descending aorta with a standardized left heart bypass technique. *J Thorac Cardiovasc Surg* 1994; 107: 126-33.

9 Svensson LG, Crawford ES, Hess KR et al. Variables predictive of outcome in 832 patients undergoing repairs of the descending thoracic aorta. *Chest* 1993; 104: 1248-253.

10 Verdant A. Descending thoracic aortic aneurysms: surgical treatment with the Gott shunt. *Can J Surg* 1992; 35: 493-96.

11 Kouchoukos NT, Masetti P, Rokkas CK et al. Safety and efficacy of hypothermic cardiopulmonary bypass and circulatory arrest for operations on the descending thoracic and thoracoabdominal aorta. Ann Thorac Surg 2001; 72: 699-707.

12 Fehrenbacher JW, Hart DW, Huddleston E et al. Optimal end-organ protection for thoracic and thoracoabdominal aortic aneurysm repair using deep hypothermic circulatory arrest. *Ann Thorac Surg* 2007; 83: 1041-1046.

13 Isma'eel H, Hamirani YS, Mehrinfar R et al. Optimal phase for coronary interpretations and correlation of ejection fraction using late-diastole and end-diastole imaging in cardiac computed tomography angiography: implications for prospective triggering. *Int J Cardiovasc Imaging* 2009; 25: 739-749.

14 National Kidney Foundation. K/DOQI clinical practice guidelines for chronic kidney disease: evaluation, classification and stratification. *Am J Kidney Dis* 2002; 39: S1-S266.

15 Marrocco-Trischitta MM, Melissano G, Kahlberg A et al. Chronic kidney disease classification stratifies mortality risk after elective stent graft repair of the thoracic aorta. *J Vasc Surg* 2009; 49: 296-301.

16 Coselli JS, Lemaire SA, Köksoy C et al. Cerebrospinal fluid drainage reduces paraplegia after thoracoabdominal aortic aneurysm repair: results of a randomized clinical trial. *J Vasc Surg* 2002; 35: 631-639.

17 Coselli JS, LeMaire SA. Left heart bypass reduces paraplegia rates following thoracoabdominal aortic aneurysm repair. *Ann Thorac Surg* 1999; 67: 1931-1934.

18 Chiesa R, Melissano G, Marrocco-Trischitta MM et al. Spinal cord ischemia after elective stent-graft repair of the thoracic aorta. *J Vasc Surg* 2005; 42: 11-17.

19 Bavaria JE, Appoo JJ, Makaroun MS et al. Endovascular stent grafting versus open surgical repair of descending thoracic aortic aneurysms in low-risk patients: a multicenter comparative trial. *J Thorac Cardiovasc Surg* 2007; 133: 369-377.

20 Wheatley GH III, Gurbuz AT, Rodriguez-Lopez JA et al. Midterm outcome in 158 consecutive Gore TAG thoracic endoprostheses: single center experience. *Ann Thorac Surg* 2006; 81: 1570-577.

21 Ricco JB, Cau J, Marchand C et al. Stent-graft repair for thoracic aortic disease: results of an independent nationwide study in France from 1999 to 2001. *J Thorac Cardiovasc Surg* 2006; 131: 131-37.

22 Glade GJ, Vahl AC, Wisselink W et al. Mid-term survival and costs of treatment of patients with descending thoracic aortic aneurysms; endovascular versus open repair: a case-control study. *Eur J Vasc Endovasc Surg* 2005; 29: 28-34.

23 Greenberg RK, O'Neill S, Walker E et al. Endovascular repair of thoracic aortic lesions with the Zenith TX1 and TX2 thoracic grafts: intermediate-term results. *J Vasc Surg* 2005; 41: 589-596.

24 Riesenman PJ, Farber MA, Mendes RR et al. Endovascular repair of lesions involving the descending thoracic aorta. *J Vasc Surg* 2005; 42: 1063-074.

25 Bortone AS, De Cillis E, D'Agostino D et al. Endovascular treatment of thoracic aortic disease: four years of experience. *Circulation* 2004; 110: II262-7.

26 Czerny M, Cejna M, Hutschala D et al. Stent-graft placement in atherosclerotic descending thoracic aortic aneurysms: midterm results. *J Endovasc Ther* 2004; 11: 26-32.

27 Neuhauser B, Perkmann R, Greiner A et al. Mid-term results after endovascular repair of the atherosclerotic descending thoracic aortic aneurysm. *Eur J Vasc Endovasc Surg* 2004; 28: 146-53.

28 Bell RE, Taylor PR, Aukett M et al. Mid-term results for second-generation thoracic stent grafts. *Br J Surg* 2003; 90: 811-817.

29 Bergeron P, De Chaumaray T, Gay J et al. Endovascular treatment of thoracic aortic aneurysms. *J Cardiovasc Surg (Torino)* 2003; 44: 349-361.

30 Chabbert V, Otal P, Bouchard L et al. Midterm outcomes of thoracic aortic stent-grafts: complications and imaging techniques. *J Endovasc Ther* 2003; 10: 494-504.

31 Marin ML, Hollier LH, Ellozy SH et al. Endovascular stent graft repair of abdominal and thoracic aortic aneurysms: a ten-year experience with 817 patients. *Ann Surg* 2003; 238: 586-595.

32 Orend KH, Scharrer-Pamler R, Kapfer X et al. Endovascular treatment in diseases of the descending thoracic aorta: 6-year results of a single center. *J Vasc Surg* 2003; 37: 91-99.

33 Schoder M, Cartes-Zumelzu F, Grabenwoger M et al. Elective endovascular stent-graft repair of atherosclerotic thoracic aortic aneurysms: clinical results and midterm follow-up. *AJR Am J Roentgenol* 2003; 180: 709-715.

34 Criado FJ, Clark NS, Barnatan MF. Stent graft repair in the aortic arch and descending thoracic aorta: a 4-year experience. *J Vasc Surg* 2002; 36: 1121-128.

35 Mitchell RS, Miller DC, Dake MD et al. Thoracic aortic aneurysm repair with an endovascular stent graft: the "first generation". *Ann Thorac Surg* 1999; 67: 1971-4;discussion 1979-980.

36 Ricco JB, Goeau-Brissonniere O, Rodde-Dunet MH et al. Use of abdominal aortic endovascular prostheses in France from 1999 to 2001. *J Vasc Surg* 2003; 38: 1273-81; discussion 1282.

37 Taylor PR, Gaines PA, McGuinness CL et al. Thoracic aortic stent grafts—early experience from two centres using commercially available devices. *Eur J Vasc Endovasc Surg* 2001; 22: 70-76.

38 Willinsky RA, Taylor SM, TerBrugge K et al. Neurologic complications of cerebral angiography: prospective analysis of 2,899 procedures and review of the literature. *Radiology* 2003; 227: 522-528.

39 Greenberg R, Resch T, Nyman U et al. Endovascular repair of descending thoracic aortic aneurysms: an early experience with intermediate-term follow-up. *J Vasc Surg* 2000; 31: 147-156.

40 Gravereaux EC, Faries PL, Burks JA et al. Risk of spinal cord ischemia after endograft repair of thoracic aortic aneurysms. *J Vasc Surg* 2001; 34: 997-1003.

41 Chiesa R, Melissano G, Marrocco-Trischitta MM et al. Spinal cord ischemia after elective stent-graft repair of the thoracic aorta. *J Vasc Surg* 2005; 42: 11-17.

42 Chaikof EL, Blankensteijn JD, Harris PL, et al. Reporting standards for endovascular aortic aneurysm repair. *J Vasc Surg* 2002; 35: 1048-060.

43 Malina M, Lindblad B, Ivancev K et al. Endovascular AAA exclusion: will stents with hooks and barbs prevent stent-graft migration? *J Endovasc Surg* 1998; 5: 310-317.

44 Volodos' NL, Karpovich IP, Shekhanin VE et al. A case of distant transfemoral endoprosthesis of the thoracic artery using a self-fixing synthetic prosthesis in traumatic aneurysm. *Grudn Khir* 1988; 84-86.

45 Parodi JC, Palmaz JC, Barone HD. Transfemoral intraluminal graft implantation for abdominal aortic aneurysms. *Ann Vasc Surg* 1991; 5: 491-499.

46 Dake MD, Miller DC, Semba CP et al. Transluminal placement of endovascular stent-grafts for the treatment of descending thoracic aortic aneurysms. *N Engl J Med* 1994; 331: 1729-734.

47 Makaroun MS, Dillavou ED, Wheatley GH et al. Gore TAG Investigators. Five-year results of endovascular treatment with the Gore TAG device compared with open repair of thoracic aortic aneurysms. *J Vasc Surg* 2008; 47: 912-918.

12

BEST PRACTICE IN THORACO-ABDOMINAL AORTIC ANEURYSM REPAIR

STÉPHAN HAULON, GEERT-WILLEM SCHURINK, NOEL O'BRIEN, MICHAEL JACOBS

In 1954 the first thoraco-abdominal aortic aneurysm (TAAA) repair was performed by Etheredge et al. [1] using a temporary shunt from the distal thoracic aorta to the distal abdominal aorta and a homograft with reimplantation of the visceral vessels. Since that time, treatment has been changed by the introduction of Dacron grafts by Michael E. DeBakey et al. [2]. Aortic cross-clamp time was the most important predictor of end-organ damage and post-operative paraplegia during TAAA repairs. Several adjuncts have since been developed to allow a longer cross-clamp time and improve outcome, e.g. profound hypothermia, neuroprotective medication, epidural cooling, and cerebrospinal fluid (CSF) drainage.

Because of high morbidity and mortality in a high-risk patient group, alternatives to open repair have been introduced. The hybrid approach combines visceral bypass surgery with a straight endovascular procedure. Total endovascular repair includes careful patient selection, precise stent-graft design (with incorporation of fenestration and/or branches) and procedure planning. Both hybrid and total endovascular approaches are becoming more widely accepted. In this chapter all three treatment options will be discussed in the context of current best practice.

General aspects of TAAA

Epidemiology

The true incidence of thoraco-abdominal aneurysms is unknown. The incidence of thoraco-abdominal aneurysms appears to be much lower than the incidence of infra-renal abdominal aortic aneurysms. In a population based study, the incidence of all new thoracic aneurysms was 5.9 per 100 000 person-years and the incidence of thoraco-abdominal aneurysms was around 2.2 per 100 000 person-years [3]. However, the continued growth of the elderly population and the widespread use of diagnostic imaging modalities is likely to cause increased numbers in the near future.

Classification

The location and extent of the thoracic and thoraco-abdominal aneurysm is important for predicting patient outcomes. For this reason, classification systems for TAAA exist, enabling surgeons to tailor the extent of the incision and to use various operative techniques and adjunctive measures for the individual patient. Furthermore it allows more appropriate comparison of surgical outcome of the different types of repair of thoraco-abdominal aneurysms using different surgical techniques and adjunctive measures. The Crawford classification of thoraco-abdominal aneurysms consists of four types [4]. In type I the aneurysm includes the total descending thoracic aorta and the proximal abdominal aorta until the level of the renal arteries. A type II TAAA starts at the level of the left subclavian artery and ends at the aortic bifurcation. In many patients, mainly with post-dissection aneurysms, the iliac arteries are also affected. In a type III TAAA , the aneurysm includes variable lengths of the more distal thoracic and ends at the aortic bifurcation or lower. Type IV TAAA includes the total abdominal aorta starting at the level of the diaphragm until the aortic bifurcation or lower.

In open surgery, only the affected part of the aorta is replaced, while in endovascular treatment a "healthy" part of the aorta proximal and distal to the aneurysm is also covered, occluding more segmental arteries than in open repair. This leads to the situation that in an endovascularly treated type IV TAAA, segmental arteries are covered comparable to a type III TAAA repaired by open surgery (and type III comparable to a type II). When comparing results from the literature, it is important to know whether the original aneurysm extent is reported or the segment of aorta treated. Often thoracic aortic aneurysms ending at the level of the celiac trunk are referred to as type I TAAA because some of the visceral vessels are in the distal sealing zone of the stent-graft and are treated with fenestrations or branches.

Indications and contra-indications

Most patients with TAAA are asymptomatic. The decision to treat the aneurysm is usually based on the size, extent and expansion rate of the aneurysm.

For patients with degenerative or post-dissection aneurysms without history of connective tissue disease, elective treatment is usually recommended if the diameter exceeds 6 cm [5,6]. Beside diameter and pain, also age, chronic obstructive pulmonary disease, renal insufficiency, extent of the aneurysm and expansion rate of the aneurysm are independent risk factors for rupture [7-9]. Because of the higher incidence of dissection and rupture in Marfan patients, the recommended threshold for repair is an aneurysm diameter of 5.0-5.5 cm [10].

Contra-indications for treatment of TAAA are mainly influenced by elevated operative risk factors like age, impaired cardiac and pulmonary function, poor functional status and renal insufficiency. Anatomic considerations such as previous thoracotomy and abdominal stoma can pose excessive operative risk. Both the operative risk factors and the anatomical considerations will influence the choice between open versus hybrid versus endovascular repair.

Best practice in open TAAA repair

Technique

The operative technique in TAAA surgery has not changed much over the last decades. Most degenerative aneurysms are repaired from proximal to distal, while most surgeons start distally in a post-dissection aneurysm, because visceral perfusion by the distal aortic perfusion is better maintained this way. The incision is tailored to the extent of the TAAA. Most thoracotomies are performed through the 6th intercostal space. This incision can be extended to the pubic bone, in case of iliac involvement. The costal margin is divided and the abdominal aorta is approached lateral from the descending colon and dorsal to the spleen and left kidney which is rotated anteriorly out of its bed. The diaphragm can be completely divided or only be cut at the anterior, muscular part, avoiding injury to the branches of the phrenic nerve. The latter approach is associated with better post-operative pulmonary function as compared to complete division. The crus of the diaphragm is opened longitudinally. The left renal artery is identified and, in our experience with type II, III and IV TAAA, always treated with a selective 8 mm polyester graft. Location for proximal and distal aortic cross-clamping are prepared and, if feasible, also one or two cross-clamp locations in between for sequential clamping. The proximal (thoracic) aorta is always completely cut and freed from the esophagus to prevent fistula formation. Standard treatment for the mesenteric arteries and right renal artery is re-implantation, as an island, in the aortic tube graft. In the case of connective tissue disease, e.g. Marfan's syndrome, as little as possible native aortic tissue is left behind or even individual bypasses to the visceral arteries are preferred. This is to prevent island aneurysm formation in the future. The level of the distal anastomosis is usually by inlay technique and depends on the extent of TAAA .

Following the initial period of the "clamp-and sew"-technique, several adjunctive measures were introduced to reduce complications related to end-organ ischemia, such as renal insufficiency, visceral ischemia and paraplegia.

By using a technique of distal aortic perfusion (e.g. left heart bypass or total extracorporeal circulation) and sequential aortic cross clamping, blood flow to the intestines, kidneys and spinal cord is maintained during repair of the thoracic segment of the aorta. Distal aortic pressure should be approximately 60 mmHg, but can be adjusted according to urine production and spinal cord function monitoring tests (when used) [11]. During repair of the mesenteric segment selective antegrade perfusion helps to reduce end-organ ischemia. Also other techniques, like the Gott shunt [12] and the in-line mesenteric shunt technique [13] can be used to reduce end-organ ischemia. Besides distal aortic perfusion, two protective measures have proven their clinical value in renal protection: cold crystalloid perfusion and normothermic blood perfusion [14].

Paraplegia due to spinal cord ischemia remains the most devastating complication after open TAAA repair. Strongest risk factors include type II TAAA and prolonged aortic cross-clamp times [15-17]. Many segmental arteries are already occluded by mural thrombus resulting in collateral feeding of the anterior spinal artery. Pre-operative knowledge of this altered circulation to the spinal cord can influence the operative strategy [18]. During open repair, several adjunctive measures can be used to prevent paraplegia. Some actions try to preserve cord blood supply (e.g. CSF drainage, segmental artery re-implantation), others are neuroprotective adjuncts such as local or systemic hypothermia, and endorphin receptor blockage [19].

Adequate spinal cord circulation can be assessed by monitoring spinal cord function by means of somatosensory evoked potentials (SSEP) and motor evoked potentials (MEP). After stimulating the dorsal tibial nerve in SSEP monitoring, the signal is conducted through the dorsal columns of the spinal cord and is recorded from the scalp. MEP can be induced by electrical or magnetic transcranial stimuli and are typically recorded at the level of the anterior tibial muscle and compared to the recordings at the thenar muscles, which are independent of the spinal cord blood supply [20].

Spinal cord function monitoring, segmental artery reimplantation, distal aortic perfusion, CSF drainage and systemic or local hypothermia are the main adjuncts used in up to date practice to reduce spinal cord ischemia.

RESULTS

The majority of published experiences in open TAAA procedures come from specialized centers, not representing common surgical practice of these complex aneurysms. When looking at nationwide databases, results of TAAA repair are quite disappointing. In electively operated patients in the state of California, 30-day and one-year mortality for TAAA repair was 19% and 31%, respectively [21]. Mortality rates from individual high volume centers show better outcome and vary between 6% and 10% [6,22-24].

Post-operative cardiac complications, reported in 12%-25% of patients, include myocardial infarction, arrhythmia, congestive heart failure and unstable angina.

Respiratory failure is the most common complication and is probably inevitable following this operation. Overall pulmonary complications in the most recent studies range between 32% and 49% [22,25]. The main risk factors for developing renal failure include aneurysm extent, ischemic time and pre-operative renal impairment. Any form of post-operative renal failure is reported in 20% and renal failure requiring dialysis in 5% after TAAA surgery [22].

Overall gastro-intestinal complications occurred in 7% of patients and was strongly correlated with mortality.

Post-operative paraplegia is strongly related to the simple clamp-and-sew technique, especially when exceeding 30 minutes clamp time. Accordingly, most centers use one or more of the afore mentioned adjunctive measures. Using these techniques in centers of excellence, paraplegia rate in type II TAAA is reduced to 3%-5% [20,24,25]. In all other types of TAAAs paraplegia rate is even lower.

Best practice in hybrid TAAA repair

Technique

Because open TAAA repair is associated with significant morbidity and mortality, alternative treatment options have been explored for patients with advanced age or significant co-morbidities. Thoracic stent-grafting is a less invasive treatment, but is limited to the thoracic aorta. If the aneurysm extents to or involves the visceral arteries, simple endovascular treatment is not an option. However, if this treatment is preceded by surgical debranching of the visceral vessels, endovascular treatment becomes a viable option.

This treatment was first described in 1999 [26] and experienced a rapid increase during the last decade. Several centers use this technique as the first choice in all TAAA patients, including young patients and those with good anesthetic risk.

Through a mid-line laparotomy, adequate exposure of the abdominal aorta and/or iliac arteries (depending on the chosen in-flow site of the bypasses), the origins of the renal arteries, the superior mesenteric artery (SMA) and the common hepatic artery (or celiac trunk [CX]) can be obtained. By using two bifurcated grafts or one bifurcated graft with additional side branches, a four-branched conduit is created which is anastomosed to either distal abdominal aorta or common iliac artery (depending on the extent of the aneurysm and the distal sealing zone required for the stent-graft). The branches are anastomosed either end-to-end or end-to-side (with proximal ligation of the native vessel to prevent type II endoleak) to the renal arteries and SMA. The last limb is tunnelled behind the pancreas and anastomosed to either the common hepatic artery or CX (with proximal ligation of the CX). For the introduction of the stent-graft, either the common femoral artery can be chosen or introduction through the (contralateral) common iliac artery may be preferred. After stent-graft deployment, completion angiography is used to confirm both exclusion of the aneurysm and patency of the retrograde visceral bypasses. Special attention should be given to possible type II endoleaks from the visceral vessels.

Results

In 2007, Donas et al. [27] reported the clinical data from the literature up until then. In total, 58 patients underwent a visceral debranching and thoraco-abdominal stent-grafting procedure. The 30-day mortality was 10.7% (but varied greatly between 0% and 33%). Patency of the bypasses was good (98% open after 14 months). Paraplegia was not reported in this series.

The largest series is the combined experience from St. Mary's Hospital (London, UK), University of Heidelberg (Germany) and the Technical University of Munich (Germany) , including 107 urgent and elective high-risk patients [28]. The 30-day mortality rate was 15%. Twelve percent of the patients suffered from spinal cord ischemia which was complete and permanent in 8.4%. Permanent renal failure requiring dialysis and bowel infarction requiring resection was seen in 3.7% and 2.8%, respectively.

Best practice in endovascular TAAA repair

Indications for endovascular repair of TAAA are the same as those for open TAAA repair but because of the lack of long-term outcome data this approach is currently usually reserved for patients who are unfit to undergo open repair. Certain patient factors, however, such as the presence of a stoma or previous thoracotomy/laparotomy may make an endovascular approach more desirable. Other factors may make an endovascular approach more difficult or indeed may preclude it altogether including:

- Collateral flow to the spinal cord via the left subclavian and internal iliac vessels means that covering these vessels should be avoided. Debranching may be necessary to avoid spinal cord ischemia.
- Emergencies: it generally takes between 6 and 8 weeks to manufacture a custom designed branched/fenestrated endograft which precludes its use in the emergency setting. Much interest is currently focused on the production of an "off the shelf" branched graft which would conform to the anatomy of most TAAAs [29].

- Inadequacy of access vessels can usually be overcome by means of an iliac conduit [30].
- Extreme neck angulation makes manipulation and accurate placement of the device very difficult, which in turn may compromize target vessel perfusion. This is also a problem in the setting of aneurysms secondary to aortic dissection where the true lumen may be quite narrowed.
- Target vessels need to be of an appropriate length and luminal diameter to allow bridging stents to be deployed adequately. Generally a landing zone of at least 20 mm is required, while vessels with a diameter of < 4 mm tend to occlude rapidly after stenting.
- There is a requirement for an adequate distal sealing zone (> 3 stent overlap) in the distal part of the branched component which can be a problem when the distance from the lowest renal artery to the aortic bifurcation is short. This can be usually overcome by means of an inverted limb in the bifurcated component.

TECHNIQUE

A detailed description of TAAA endograft design and implantation technique was provided in the EVC 2008 text book [31], which can be briefly summarized as follows:

Currently, the only CE approved fenestrated and branched endografts are manufactured by Cook Inc. (Bloomington, Indiana, USA). A wide range of custom-endografts combining fenestrations and/or branches can be manufactured to match the anatomy of most complex aortic aneurysms using the following general principles.

- The proximal and distal sealing zones of the endograft will be positioned over healthy arterial segments (> 20 mm in length).
- Any ostium (visceral or internal iliac = target vessels) covered by the fabric of the endograft will be perfused by a bridging stent-graft positioned through a fenestration or a branch. When the anticipated gap between the wall of the deployed graft and the vessel orifice is less than 10 mm a fenestration is used and if it is longer than 10 mm a branch is designed.
- When catheterization of the target vessel from a femoral access is anticipated to be challenging (e.g.; when the angle of the target vessel to the aortic wall is < 60 degrees), the diameter of the aortic endograft can ultimately be reduced to allow the addition of a branch that will facilitate access to the target vessel from a brachial approach.
- It is mandatory to design large overlap segments between the various modular components of the aortic endografts and between the bridging stent-grafts and the fenestrations or branches.

The endograft design to exclude most type IV thoraco-abdominal aneurysms is a 3-component system. A proximal tubular endograft is customized with fenestrations to match the patient-specific orientation of the visceral vessels. A bifurcated endograft is subsequently implanted inside the tubular component with an optimal 3-stent overlap. The addition of a limb extension usually completes the implant. The proximal sealing zone will be located above the origin of the celiac trunk. Small fenestrations will usually perfuse the renal arteries, a large strut free fenestration the SMA, and a scallop or a second large strut free fenestration the celiac trunk.

Patients with type I, II and III thoraco-abdominal aneurysms are also potential candidates for an endovascular repair. The choice between a fenestration and a branch to perfuse the visceral arteries in the aneurysm sac primarily depends on the anatomy of these vessels and the diameter of the aortic lumen. It is crucial to assess the anatomy of the aortic arch when a branch is designed since compromizing of the left subclavian may predispose to the development of spinal cord ischemia. If necessary a carotid-subclavian bypass can be performed as a protective measure.

PRE-OPERATIVE IMAGING

Designing a device which will accommodate the aortic branches is complex. Critical end organs depend on blood flow through the fenestrations or branches of the endograft. Inappropriate orientation of the visceral branches and fenestrations will preclude successful endovascular repair. Essential information needed for pre-operative assessment of aortic aneurysms includes the relationship of the aneurysm to the aortic branches, the degree of iliac arterial involvement with the aneurysm, the presence of other co-existing iliac arterial or aortic aneurysms, the presence of accessory or aberrant aortic branches and the presence of associated iliac arterial occlusive disease. Thus, high resolution spiral computed tomography (CT) scans (0.75 mm reconstructions) and 3D workstations are mandatory for designing complex aortic endografts. Curved planar reconstruction (CPR) assesses the true cross-sectional diameters and is mandatory to accurately assess lengths in a curved aorta. CPR is performed following an automated vessel centerline extraction between two points selected proximal and distal to the aneurysm. Various vessel view layouts are then required to analyse diameters and lengths in support of an accurate endograft design (Figs. 1,2).

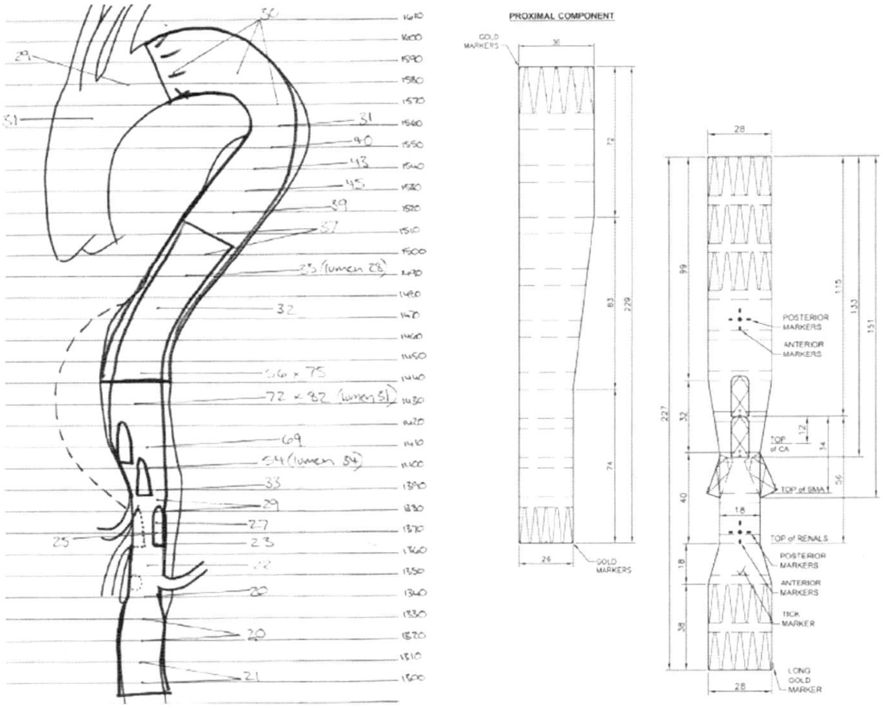

FIG. 1 Drawing of a type I TAAA (left) and the planning of two stent-grafts (right). The distal component contains four side branches for the visceral arteries.

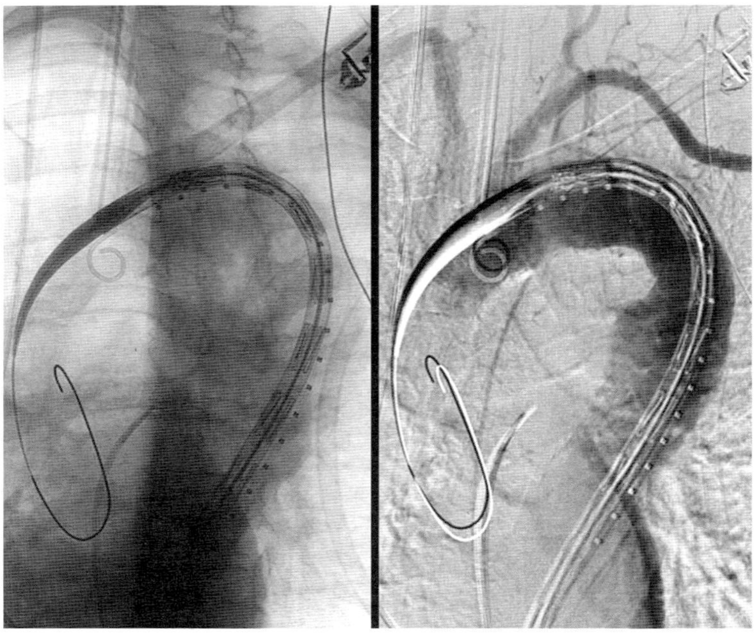

FIG. 2 The proximal stent-graft will be deployed just distal to the left subclavian artery.

PROCEDURE DESCRIPTION

Open or percutaneous access is required to both common femoral arteries. On one side, the main body of the graft is introduced and on the contralateral side, a 20 or 24 Fr sheath is inserted over a stiff wire. The stiff wire is retrieved, and three or four 5 Fr sheaths are introduced through the valve of the large sheath. An angiography catheter is advanced over a guide wire through one 5 Fr sheath to a suitable position in the aorta (above the target vessels). Under fluoroscopy the fenestrations, branches and the associated markers are recognized and the orientation of the main body of the device is checked. On the ipsilateral side, a stiff guide wire is advanced to the level of the aortic arch. The fenestrated/branched body is inserted over this stiff wire to the required position so that the appropriate fenestrations are correctly aligned with their matching target vessels (checked by repeated angiographies with small volumes of contrast) (Fig. 3). The outer sheath of the delivery system is withdrawn. The diameter reducing ties restrain the endograft partially. It can therefore still be rotated, advanced or pulled back as necessary. Through a contralateral 5 Fr sheath, access to the lumen of the endograft is obtained. A side branch access sheath is then advanced on this wire and catheterization of a target vessel through its appropriate fenestration performed. The access sheath is subsequently advanced into the vessel over a stiff wire. The maneuver is repeated for each target vessel and its fenestration. Appropriate covered stents are advanced through the access sheaths into the target vessels. If the endograft's design includes one or more downward branches, a hydrophilic wire is advanced in the branch-preloaded catheter until it is in the descending thoracic aorta. A 7 Fr sheath is also positioned into the descending aorta from a brachial artery. A snare is advanced through this sheath to capture the wire from the preloaded catheter, to create through and through access from the groin to the brachial artery. Over this wire, the brachial sheath is advanced into the endograft and ultimately into the side branch (Fig. 4). The target vessel is then selectively catheterized. When a stiff wire has been positioned in the target vessel, the through and through wire is retrieved. This latter maneuver is necessary to advance the brachial sheath and subsequently the bridging stent-graft into the target vessel. Once the bridging stent-grafts are all positioned in their target vessels, the diameter reducing ties of the endograft are released. For each target vessel, the C-arm tube is oriented tangential to the fenestration. The bridging stent is positioned with 3-4 mm protruding in the aorta and expanded once the access sheath has been withdrawn. The aortic extremity of the bridging stent is then flared with a 12 mm-diameter 2 cm-long balloon. The fenestrated/branched component is then connected to

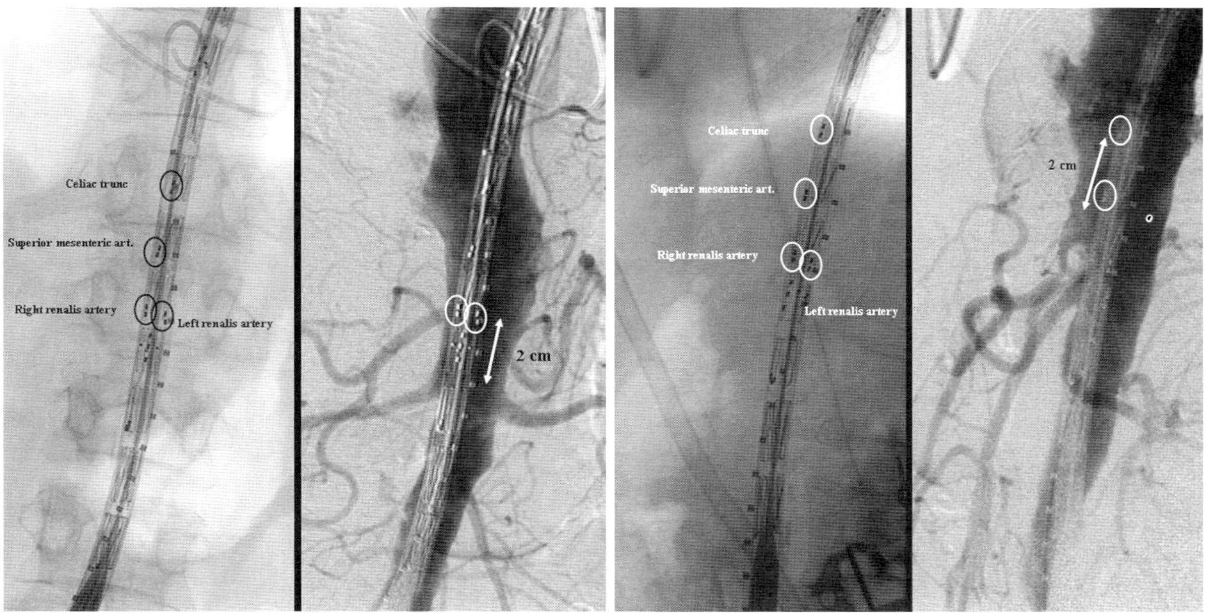

FIG. 3 AP (left) and lateral (right) X-ray and angiography. Each side branch can be identified by two gold markers (black/white circle) which will be positioned two centimeters above the target vessel.

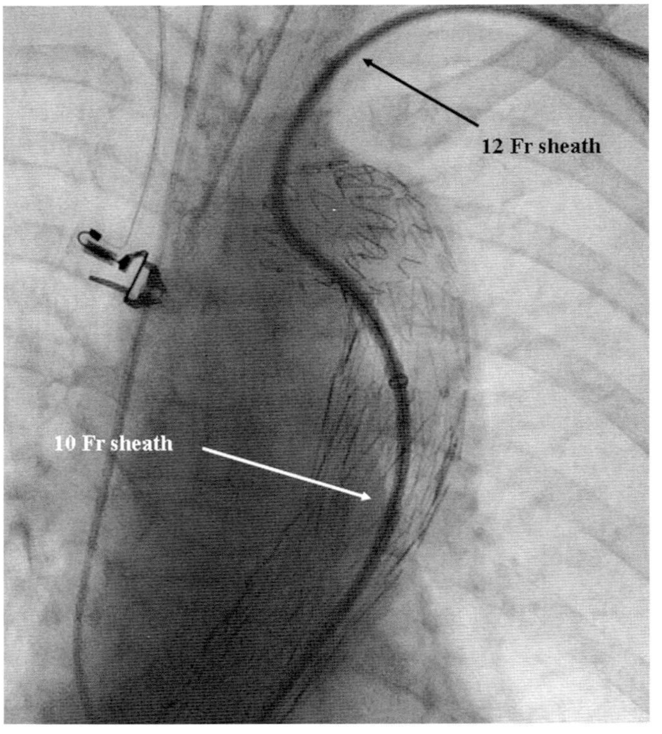

FIG. 4 After deployment of the branched stent-graft axillary access will be obtained. The first 12 Fr sheath will have a stable position in the aortic arch minimizing the change on cerebral embolization. The 10 Fr sheath will be positioned in each side branch to facilitate branch extension.

other aortic components as planned, being careful not to dislodge or disrupt the existing device, or the fenestration stents.

If the endograft is designed with caudally-directed branches only, one femoral artery access is necessary because the large 20 Fr controlateral sheath is not required. It is recommended in this latter setting to start the procedure by connecting the branched endograft to the other aortic components. Once this has been achieved, the femoral artery can be closed and flow to the lower limbs restored. Catheterization of the branches from a brachial access and ultimately bridging stent implantation are then performed (Fig. 5). This technique limits pelvic and lower limb ischemia caused by the presence of large sheaths in the iliac vessels over a prolonged time and accordingly probably reduces the spinal cord ischemia rate.

On-table angiography completes the procedure and is used to confirm the absence of any significant endoleak (Fig. 6). CT angiography is carried out prior to discharge and follow-up with duplex ultrasound, CT angiography and chest/abdominal radiography performed at 1, 6, 12, 18 and 24 months and yearly thereafter (Figs. 7,8).

Results

It was not until 2001 that the first case report concerning a TAAA endovascular repair using a multibranched endograft emerged [32]. Following this report, a limited number of centers with extensive EVAR experience have launched TAAA endovascular repair programs, and published early results. Because of the relative rarity of the pathology, and the experience required to implant such complex endografts, no multicenter trials have been initiated. At present, analysis is restricted to the experience of single center series.

The Cleveland Clinic Foundation published a single center retrospective series of 724 patients treated over a 5-year period (2001-2006) [33]. They compared open (n = 372) and endovascular (n = 352) repair. The report included patients treated for TAAA (open = 236; endovascular = 189) and thoracic aortic aneurysm (TAA) (open = 136; endovascular = 163). Importantly, this study clas-

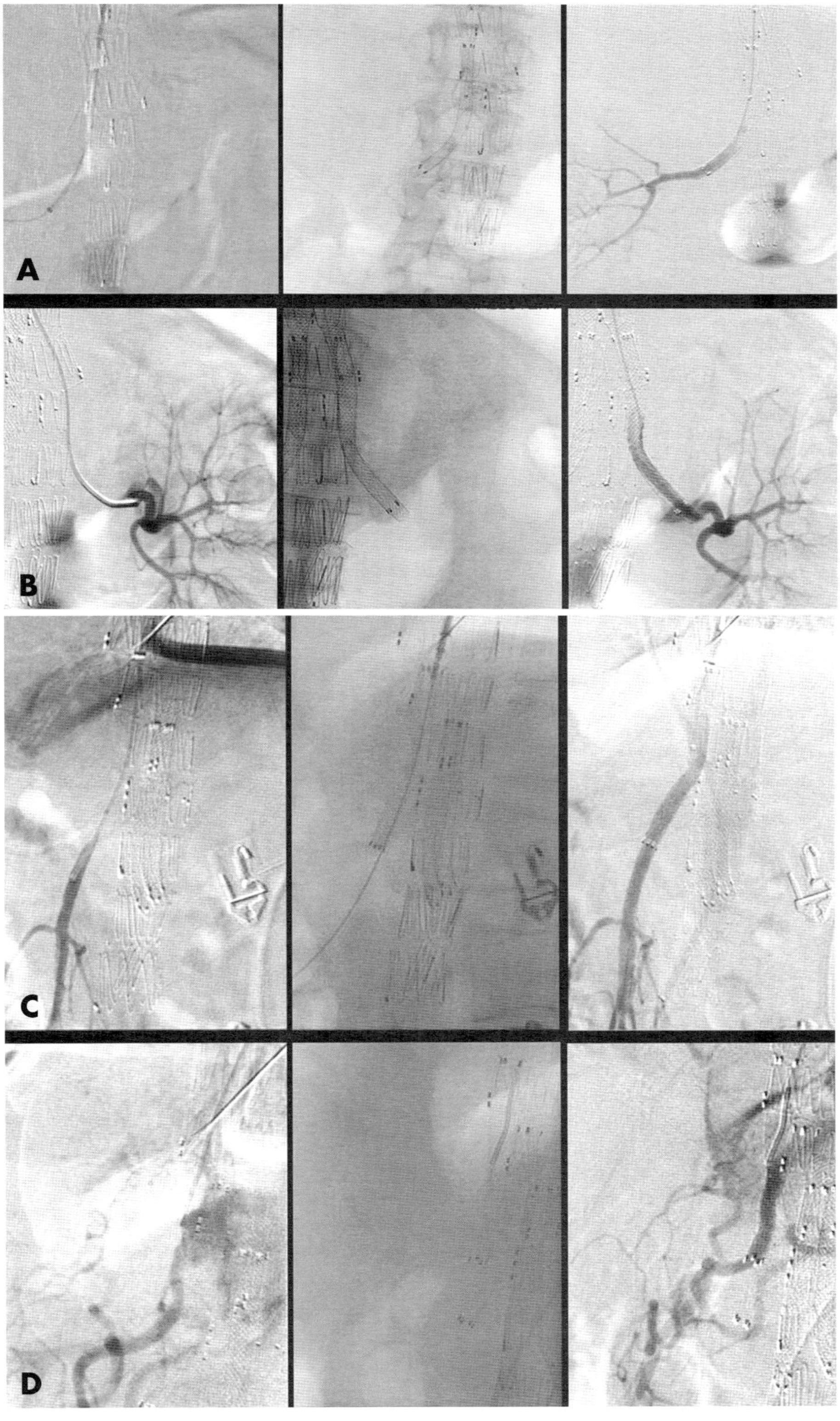

FIG. 5 From bottom to top each side branch and target vessel is cannulated and confirmed (left), stented (middle) and checked on patency (right). In this patient, the side branch for the left (A) and right renal arteries (B), superior mesenteric artery (C) and celiac trunk (D) were extented using Fluency stent-grafts and Wallstents.

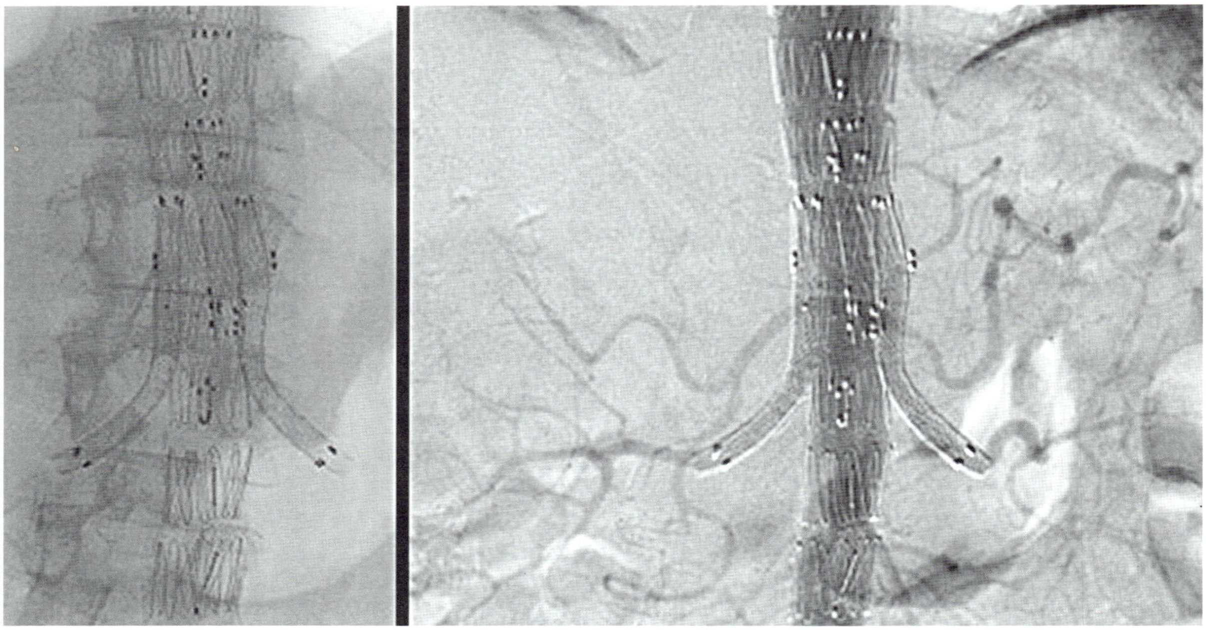

FIG. 6 Final X-ray and angiography of the visceral segment.

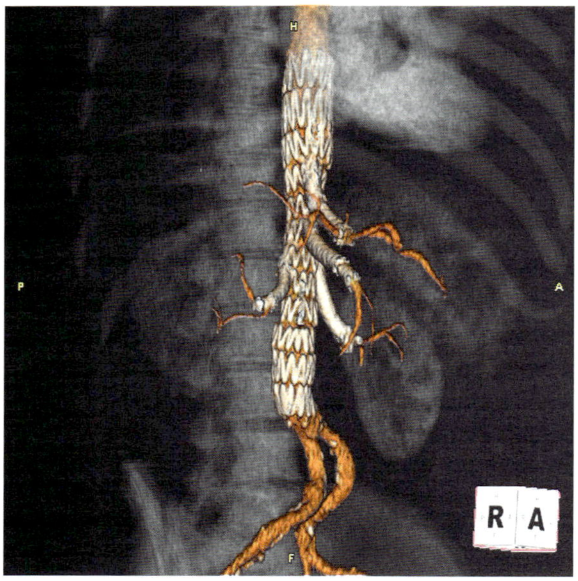

FIG. 7 Post-operative CT reconstruction of four branched stent-graft for type II/IV TAAA.

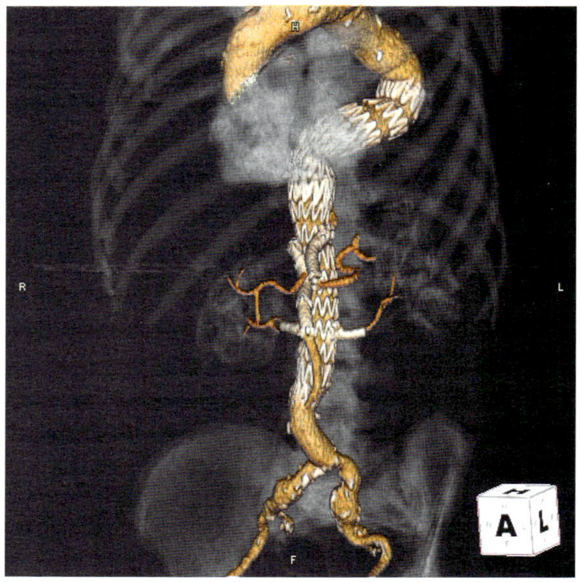

FIG. 8 Post-operative CT reconstruction of stent-graft for a recurrent aneurysm at the level of the visceral aortic segment after previous open TAA and AAA repair. The stent-graft consists of two mesenteric helical branches and two renal fenestrations.

sified the type of repair performed based on the final extent of aortic coverage after the graft was implanted and hence compared "like with like", overcoming the criticism levelled by some authors that reports on endovascular repair often did not account for the extra aortic coverage required for proximal and distal sealing zones. Compared to the open group, endovascular patients were significantly older, suffered more co-morbidities, and a greater proportion underwent aortic repair previously. The 30-day mortality rate was 5.7% (20/352) in the endovascular repair (ER) group and 8.3%

in the open repair (OR) group. One-year mortality rates were 15.6% for ER and 15.9% for OR. Spinal cord injury (SCI) was reported in 4.3% ER patients and 7.5% OR patients. The vast majority of SCI had a delayed onset (> 24 hours). The development of SCI was strongly related to the extent of the aneurysm repair and to prior distal aortic repair in the ER group. No ruptures or conversions occurred during the follow-up period. In this study, the authors did not report either the endoleak or target vessel patency rates. A publication by Roselli et al. [34] from the same institution looked at a subgroup (n = 73) of the patients who were at high risk for open repair and who underwent endovascular repair of TAAA as part of a prospective trial evaluating the safety of the Cook device. 28 type I, II or III TAAAs and 45 type IV TAAAs were treated. Failure to cannulate a branch or fenestration occurred in 4 cases. The 30-day mortality rate was 5.5% (4/73) and two further patients died from complications related to peri-operative spinal cord ischemia later than 30 days from their procedure. The SCI rate was 2.7% (2/73) and both patients died. There were 13 secondary interventions for a rate of 18% including procedures to treat 3 type I, 2 type II and 4 type III endoleaks. In total 15 endoleaks were detected; 3 type I, 7 type II and 5 type III.

A Dutch experience [35] comprised 30 patients (8 type I TAAA, 5 type II; 12 type III and 5 type IV) deemed unfit for conventional open surgery (ASA > 3 in 90% of cases). The mean follow-up was 12 months. The 30-day mortality rate was 6.7% (aortic arch rupture followed by multi-organ failure in one patient and massive gastro-intestinal hemorrhage associated with esophageal ischemia in another). A total of 97 target vessels were perfused via branches or fenestrations. The early target vessel patency rate was 98% (failed access to one celiac trunk and rupture of a renal artery). Three additional target vessels occluded (both renal arteries in one patient who went on to require dialysis, and an asymptomatic occlusion of a celiac scallop) during the follow-up period. The SCI rate was 16.7% (5/30). These instances of paraplegia all resolved early in the postoperative period apart from the patient who died of hemorrhage on day 8. In common with the Cleveland Clinic experience, Verhoeven et al. [35] indicated that the mean operative and fluoroscopy times reduced with increasing experience.

In 2008, Chuter et al. [36] published a series of 22 patients (81 target vessels) treated between 2006 and 2008. The 30-day mortality rate was 9.1% (2/22) and there were no conversions or late aneurysm ruptures. The early postoperative and follow-up visceral vessel patency rates were 100% and 98.8 %, respectively. Reinterventions were required in two patients (9.1%). Hypotension was thought to be responsible for transient SCI in three patients (13.6%), but all recovered without residual neurological sequelae.

The St-Mary's Hospital group that pioneered the hybrid treatment of complex TAAA [37], has now moved towards the totally endovascular approach. They recently published their experience with the endovascular repair of TAAA [38]. They reported 8 patients (2 type I; 2 type III, and 4 type IV) treated since 2005 with a median follow-up of 12 months. In this high-risk cohort there were no deaths. The early visceral vessel patency rate was 98%. One patient underwent conversion to open repair and one patient presented with delayed onset paraplegia (type III TAAA) but experienced full neurological recovery. During follow-up, they identified one type 2 and two type 3 endoleaks (the latter were successfully treated percutaneously).

In our unit (Department of Vascular Surgery, University Hospital of Lille), between August 2006 and October 2009, we have treated 42 high risk patients deemed unfit for open surgery (2 type I TAAA I, 9 type II, 16 type III and 15 type IV) [39]. The median age of our patients was 69 years (range, 50 to 83 years). A previous aortic repair had been performed in 16 (38%). The ASA score was > 3 in 33 (79%). The median maximal aneurysm diameter was 66 mm (range, 55 to 100 mm). The median follow-up is 7 months (range, 1 to 34 months). The early target vessel patency rate was 99%. The in-hospital mortality rate was 12% (5/42). The SCI rate was also 12 % (5/42). In 4/5 cases the paraparesis resolved during the recovery period. The other patient had permanent paraplegia. During follow-up, two patients died from non aneurysm related causes (myocardial and cerebral infarctions). The endoleak rate was 22% (8/37) with 7 type 2 and 1 type 3 endoleaks (located at the joint between the SMA stent-graft and its fenestration). Only the latter was treated (the sole secondary intervention to date).

To date, none of the series have reported instances of delayed aortic aneurysm rupture and Roselli's series reports aneurysm sac shrinkage of at least 5mm in all patients reaching one-year follow-up. Device migration has not been reported.

The main outcome measures in the afore mentioned publications are summarized in the Table.

Table PRINCIPLE OUTCOME MEASURES FROM THE SERIES OF ENDOVASCULAR TAAA REPAIR PUBLISHED TO DAE

First author (ref.)	*Year*	*Number*	*TAAA I,II, III*	*TAAA IV*	*30 day mortality*	*Spinal cord ischemia*	*Dialysis (including transient)*	*Endoleak*	*Secondary intervention*	*Early stent patency*	*Follow-up months*
Roselli [34]	2007	73	28/73 [38%]	45/73 [62%]	5.5%	2.7%	1.4%	20.5%	18%	NA	> 12
Chuter [3]	2008	22	NA	NA	9.1%	13.6%	9.1%	9.1%	10%	100%	NA
Greenberg [33]	2008	352	120/352 [34%]	69/352 [20%]	5.7%	9.4%	NA	NA	0.5%	NA	NA
Verhoeven [35]	2009	30	25/30 [83%]	5/30 [17%]	6.7%	16.7%	6.7%	NA	7%	97%	12
Bicknell [38]	2009	8	4/8 [50%]	4/8 [50%]	0%	12.5%	12.5%	37.5%	37.5%	97%	12
Haulon [39]	2009	42	27/42 [64%]	15/42 [36%]	12%	12%	7%	22%	3%	98%	7

NA: not available

Choosing between approaches

While long-term follow-up data is awaited for endovascular treatment of TAAA, it is apparent that the early data currently available compare favourably with the results obtained with open TAAA surgery. In the absence of randomized trials, it is worth bearing in mind that there are two significant biases against the endovascular approach when comparing the available data for the two procedures. Firstly, the published endovascular series include the initial learning curve at each institution and results are likely to further improve with more experience of the technique. Secondly, the published series have generally featured patients deemed unfit for open TAAA repair who are an inherently sicker population than those studied in the series of open repair. To counter this argument it is reasonable to also point out that single center series of open repair from high volume centers often have excellent results when compared to the registry data for open repair and that it is entirely possible that any benefits currently attainable with an endovascular approach might not be reproducible if and when the technique is practiced more widely (outside of the reference centers currently performing the procedure). To this end we feel it is imperative that centers considering endovascular repair of complex aneurysms possess the necessary personnel (surgeons and anesthetists skilled in endovascular and open techniques), equipment (imaging and endovascular operating room), and infrastructure (Intensive care facilities, dialysis etc.). Centers performing endovascular procedures need to have experience in performing open procedures also in order to avoid selection bias and to be able to convert in the situation of failure of the endovascular approach. There are now very few absolute anatomic contra-indications for an endovascular approach, largely due to the rapid evolution of techniques to overcome anatomic challenges. This fact means that the "hybrid technique" of full visceral debranching and subsequent aortic re-lining is now very rarely required. Certainly, however, it is worth considering partial debranching procedures to favourably manipulate the anatomy of the visceral aortic segment to allow an endovascular approach such as the use of hepato-renal bypass or spleno-renal bypass [40]. As mentioned earlier there is considerable interest in the development of "off the shelf" multi-branched devices [29] which would allow the majority of TAAAs to be treated in the emergency setting. Such devices are in fact already available for use in iliac aneurysms. Critics of endovascular approaches have suggested that follow-up protocols are cumbersome and secondary interventions frequent. It is interesting to note that in the more recent larger series of endovascular TAAA repair, the secondary intervention rate has generally been 10% or less, all such interventions being performed by endovascular means (Table).

As well as the huge advances seen in endovascular techniques, there have been a number of advances in techniques utilized in open repair also. These include the use of distal aortic perfusion, spinal fluid drainage and other adjunctive measures to minimize visceral and spinal ischemia risks. Nonetheless, despite these significant advances, the outcome data of open and endovascular approaches are broadly similar despite the physiological differences in the patient groups studied. Assuming that the medium and long-term follow-up data for endovascular repair is satisfactory, it is likely that patient preference will dictate that the role of endovascular approaches will continue to expand in the future. For the moment, however, there remains insufficient data to recommend endovascular surgery over open surgery in patients who are fit to undergo open repair and open surgery therefore remains the gold standard when possible.

REFERENCES

1 Etheredge SN, Yee J, Smith JV et al. Successful resection of large aneurysm of the upper abdominal aorta and replacement with homograft. *Surgery* 1955; 38: 1071-1081.

2 DeBakey ME, Cooley DA, Crawford ES et al. Clinical application of a new flexible knitted dacron arterial substitute. *Am Surg* 1958; 24: 862-869.

3 Bickerstaff LK, Pairolero PC, Hollier LH et al. Thoracic aortic aneurysms: a population-based study. *Surgery* 1982; 92: 1103-1108.

4 Crawford ES,Coselli JS. Thoracoabdominal aneurysm surgery. *Semin Thorac Cardiovasc Surg* 1991; 3: 300-322.

5 Kouchoukos NT, Dougenis D. Surgery of the thoracic aorta. *N Engl J Med* 1997; 336: 1876-1888.

6 Jacobs MJ, Mommertz G, Koeppel TA et al. Surgical repair of thoracoabdominal aortic aneurysms. *J Cardiovasc Surg (Torino)* 2007; 48: 49-58.

7 Pitt MP, Bonser RS. The natural history of thoracic aortic aneurysm disease: an overview. *J Card Surg* 1997; 12: 270-178.

8 Juvonen T, Ergin MA, Galla JD et al. Risk factors for rupture of chronic type B dissections. *J Thorac Cardiovasc Surg* 1999; 117: 776-786.

9 Perko MJ, Norgaard M, Herzog TM et al. Unoperated aortic aneurysm: a survey of 170 patients. *Ann Thorac Surg* 1995; 59: 1204-1209.

10 Coady MA, Rizzo JA, Hammond GL et al. What is the appropriate size criterion for resection of thoracic aortic aneurysms? *J Thorac Cardiovasc Surg* 1997; 113: 476-491.

11 Jacobs MJ, Eijsman L, Meylaerts SA et al. Reduced renal failure following thoracoabdominal aortic aneurysm repair by selective perfusion. *Eur J Cardiothorac Surg* 1998; 14: 201-205.

12 Verdant A, Cossette R, Page A et al. Aneurysms of the descending thoracic aorta: three hundred sixty-six consecutive cases resected without paraplegia. *J Vasc Surg* 1995; 21: 385-391.

13 Cambria RP, Davison JK, Giglia JS et al. Mesenteric shunting decreases visceral ischemia during thoracoabdominal aneurysm repair. *J Vasc Surg* 1998; 27: 745-749.

14 Koksoy C, LeMaire SA, Curling PE et al. Renal perfusion during thoracoabdominal aortic operations: cold crystalloid is superior to normothermic blood. *Ann Thorac Surg* 2002; 73: 730-738.

15 Cambria RP, Clouse WD, Davison JK et al. Thoracoabdominal aneurysm repair: results with 337 operations performed over a 15-year interval. *Ann Surg* 2002; 236: 471-479.

16 Estrera AL, Miller CC 3rd, Huynh TT et al. Neurologic outcome after thoracic and thoracoabdominal aortic aneurysm repair. *Ann Thorac Surg* 2001; 72: 1225-1230.

17 Jacobs MJ, Meylaerts SA, de Haan P et al. Strategies to prevent neurologic deficit based on motor-evoked potentials in type I and II thoracoabdominal aortic aneurysm repair. *J Vasc Surg* 1999; 29: 48-57.

18 Nijenhuis RJ, Jacobs MJ, Schurink GW et al. Magnetic resonance angiography and neuromonitoring to assess spinal cord blood supply in thoracic and thoracoabdominal aortic aneurysm surgery. *J Vasc Surg* 2007; 45: 71-77.

19 Cambria RP, Giglia JS. Prevention of spinal cord ischaemic complications after thoracoabdominal aortic surgery. *Eur J Vasc Endovasc Surg* 1998; 15: 96-109.

20 Jacobs MJ, de Mol BA, Elenbaas T et al. Spinal cord blood supply in patients with thoracoabdominal aortic aneurysms. *J Vasc Surg* 2002; 35: 30-37.

21 Rigberg DA, McGory ML, Zingmond DS et al. Thirty-day mortality statistics underestimate the risk of repair of thoracoabdominal aortic aneurysms: a statewide experience. *J Vasc Surg* 2006; 43: 217-222.

22 Conrad MF, Crawford RS, Davison JK et al. Thoracoabdominal aneurysm repair: a 20-year perspective. *Ann Thorac Surg* 2007; 83: S856-S862.

23 Coselli JS, Conklin LD, LeMaire SA. Thoracoabdominal aortic aneurysm repair: review and update of current strategies. *Ann Thorac Surg* 2002; 74: S1881-S1884.

24 Kouchoukos NT, Masetti P, Murphy SF. Hypothermic cardiopulmonary bypass and circulatory arrest in the management of extensive thoracic and thoracoabdominal aortic aneurysms. *Semin Thorac Cardiovasc Surg* 2003; 15: 333-339.

25 Coselli JS, Bozinovski J, LeMaire SA. Open surgical repair of 2286 thoracoabdominal aortic aneurysms. *Ann Thorac Surg* 2007; 83: S862-S864.

26 Quinones-Baldrich WJ, Panetta TF, Vescera CL et al. Repair of type IV thoracoabdominal aneurysm with a combined endovascular and surgical approach. *J Vasc Surg* 1999; 30: 555-560.

27 Donas KP, Czerny M, Guber I et al. Hybrid open-endovascular repair for thoracoabdominal aortic aneurysms: current status and level of evidence. *Eur J Vasc Endovasc Surg* 2007; 34: 528-533.

28 Drinkwater SL, Bockler D, Eckstein H et al. The Visceral Hybrid Repair of Thoraco-abdominal Aortic Aneurysms - A Collaborative Approach. *Eur J Vasc Endovasc Surg* 2009; 38: 578-585.

29 Sweet MP, Hiramoto JS, Park KH et al. A standardized multi-branched thoracoabdominal stent-graft for endovascular aneurysm repair. *J Endovasc Ther* 2009; 16: 359-364.

30 Batt M, Haulon S, Bouillanne PJ et al. Iliac conduit for renal and visceral artery access during endovascular repair of a pararenal aneurysm with a fenestrated stent-graft. *J Endovasc Ther* 2007; 14: 416-420.

31 Haulon S, Azzaoui R, Jean-Baptiste E et al. Branched and fenestrated endografts: technology,planning process and implantation technique. In: Branchereau A, Jacobs M, editors. *Endovascular aortic repair; the state of the art.* Turin: Edizioni Minerva Medica; 2008. pp. 115-122.

32 Chuter TA, Gordon RL, Reilly LM et al. Multibranched stent-graft for type III thoracoabdominal aortic aneurysm. *J Vasc Interv Radiol* 2001; 12: 391-392.

33 Greenberg RK, Lu Q, Roselli EE et al. Contemporary analysis of descending thoracic and thoracoabdominal aneurysm repair: a comparison of endovascular and open techniques. *Circulation* 2008; 118: 808-817.

34 Roselli EE, Greenberg RK, Pfaff K et al. Endovascular treatment of thoracoabdominal aortic aneurysms. J Thorac Cardiovasc Surg 2007; 133: 1474-1482.

35 Verhoeven EL, Tielliu IF, Bos WT et al. Present and future of branched stent grafts in thoraco-abdominal aortic aneurysm repair: a single-centre experience. *Eur J Vasc Endovasc Surg* 2009; 38: 155-161.

36 Chuter TA, Rapp JH, Hiramoto JS et al. Endovascular treatment of thoracoabdominal aortic aneurysms. *J Vasc Surg* 2008; 47: 6-16.

37 Black SA, Wolfe JH, Clark M et al. Complex thoracoabdominal aortic aneurysms: Endovascular exclusion with visceral revascularization. *J Vasc Surg* 2006; 43: 1081-1089.

38 Bicknell CD, Cheshire NJ, Riga CV et al. Treatment of complex aneurysmal disease with fenestrated and branched stent grafts. *Eur J Vasc Endovasc Surg* 2009; 37: 175-181.

39 Haulon S, D'Elia P, O'Brien N et al. Endovascular repair of thoracoabdominal aortic aneurysms. *Eur J Vasc Endovasc Surg* 2009; [Epub ahead of print].

40 Lerussi G, O'Brien N, Sessa C et al. Hepatorenal bypass allowing fenestrated endovascular repair of juxtarenal abdominal aortic aneurysm: a case report. *Eur J Vasc Endovasc Surg* 2009; [Epub ahead of print].

13

OPEN REPAIR OF INFRA- AND SUPRARENAL AORTIC ANEURYSMS

BARBARA RANTNER, GUSTAV FRAEDRICH

Ever the predicted risk of rupture exceeds the predicted risk of surgery, indication for surgical aneurysm repair is given.

The concept of screening for abdominal aortic aneurysms via ultrasound scanning is common since many years; meanwhile three large controlled randomized trials have shown, that screening men aged 65 to 74 years reduced the mortality from abdominal aortic aneurysm by at least 40% [1-6].

Patient selection

Because aneurysm size is the best indicator for the risk of rupture, it is the dominant factor in selecting patients for elective aneurysm repair. The UK small aneurysm trial (UKSAT) [7] and the American Aneurysm Detection and Management trial (ADAM) both concluded, that early elective open surgery was not justified in patients with abdominal aortic aneurysms < 5.5 cm in diameter [8-11]. These trials demonstrated a 30-day operative mortality for elective open repair ranging from 2.7% to 5.5%. Furthermore, both trials indicated that the rupture rate of small aneurysms ranged at less than 1% per year. In patients considered to be at good surgical risk and presenting with an aneurysm size between 5 and 6 cm, the 5-year risk of rupture in about 20%-25% favours aneurysm repair. In contrast, high risk patients should be observed by serial noninvasive imaging of the aneurysm at 6-months intervals [12-14]. The recently conducted CEASAR trial found also no benefit for treating small aneurysms via endovascular technique. The authors also assume that close surveillance guarantees low mortalitity levels. Among their study population only 2/178 patients experienced aneurysm rupture in a follow up of 36 months [15].

Enlargement to > 6 cm is an indication for aneurysm treatment even in the high risk group, since the risk of rupture exceeds the risk of surgery in all but the sickest patients. Otherwise, the onset of symptoms or signs of relevant aneurysm expansion (> 0.5 cm enlargement within 6 months, growth of thrombus formation) or an excentric shape should prompt therapy [12-14].

The evaluation of a patient for elective aneurysm repair is not standardized and the term "fit for surgery" is widely and diversely used. Several pre-operative fitness scoring systems have been developed and validated. The Goldman Cardiac Index may not be applicable to patients undergoing aneurysm repair since it mainly focuses on cardiac risk [16]. The other scoring systems have been validated in patients undergoing aortic aneurysm repair, each scoring included different pre-operative variables. The Leiden Risk Score requires most details and is especially useful for identifying low-risk patients [17]. The Customized Probability Index and the Glasgow Aneurysm Score are simpler and very similar; both include a component for cerebrovascular disease, but the Glasgow Aneurysm Score does not take the respiratory status into account [18-20]. The Customized Probability Index has been validated for all vascular surgery patients, is simple to calculate, and includes components for the three most commonly cited factors associated with the outcome after aneurysm repair, namely cardiac, respiratory, and renal function [18,19]. The method of calculation of the Customized Probability Index is shown in the Table, with low scores indicating good fitness [21].

Table CALCULATION OF THE MODIFIED CUSTOMIZED PROBABILITY INDEX [21]

Component	*Points*
Cardiovascular disease	
– Previous history of myocardial infarction, cardiac revascularization, angina, severe valve disease or signifacnt arrhythmia	+13
– Uncontrolled congestive heart failure	+14
– Receiving treatment for hypertension	+7
Respiratory dysfunction	
– < 60% for ratio of observed to expected FEV1	+7
Renal dysfunction	
– Serum creatinine ≥ 180 mol/L	+16
– Medication status (protective)	
– Beta-blocker use	-15
– Statin use	-10

Operative technique

Transperitoneal approach

The preferred and most frequently used method is the transperitoneal approach for the repair of infra-renal aortic aneurysms. The patient is placed in the supine position, and the skin of the lower chest, entire abdomen and both groins is prepared. Pre-operative identification of lower extremity pulses is helpful assessing post-operative distal perfusion. The speed of incision and closure, the impact of post-operative pain, the extend of the aneurysm, the degree of obesity, and the coexistence of chronic pulmonary disease determine the choice of incision in individual patients. Either a long midline incision or a wide transverse incision can be made. The operating surgeon may stand on either side of the patient, in case of a limited number of assistants, the left side may allow a better access to the aorta.

An initial abdominal exploration should always be carried out since the probability of a coexisting malignant tumor or other intra-abdominal pathologies is substantial in this age group. Simultaneously, the position of the nasogastric tube should be checked at the time of laparotomy.

Retracting the transverse colon superiorly and holding the small bowel to the right allows good access to the peritoneum where a longitudinal incision is made at the left of the base of the small bowel mesentery to expose the aneurysm. This incision is then extended in both direction, upwards to the ligament of Treitz and the superior and medial duodenal attachments and down to the ilica arteries. Care must be taken to the crossing ureters. The parasympathetic nerves stretch anterior to the proximal part of the left common iliac artery on their way to the pelvis and should be retracted with the peritoneum rather than incised in order to reduce sexual dysfunction. After mobilization, the small intestine is either packed into the right upper portion of the abdomen or viscerated and retracted rightward after placing it in a plastic bag to reduce fluid loss.

The extend of the aneurysm, especially its upper and lower limits, the condition of the major adjacent arteries, particularly the renal and common iliac arteries, are determined by palpation. Extensive manipulation of the aneurysms should, however, be avoided until proximal and distal control are established.

In order to obtain adequate control of the aneurysm, the exposure of the left renal vein is often necessary. In large aneurysms it might be useful to retract the vein superiorly after careful ligation of the caudal side branches. The upper part of the dissection is pursued until full control of the neck of the aneurysm is achieved. First dissecting close to the anterior surface of the aortic segment immediately proximal to the aneurysm, and then staying in this inner layer as one proceeds laterally and posteriorly around the circumference of the aorta, control can quickly and easily be obtained. Before further dissection or manipulation is done, control of the iliac arteries is gained in a similar way. The iliac arteries can be evaluated and the decision whether a tube or bifurcated graft should be placed, made. Extended circumferential preparation does not seem necessary to control the iliac arteries and helps to avoid injury of the underlying veins.

If the inferior mesenteric artery is not already occluded, it may be controlled temporarily with a small vascular clamp or a double vesselloop. The inferior mesenteric artery should never be ligated until the aneurysm is opened and backbleeding is assessed, particularly if the hypogastric arteries are involved in the aneurysmal process.

There are several prosthetic grafts available for aortic replacement: knitted or woven Dacron, impregnated with collagen or gelatine if needed, and polytetrafluoroethylene. Before cross-clamping, heparin is given intravenously (5 000 IE bolus). To avoid peripheral embolization, the iliac arteries are clamped first.

The aneurysm is opened longitudinally in the anterior wall, at the upper end just at the neck of the aneurysm, the wall is incised horizontally to form a distinct ring for the upper anastomosis. The posterior part of the aortic wall is not necessarily divided, although some surgeons prefer to completely transect the aorta. Depending on the degree of aneurysm formation the incision is continued distal into the iliac arteries. After clearing the aneurysmal sac of its thrombotic content, bleeding from lumbar arteries is controlled by deep sutures. Thereafter the upper anastomosis can be started. The suture begins at the posterior midline, deep bites are taken in order to create a double layer of the posterior wall for extra strength. The anterior half of the suture line is then completed with continuous deeply placed sutures. For extremely friable walls pledgets might be incorporated into the suture line. After completing the upper anastomosis, the aortic clamp is released to check for suture line bleeding. Particular attention needs to be taken to the posterior wall since it is difficult to be reached after the performance of the distal anastomosis.

If the iliac arteries are of normal diameter, only a tube graft is needed. A similar technique is used right at the bifurcation, suturing from within the lumen and encompassing both iliac artery orifices within the suture line. In case of iliac artery aneurysms, they are incised anteriorly. This allows the suture of the limbs of a bifurcated graft into an oblique ellipse that enclose the orifices of both the internal and external iliac arteries. If the ureters are in the field, the graft should be placed beneath them before the anastomoses are performed. As soon as one iliac anastomosis is finished, the flow into the extremity should be restored. Declamping needs to be performed slowly to avoid hypotension. If an adequate volume regimen has been maintained by the anesthesiologists the declamping shock with the reperfusion of the lower legs can be avoided. Reclamping and restoring further volume should in case be done rather than resorting to vasopressors. Distal perfusion needs to be evaluated by pulse acquisition in the groins.

After hemostasis is achieved, the bowels and in particular the left colon needs to be inspected for any signs of ischemia. In the rare circumstances when sigmoid colon perfusion appears marginal, which is more often the case if the hypogastric arteries are diseased, reimplantation of the inferior mesenteric artery to the left side of the graft should be performed.

As a last step the aneurysmal wall is trimmed and sutured around the graft to serve as a natural tissue barrier and to prevent the formation of a fistula. The retroperitoneum is closed to surely separate the graft from the overlying duodenum.

RETROPERITONEAL APPROACH

In contrast to earlier reports that the retroperitoneal approach offers advantages concerning pulmonary complications, paralytic ileus and shortens the duration of hospital stay, recent trials showed that the only advantage is the more rapid return of gastrointestinal function [22-25]. There is little evidence to support the superiority of one approach over the other for routine aneurysm repair.

Among the advantages of the transperitoneal approach we find that:

- the opening and closing of the incision is faster and easier;

- It allows the exploration of intraperitoneal pathologies;
- It provides easier access to the right iliac artery;
- It offers a better access to the right renal artery;

The retroperitoneal approach offers advantages in case of:

- dense intraperitoneal adhesions from prior operations;
- colostomy or ileostomy;
- inflammatory aneurysms because adhesions between the aneurysm and the duodenum do not restrict access to the aorta;
- a horseshoe kidney, since it allows easier avoidance of the multiple and accessory renal arteries;
- juxtarenal aneurysm formation;
- infection of a pre-existing aortic graft with the need of replacement.

Body positioning is much more essential in achieving optimal exposure with the retroperitoneal approach: the patient's left shoulder is elevated to a 45° to 60 ° angle relative to the table while the pelvis is positioned as near horizontal as possible. The left-sided incision is started at the 12th rib, for higher exposure at the 10th rib.

Beginning at the lateral border of the left rectus muscle midway between the symphysis and the umbilicus, the skin incision is carried superiorly and then curved laterally up to the tip of the 12th rib. The underlying muscles are divided, delivering access to the underlying peritoneum. The infrarenal aorta is exposed after dissecting between the preperitoneal fat and the peritoneum. The ureter can be mobilized from the bifurcation of the common iliac artery to the ureteropelvic junction if necessary. Medial mobilization of the peritoneum exposes the inferior mesenteric artery, which, when ligated close to the aorta, permits access to the right side of the aorta and the confluence of the left renal vein and the inferior vena cava. Inferior and medial mobilization of the peritoneal sac provides exposure of the right iliac artery when necessary. Aneurysm repair follows as mentioned above after adequate exposure.

One disadvantage of the retroperitoneal approach, however, is that bowel viabilitiy cannot be easily assessed without incising the peritoneum.

Suprarenal aortic aneurysms

For exposure of suprarenal aortic aneurysms either a left-sided retroperitoneal approach can be choosen (see above) or a transperitoneal laparotomy with a medial visceral rotation.

After a midline abdominal laparotomy, the small bowel is placed in an intestinal bag and displaced to the right. After incision of the lateral peritoneal reflection the sigmoid and descending colon are mobilized. The peritoneal incision is carried through the phrenocolic and lienorenal ligaments and a plane is developed between the pancreas and the Gerota´s fascia. The descending colon, pancreas, and spleen are rotated anteriorly and medially, leaving the left kidney in situ. After reflection of the peritoneum from the left crus of the diaphragm the aorta is clearly in view, crossed only by the left renal vein, the autonomic ganglia tissue, and the left crus of the diaphragm.

Exposure of the upper abdominal aorta requires circumferential dissection of the left renal vein to its junction with the inferior vena cava, so that it can be widely displaced as needed. The superior mesenteric artery and celiac axis are exposed by excising the dense autonomic ganglia on the left lateral surface of the aorta, and by incising the left crus of the diaphragm. These vessels can then be circumferentially dissected. Resection of the median arcuate ligament and separation of the muscle fibers of the diaphragm exposes the supraceliac abdominal aorta and distal thoracic aorta [26]. Aneurysm repair is performed as mentioned above with replanation of the side-branches as needed.

REFERENCES

1 Ashton HA, Gao L, Kim LG et al. Fifteen-year follow-up of a randomized clinical trial of ultrasonographic screening for abdominal aortic aneurysms. *Br J Surg* 2007; 94: 696-701.

2 Ashton HA, Buxton MJ, Day NE et al. The Multicentre Aneurysm Screening Study (MASS) into the effect of abdominal aortic aneurysm screening on mortality in men: a randomised controlled trial. *Lancet* 2002; 360: 1531-1539.

3 Scott RA, Ashton HA, Kay DN. Abdominal aortic aneurysm in 4237 screened patients: prevalence, development and management over 6 years. *Br J Surg* 1991; 78: 1122-1125.

4 Scott RA, Vardulaki KA, Walker NM et al. The long-term benefits of a single scan for abdominal aortic aneurysm (AAA) at age 65. *Eur J Vasc Endovasc Surg* 2001; 21: 535-540.

5 Wilmink TB, Quick CR, Hubbard CS et al. The influence of screening on the incidence of ruptured abdominal aortic aneurysms. *J Vasc Surg* 1999; 30: 203-208.

6 Earnshaw JJ, Shaw E, Whyman MR et al. Screening for abdominal aortic aneurysms in men. *BMJ* 2004; 328: 1122-1124.

7 Lederle FA, Wilson SE, Johnson GR et al. Immediate repair

compared with surveillance of small abdominal aortic aneurysms. *N Engl J Med* 2002; 346: 1437-1444.

8 Ballard DJ, Filardo G, Fowkes G et al. Surgery for small asymptomatic abdominal aortic aneurysms. *Cochrane Database Syst Rev* 2008; CD001835.

9 Greenhalgh RM, Forbes JF, Fowkes FG et al. Early elective open surgical repair of small abdominal aortic aneurysms is not recommended: results of the UK Small Aneurysm Trial. Steering Committee. *Eur J Vasc Endovasc Surg* 1998; 16: 462-464.

10 Brown LC, Thompson SG, Greenhalgh RM et al. Fit patients with small abdominal aortic aneurysms (AAAs) do not benefit from early intervention. *J Vasc Surg* 2008; 48: 1375-1381.

11 Lederle FA, Powell JT, Greenhalgh RM. Repair of small abdominal aortic aneurysms. *N Engl J Med* 2006; 354: 1537-1538.

12 Brewster DC, Cronenwett JL, Hallett JW Jr et al. Guidelines for the treatment of abdominal aortic aneurysms. Report of a subcommittee of the Joint Council of the American Association for Vascular Surgery and Society for Vascular Surgery. *J Vasc Surg* 2003; 37: 1106-1117.

13 Hirsch AT, Haskal ZJ, Hertzer NR et al. ACC/AHA 2005 Practice Guidelines for the management of patients with peripheral arterial disease (lower extremity, renal, mesenteric, and abdominal aortic): a collaborative report from the American Association for Vascular Surgery/Society for Vascular Surgery, Society for Cardiovascular Angiography and Interventions, Society for Vascular Medicine and Biology, Society of Interventional Radiology, and the ACC/AHA Task Force on Practice Guidelines (Writing Committee to Develop Guidelines for the Management of Patients With Peripheral Arterial Disease): endorsed by the American Association of Cardiovascular and Pulmonary Rehabilitation; National Heart, Lung, and Blood Institute; Society for Vascular Nursing; TransAtlantic Inter-Society Consensus; and Vascular Disease Foundation. *Circulation* 2006; 113: e463-e654.

14 Kent KC, Zwolak RM, Jaff MR et al. Screening for abdominal aortic aneurysm: a consensus statement. *J Vasc Surg* 2004; 39: 267-269.

15 Ouriel K. Randomized clinical trials of endovascular repair versus surveillance for treatment of small abdominal aortic aneurysms. *J Endovasc Ther* 2009; 16 (Suppl 1): I94-105.

16 Lee TH, Marcantonio ER, Mangione CM et al. Derivation and prospective validation of a simple index for prediction of cardiac risk of major noncardiac surgery. *Circulation* 1999; 100: 1043-1049.

17 Steyerberg EW, Kievit J, de Mol Van Otterloo JC et al. Perioperative mortality of elective abdominal aortic aneurysm surgery. A clinical prediction rule based on literature and individual patient data. *Arch Intern Med* 1995; 155: 1998-2004.

18 Kertai MD, Boersma E, Westerhout CM et al. A combination of statins and beta-blockers is independently associated with a reduction in the incidence of perioperative mortality and nonfatal myocardial infarction in patients undergoing abdominal aortic aneurysm surgery. *Eur J Vasc Endovasc Surg* 2004; 28: 343-352.

19 Kertai MD, Boersma E, Klein J et al. Optimizing the prediction of perioperative mortality in vascular surgery by using a customized probability model. *Arch Intern Med* 2005; 165: 898-904.

20 Biancari F, Hobo R, Juvonen T. Glasgow Aneurysm Score predicts survival after endovascular stenting of abdominal aortic aneurysm in patients from the EUROSTAR registry. *Br J Surg* 2006; 93: 191-194.

21 Brown LC, Greenhalgh RM, Howell S et al. Patient fitness and survival after abdominal aortic aneurysm repair in patients from the UK EVAR trials. *Br J Surg* 2007; 94: 709-716.

22 Sicard GA, Reilly JM, Rubin BG et al. Transabdominal versus retroperitoneal incision for abdominal aortic surgery: report of a prospective randomized trial. *J Vasc Surg* 1995; 21: 174-181.

23 Davidson BR, Gardham R. Selective use of a right retroperitoneal approach to abdominal aortic aneurysm. *Br J Surg* 1992; 79: 639-640.

24 Davidson BR, Gardham R. Left retroperitoneal approach for inflammatory abdominal aortic aneurysms. *Surgery* 1992; 111: 719-720.

25 Cambria RP, Brewster DC, Abbott WM et al. Transperitoneal versus retroperitoneal approach for aortic reconstruction: a randomized prospective study. *J Vasc Surg* 1990; 11: 314-324.

26 Haimovici's vascular surgery - 5th edition. Ascher E, Hollier LH, Strandness DE, editors. Oxford: Blackwell Publishing Ltd; 2004. pp. 867-868.

14

ENDOVASCULAR REPAIR OF INFRA- AND SUPRARENAL ANEURYSMS

TIM RESCH, BJÖRN SONESSON, NUNO DIAS, MARTIN MALINA

Endovascular repair of abdominal aortic aneurysm (EVAR) was introduced almost 20 years ago as an alternative to open aneurysm repair (OR) and has since become an established treatment option for abdominal aortic aneurysm (AAA). After the initial years of early aortic endografts and steep learning curves, EVAR became established in the late 1990s and large randomized trials were performed in the UK and the Netherlands that indicated at least a short-term benefit for EVAR versus OR [1,2]. The long-term outcome of these trials as well as some more up-to-date randomized trials will determine the ultimate place for EVAR when treating infra-renal aortic aneurysms. It is, however, clear that EVAR has a definite role in AAA treatment. Even though the results of EVAR early on showed great promise, several areas of concern were identified, that might jeopardize EVAR outcome. Much focus was centered on the proximal and distal fixation and sealing zones of the aneurysm as these were critical to treatment success. Whereas excellent results have been achieved in patients with favorable anatomy, several adverse anatomical factors clearly dampen this success. Despite this, considering the appeal of EVAR, treatment has been extended to anatomically unfavorable candidates, resulting in correspondingly worse outcomes. In addition, some data suggest that unfavorable EVAR anatomy might indeed indicate a higher risk of AAA rupture and therefore a stronger indication for AAA repair, and this group of patients might benefit from EVAR as well [3]. These results led to an early development of customized or semi-customized aortic endografts to be able to extend EVAR to more patients. Customization included both the distal, iliac arteries (i.e. iliac branch grafts) as well as the pararenal aortic segment (fenestrated aortic stent-grafts). These techniques have become increasingly utilized over the past ten years and have expanded the scope of EVAR considerably.

The aim of this chapter is to review the current status and development of EVAR for infra-renal as well as suprarenal aneurysm including those with adverse iliac anatomy.

Infra-renal aneurysm repair

When considering the results of EVAR for infra-renal aneurysm it is important to take into account the complexity of the aneurysm treated as this will directly impact the outcome of EVAR both in the long- and short-term. Unfavorable aneurysm neck anatomy (i.e. short, angled, conical, wide, thrombus lined) is often a sign of aneurismal disease extending into the aneurysm neck, which might lead to difficulties in achieving a seal of the aneurysm during the endograft implantation [4]. In the short-term this can often be dealt with by adjunctive maneuvers such as additional angioplasty, stenting or endograft extension but in the mid- to long-term such adverse anatomy will affect the outcome and lead to endograft migration, endoleaks as well as late rupture all of which require secondary interventions to the detriment of the patient.

In the iliac segment of the aneurysm, the same holds true. Ectasia or aneurysms in the common iliac arteries make this region less suitable for endograft implantation. Oftentimes the stent-graft can be customized with e.g. flared distal limbs, to achieve a distal seal in the iliacs, but in the long-term such unfavorable morphology will have a higher risk of failure just as in the proximal aneurysm neck [5]. Occlusion of the internal iliac arteries with extension of the stent-graft limbs into the external iliac arteries is an often-utilized option to achieve aneurysm seal in the setting of poor landing zones in the common iliac arteries. This is however, in many series, at the cost of a significant, degree of patient morbidity (e.g. buttock claudication, sexual dysfunction as well as bowel ischemia) [6] and increased risk of stent-graft failure due to kinking and occlusion in the often tortuous external iliac arteries [7].

The abovementioned factors are critical to consider when analyzing the outcome of "standard" infra-renal EVAR and in fact often explain the major differences in outcome between the large, multicenter, often industry-supported trials and the single-center and register experiences reported.

Outcome of EVAR in the "instruction for use" setting

The instruction for use (IFU) for commercially available AAA stent-grafts defines the anatomical limitations of the specific graft. The results for a specific graft are therefore dependent on staying within the limits of the IFU. For all practical purposes this means that a good quality infra-renal neck (minimal thrombus, moderate angulation, not conical) of at least 10-15 mm in length must be present to achieve an adequate fixation and seal. The distal implantation sites entail common iliac arteries of < 16-20 mm in diameter with a landing segment of at least 15-20 mm in length. Access must be adequate to ensure stent-graft delivery i.e. external iliac arteries > 6-7 mm in diameter without excessive tortuosity or calcifications. It is of paramount importance that these factors are kept in mind when extrapolating the results of EVAR to patients with adverse anatomy. Table I summarizes some results from currently available stent-grafts in patients adhering to IFU criteria.

Table I Results of infrarenal EVAR in "Instruction for use" setting with different stent-grafts

Study (ref.)	*n*	*30 d mortality*	*Re-intervention*	*Late rupture*	*5 y survival*
AneuRx [8]	1 193	0.3%	-	3.2%	60.1%
Excluder [9]	235	1.8%	13.8%	0	72%
Powerlink [10]	192	1%	13.4%	0	78.1%
Talent [11]	165	1.2%	18.8%	1	78.1%
Zenith [12]	158	0.8%	20%	0	83%*

*low risk cohort

Outcome of EVAR in the "real-life" setting

As stated, the theoretical and practical advantages of EVAR have led to a significant "stretch" of the current indications for its use. From an anatomical standpoint, previous studies have shown that only 40%-50% of AAA patients truly fulfill the IFU [7-13], yet even nationwide registries in the US indicate that more than 70% of aneurysms are treated by EVAR with very good short-term outcome. A significant number of patients that are treated outside of the IFU might in fact be non-operative candidates from a physiological standpoint and are thus offered EVAR despite unfavorable anatomy. The justification of such an approach must be individualized and is often justified by factors that might make long-term outcome less important (e.g. advanced age). When studying the individual factors that determine EVAR failure this generally falls into one of three areas: unsuitable landing zones proximally and distally, poor access and mechanical failure of the stent-graft itself.

With regards to the landing zones, the proximal neck has attracted the greatest focus. Several studies have shown that adverse neck anatomy will lead to stent-graft failure both in the short- and long-term and it is the single most important factor in preventing EVAR being performed [13]. The most significant adverse factors to consider in an aneurysm neck are length, diameter, quality (i.e. thrombus lined or heavily calcified) and angulation. The literature does not provide a clear answer as to the individual impact of all of these and this is probably a result of the often poor quality in study design. The majority of studies in this field are retrospective, single center reports with limited number of patients making results hard to interpret.

Poor iliac access is the second most common factor for not considering a patient fit for EVAR. Some studies indicate that up 50% of patients have iliac arteries unsuitable for EVAR [14]. This has led to development of smaller, more flexible and hydrophilic EVAR delivery systems to overcome the access issues. Adjunctive maneuvers such as balloon angioplasty and using vessel dilators are simple measures to improve access. If this fails, a surgical conduit can be used to facilitate access. This does add a significant operative burden to EVAR and negates some of the advantages of the procedure. We favour using so called endoconduits, or "cracking and paving technique" to allow access in hostile iliac territory [15]. In our experience, these techniques mean that virtually no patient is denied EVAR due to access issues and the placement of surgical iliac conduits have more or less lost its place in this arena at our institution.

Juxtarenal and suprarenal aneurysm repair

In the setting of an inadequate infra-renal aneurysm neck, the endovascular repair must be extended to a healthier, more proximal segment of the aorta. To achieve this, the branching visceral arteries of the aorta (i.e. the renal arteries, the superior mesenteric artery and the celiac artery) must often be incorporated into the aortic repair. Currently, the most widely used method to do this is by crafting holes, so called fenestrations, into the proximal segment of the aortic endograft. This technique was first described in the late 1990s and has been popularized by Roy Greenberg at the Cleveland Clinic Foundation, OH, USA. The technique has been described extensively in the literature and will be summarized briefly. The endovascular graft is of a modular design consisting of a main proximal body containing the fenestration, a bifurcated body extension similar to a conventional infrarenal endograft and iliac limb(s). The main fenestrated body is customized to each individual patient anatomy according to pre-operative computed tomography (CT) scanning. The importance of excellent pre-operative imaging cannot be overemphasized when planning a complex aortic endograft repair. A well timed, contrast enhanced CT reformatted in 0.75-1 mm slice thickness is desirable. This dataset is then post processed in a dedicated 3D vascular workstation to analyze the data (Fig. 1). The 3D workstation will allow for centerline analysis as well as maximum intensity projection (MIP) and multiplanar rendering (MPR) achieving accuracy in endograft planning. The position and size of the fenestrations as well as the diameters and length of the modular stentgraft are then planned [16-25].

During the procedure, the fenestrated endograft is positioned with the help of radio opaque gold markers on the stent-graft. The stent-graft is then introduced and partially deployed in the aorta after which the fenestrations are catheterized from within the endograft. Once the target vessels have been catheterized as well, bridging stents (covered

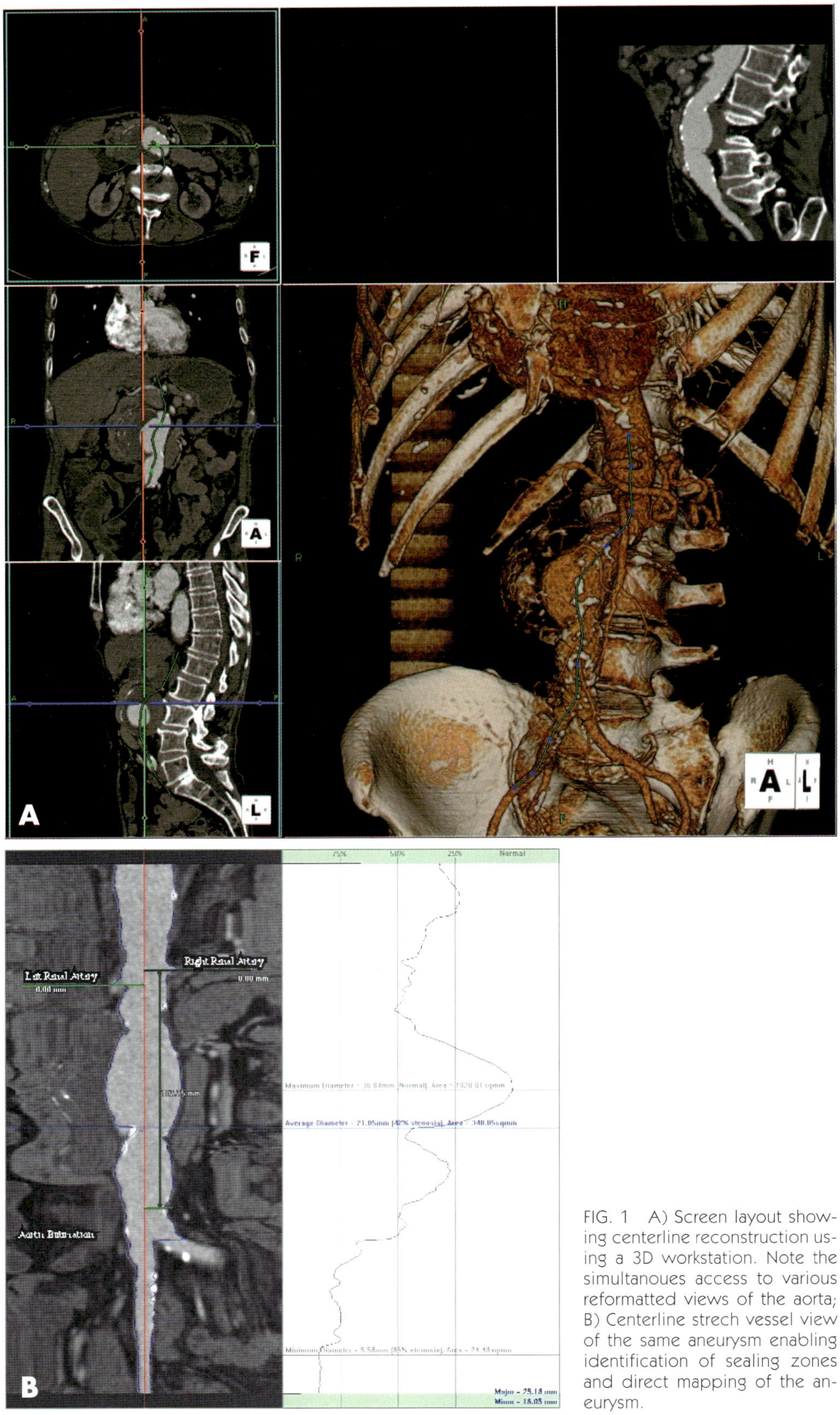

FIG. 1 A) Screen layout showing centerline reconstruction using a 3D workstation. Note the simultanoues access to various reformatted views of the aorta; B) Centerline strech vessel view of the same aneurysm enabling identification of sealing zones and direct mapping of the aneurysm.

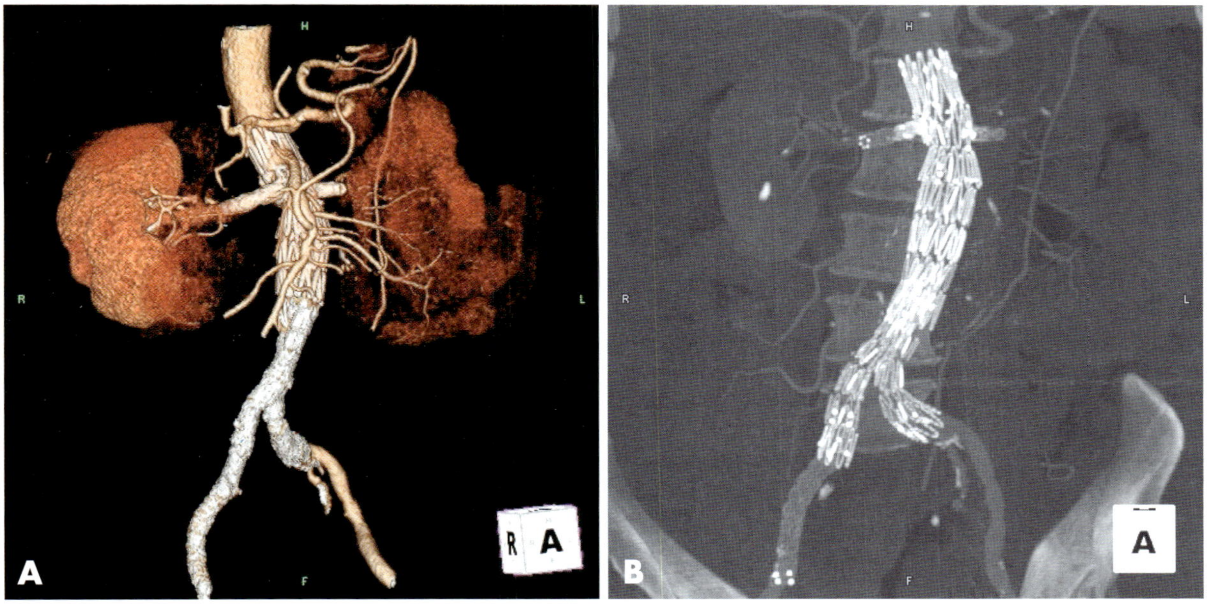

FIG. 2 A) A post-operative 3D view of fenestrated stent-graft; B) Maximum intesity projection image of same graft where the window setting has been adjusted to allow detailed analysis of the stent skeleton.

or uncovered depending on local anatomy) are deployed into the target vessels. The endovascular repair is then completed with the bifurcated and iliac portions of the composite graft (Fig. 2).

Fenestrated endografts are currently used both in situations were an infra-renal neck exists but is of poor quality or too short and were there is no neck at all. From a technical standpoint the delivery of the endograft is identical in these situations but in the latter circumstance the seal will be achieved around the fenestrations themselves by contact of the endograft fabric and a bridging covered stent. When an infra-renal neck exists, but one inadequate for a standard infra-renal EVAR, a fenestrated endograft is merely a means to fully utilize the infra-renal sealing zone without jeopardizing the branching vessels. Fenestrated endograft have also been used in the treatment of de thoraco-abdominal aneurysm and residual aneurysms after both open and endovascular repair, but the results of this are beyond the scope of this chapter.

There have been several series published describing the outcome of fenestrated endografting and these are summarized in Table II. A recent meta-analyis [26] concluded that fenestrated endografting provides superior results compared to open surgery with regards to operative mortality and that it has a definite role in the treatment of juxtarenal aneurysms. There are several problems when attempting to compare the outcome of open versus endovascular repair of this type of pathology: one is the lack of a robust classification system and another the often heterogeneous pathologies treated (including both primary and residual aneurysms, pseudoaneruysms etc). In addition, since the incidence of juxtarenal aneurysms is significantly lower than infrarenal AAA, very few institutions will acquire the technical skills and experience to be able to perform both procedures at the same level thus making any comparison more difficult and often based on historical groups. The ultimate place of endovascular repair of juxtarenal aneurysm can only be determined by randomized trials but the rarity of the condition as well as various technical aspects make this quite difficult.

EVAR in the setting of poor distal landing zones

The most commonly encountered problem in the distal sealing zones of an aneurysm is ectatic or aneurysmatic common iliac aneurysms. This occurs in roughly 20%-30% of AAA patients and represents a technical problem when considering

Table II RESULTS OF FENESTRATED AORTIC STENT-GRAFTING

First author [ref.]	*n*	*30 d mortality [%]*	*Technical success [%]*	*TVP 1year[%]*	*Re-interventions [%]*
Anderson [17]	13	0	100	97	0
Halak [18]	17	0	91	89	
Muhs [19]	28	2.6	94	92	8
O'Neill [20]	119	1	98	94	12
Semmens [21]	58	3.4	91	91	24
Ziegler [22]	63	0	97	93	21
Scurr [23]	45	2.2	67	97	13
Bicknell [24]	15	0	98	97	0
Kristmundsson [25]	54	5.5	91	96	9

TVP: target vessel patency

aneurysm repair regardless of whether this is done open or endovascularly [5]. Two main approaches exist when dealing with these issues in the context of EVAR: either blocking flow in the branching internal iliac artery and landing the endograft more distally in the external iliac artery or preserving flow in the internal iliac artery by some means. The concept of internal iliac embolization is not new; it has been used extensively in the setting of e.g. trauma and uterine embolization. Internal iliac artery blockage as a precursor to AAA exclusion is well described both after open and endovascular repair. Unilateral internal iliac occlusion is generally well tolerated in the presence of a contralateral patent internal iliac artery. In the immediate post-operative period a majority of patients will complain of buttock claudication but only 10%-15% will have persistent claudication and loss of sexual dysfunction one year after surgery. In situations where both internal iliacs are occluded there seems to be a significantly higher risk of both minor and major complications (e.g. bowel and scrotal ischemia) [27]. In the light of the increased complexity that internal iliac flow preservation adds to any aortic procedure, this means that most patients with unilateral iliac disease can and will be treated by internal iliac blockage on one side and flow preservation on the other side. There are certain circumstances when preservation of bilateral internal iliac artery flow is desired: when spinal cord flow is critical (i.e. TAAA repair, previous TAA repair), in patients with previous bowel surgery and in young patients who have concerns about sexual dysfunction [28].

When considering preservation of flow to the internal iliac artery there are several options, both open and endo, available. Internal iliac artery bypass has been well described and is a possible adjunct but it diminishes the minimally invasive approach of the aortic repair. The most common endovascular option is to use a flared limb to land in the common iliac artery. Most commercial endografts will provide limbs up to 24 mm in diameter (some even up to 28 mm) and this will allow treatment of common iliac arteries up to 20-24 mm in diameter. The immediate results of such techniques are very good and provide good immediate outcome. The mid- and long-term data is, however, more questionable. Several studies indicate that iliac arteries in excess of 16-18 mm in diameter have an increased risk of further dilatation leading to stentgraft dislocation and endoleaks necessitating secondary procedures [5]. In an attempt to overcome the problems with adverse iliac landing zones, branched stent-grafts for the iliac bifurcation have been developed. This allows for internal

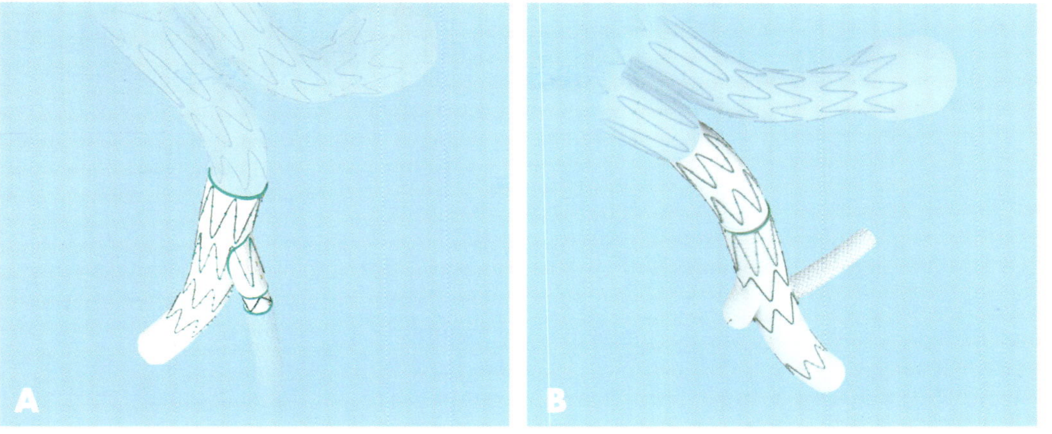

FIG. 3 A) Helical sidebranch stentgraft. Images courtesy of COOK Europe; B) ZBIS "straight" iliac sidebranch. Images courtesy of COOK Europe

iliac artery flow preservation without compromising the more proximal AAA repair utilizing standard, off-the-shelf covered stents, sheaths and wires as ancillary equipment. Currently, there are two designs for branched iliac stent-grafts: a straight design and a helical design (Fig. 3). The latter is designed to optimize flow into the internal iliac artery, ease internal iliac artery catheterization and to maximize overlap between the branched graft and the bridging covered stent into the internal iliac artery. Briefly, the branched stent-graft is introduced on the affected side and partially deployed. With the guide of an indwelling catheter in the side branch, a wire is snared from the contralateral groin, and a large sheath placed into the side branch. The internal iliac artery is catheterized via the side branch and a bridging covered stent is placed from the side branch into the internal iliac artery completing the repair. The published results on iliac side branches are summarized in Table III. The short-term technical and clinical success rates for this procedure is quite good with midterm branch patency of 89% in the published series. The definite results and indications in clinical practice remain to be answered with extended experiences and comparative trials. The study by Verzini et al. [29], which is the only one published attempting a comparison with patients undergoing iliac artery embolization, indicates similar rates of endoleaks and aneurysm shrinkage but with a lesser degree of ischemic complications in the iliac branch group. All patients underwent revascularization of at least one internal iliac in the setting of bilateral common iliac involvement — those not included in the endovascular iliac branch group underwent open revascularization of one internal iliac artery. No major ischemic complications occurred in either group.

Table III RESULTS OF BRANCHED ILIAC STENT-GRAFTS

First author [ref.]	*n*	*30d mortality [n]*	*Technical success*	*Branch patency*
Haulon [27]	52	0	49/52	43/49
Dias [28]	23	1	21/23	18/22
Verzini [29]	32	0	30/32	23/23
Ziegler [30]	46	0	30/46*	26/30

*13/16 failures occurred with 1st generation, discontinued, device.

The Malmö experience

The endovascular AAA programme started in Malmö in the early 1990s and has gradually expanded over the years. We have now treated more than 1 000 patients with EVAR and at the current time over 95% of patients are offered EVAR in the elective setting. Our results have been extensively published and several lessons have been learned over the years.

In patients with appropriate aortic morphology the results with EVAR are very favorable and at present we have a 30-day mortality of approximately 1%-1.5% in these patients. During follow-up, stent-graft migration occurs in less than 0.5% of these patients and re-interventions occur in less than 5% of patients annually. The majority of these are due to either kinks in the limbs of the endograft that are treated due to limb occlusions or to prevent an occlusion or due to endoleaks in the setting of aneurysm growth. We have had no case of immediate conversion to open surgery in over ten years and the incidence of late conversions is less than 0.5% annually.

Our follow-up paradigm for standard EVAR is under constant scrutiny and evolution and as we learn more about the impact of the immediate operative result on long-term outcome we are able to tailor our follow-up regime accordingly [31]. In standard cases where the intra-operative result is good we perform only ultrasound (to measure aneurysm size) and abdominal X-ray (to study stent-graft configuration) annually. In cases of aneurysm growth or configurational changes additional CT scanning is performed to analyze the situation further. In cases where either the anatomy is challenging or the operative result not completely satisfactory we will perform a more intensive follow-up including CT scans at 1 month and 1 year to track any issues with stent-graft performance.

In cases of poor aneurysm morphology, unsuitable for standard infrarenal EVAR, we liberally apply more complex endografts. In fact, some preliminary data from the EVAR 2 trials indicate that aneurysms with anatomy unsuitable for standard EVAR might be at higher risk of aneurysm rupture, providing a partial explanation for the lack of outcome difference between the treatment and observational arm in this trial [3]. We find the implantation of a fenestrated stent-graft in the setting of a short or otherwise poor infrarenal aneurysm neck to be a fairly straightforward procedure and we have achieved very favorable results with fenestrated stent-grafts with a 30-day mortality currently of less than 3% and a long-term target vessel patency of 95%. We currently treat between 15%-20% of aneurysms presenting to our institution with fenestrated stent-grafts and have treated more than 100 patients with this technology. Over two third of the aneurysms shrink during follow-up indicating a successful outcome. Fenestrated stent-grafts have also become a useful tool when treating residual aneurysms after open surgery or EVAR.

In elective aneurysm patients, we have also found a role for branched iliac stent-grafts. We aim at preserving at least one internal iliac artery in aneurysm patients as our experience indicates a significant level of morbidity if both internal iliac arteries are blocked. In our experience, iliac branch devices are also valuable in situations where collateral flow to the spinal cord is threatened, as is the case in thoraco-abdominal stent-grafting or in patients undergoing repair of either the abdominal or thoracic aorta where a previous aortic repair exists. Reports indicate that these patients are at a higher risk of spinal cord ischemic events and we feel that everything must be done in these situations to preserve as much collateral flow as possible. Even though iliac artery preservation adds a level of complexity to any aortic procedure the results are favorable with a technical success rate of 90% and a 3-year patency of approximately 80%.

There is always a balance to be sought when considering a patient for a more complex aortic repair. The added difficulty, cost and risk of the procedure must obviously be weighed against the clinical benefit and this is considered on an individual basis. However, we feel that both fenestrated and iliac branch technology is presently proven enough to be a very valuable addition to any aortic program.

Conclusion

EVAR for infra-renal aneurysm has proven its role as the perhaps primary treatment option and current endografts provide durable results in the 5-10-year perspective. Further technical improvements with standard stent-grafts will most likely expand the treatment indications to more adverse neck anatomy by improving the proximal flexibility and fixation and to patients with poor iliac access by reducing the profiles of delivery systems.

At present, it is important to recognize that the excellent results of EVAR for infra-renal AAA are primarily achieved in patients with favorable anatomy even though a good case can be made for extending the indication for EVAR in patients with adverse anatomy in the setting of physiological comorbidities or advanced age. The current results of complex stent-grafts in morphologically poor candidates for standard EVAR are very promising and motivate extending EVAR treatment further.

REFERENCES

1 Greenhalgh RM, Brown LC, Kwong GP et al. Comparison of endovascular aneurysm repair with open repair in patients with abdominal aortic aneurysm (EVAR trial 1), 30-day operative mortality results: randomised controlled trial. *Lancet* 2004; 364: 843-848.

2 Prinssen M, Verhoeven EL, Buth J et al. A randomized trial comparing conventional and endovascular repair of abdominal aortic aneurysms. *N Engl J Med* 2004; 351: 1607-1618.

3 Powell JT, Brown LC, Greenhalgh RM et al. The rupture rate of large abdominal aortic aneurysms: is this modified by anatomical suitability for endovascular repair? *Ann Surg* 2008; 247: 173-179.

4 Chisci E, Kristmundsson T, de Donato G et al. The AAA with a challenging neck: outcome of open versus endovascular repair with standard and fenestrated stent-grafts. *J Endovasc Ther* 2009; 16: 137-146.

5 McDonnell CO, Semmens JB, Allen YB et al. Large iliac arteries: a high-risk group for endovascular aortic aneurysm repair. *J Endovasc Ther* 2007; 14: 625-629.

6 Lin PH, Chen AY, Vij A. Hypogastric artery preservation during endovascular aortic aneurysm repair: is it important? *Semin Vasc Surg* 2009; 22: 193-200.

7 Sivamurthy N, Schneider DB, Reilly LM et al. Adjunctive primary stenting of Zenith endograft limbs during endovascular abdominal aortic aneurysm repair: implications for limb patency. *J Vasc Surg* 2006; 43: 662-670.

8 Zarins CK, White RA, Schwarten D et al. AneuRx stent graft versus open surgical repair of abdominal aortic aneurysms: multicenter prospective clinical trial. *J Vasc Surg* 1999; 29: 292-308.

9 Peterson BG, Matsumura JS, Brewster DC et al. Five-year report of a multicenter controlled clinical trial of open versus endovascular treatment of abdominal aortic aneurysms. *J Vasc Surg* 2007; 45: 885-890.

10 Wang GJ, Carpenter JP. The Powerlink system for endovascular abdominal aortic aneurysm repair: six-year results. *J Vasc Surg* 2008; 48: 535-545.

11 Torsello G, Osada N, Florek HJ et al. Long-term outcome after Talent endograft implantation for aneurysms of the abdominal aorta: a multicenter retrospective study. *J Vasc Surg* 2006; 43: 2772-2784.

12 Greenberg RK, Chuter TA, Cambria RP et al. Zenith abdominal aortic aneurysm endovascular graft. *J Vasc Surg* 2008; 48: 1-9.

13 Arko FR, Filis KA, Seidel SA et al. How many patients with infrarenal aneurysms are candidates for endovascular repair? The Northern California experience. *J Endovasc Ther* 2004; 11: 33-40.

14 Elkouri S, Martelli E, Gloviczki P et al. Most patients with abdominal aortic aneurysm are not suitable for endovascular repair using currently approved bifurcated stent-grafts. *Vasc Endovascular Surg* 2004; 38: 401-412.

15 Hinchliffe RJ, Ivancev K, Sonesson B et al. "Paving and cracking": an endovascular technique to facilitate the introduction of aortic stent-grafts through stenosed iliac arteries. *J Endovasc Ther* 2007; 14: 630-633.

16 Truijers M, Resch T, Van Den Berg JC et al. Endovascular aneurysm repair: state-of-art imaging techniques for preoperative planning and surveillance. *J Cardiovasc Surg (Torino)* 2009; 50: 423-438.

17 Anderson JL, Berce M, Hartley DE. Endoluminal aortic grafting with renal and superior mesenteric artery incorporation by graft fenestration. *J Endovasc Ther* 2001; 8: 3-15.

18 Halak M, Goodman MA, Baker SR. The fate of target visceral vessels after fenestrated endovascular aortic repair–general considerations and mid-term results. *Eur J Vasc Endovasc Surg* 2006; 32: 124-128.

19 Muhs BE, Verhoeven EL, Zeebregts CJ et al. Mid-term results of endovascular aneurysm repair with branched and fenestrated endografts. *J Vasc Surg* 2006; 44: 9-15.

20 O'Neill S, Greenberg RK, Haddad F et al. A prospective analysis of fenestrated endovascular grafting: intermediate-term outcomes. *Eur J Vasc Endovasc Surg* 2006; 32: 115-123.

21 Semmens JB, Lawrence-Brown MM, Hartley DE et al. Outcomes of fenestrated endografts in the treatment of abdominal aortic aneurysm in Western Australia (1997-2004). *J Endovasc Ther* 2006; 13: 320-329.

22 Ziegler P, Avgerinos ED, Umscheid T et al. Fenestrated endografting for aortic aneurysm repair: a 7-year experience. *J Endovasc Ther* 2007; 14: 609-618.

23 Scurr JR, Brennan JA, Gilling-Smith GL et al. Fenestrated endovascular repair for juxtarenal aortic aneurysm. *Br J Surg* 2008; 95: 326-332.

24 Bicknell CD, Cheshire NJ, Riga CV et al. Treatment of complex aneurysmal disease with fenestrated and branched stent grafts. *Eur J Vasc Endovasc Surg* 2009; 37: 175-181.

25 Kristmundsson T, Sonesson B, Malina M et al. Fenestrated endovascular repair for juxtarenal aortic pathology. *J Vasc Surg* 2009; 49: 568-575.

26 Nordon IM, Hinchliffe RJ, Holt PJ et al. Modern treatment of juxtarenal abdominal aortic aneurysms with fenestrated endografting and open repair–a systematic review. *Eur J Vasc Endovasc Surg* 2009; 38: 35-41.

27 Haulon S, Greenberg RK, Pfaff K et al. Branched grafting for aortoiliac aneurysms. *Eur J Vasc Endovasc Surg* 2007; 33: 567-574.

28 Dias NV, Resch TA, Sonesson B et al. EVAR of aortoiliac aneurysms with branched stent-grafts. *Eur J Vasc Endovasc Surg* 2008; 35: 677-684.

29 Verzini F, Parlani G, Romano L et al. Endovascular treatment of iliac aneurysm: Concurrent comparison of side branch endograft versus hypogastric exclusion. *J Vasc Surg* 2009; 49: 1154-1161.

30 Ziegler P, Avgerinos ED, Umscheid T et al. Branched iliac bifurcation: 6 years experience with endovascular preservation of internal iliac artery flow. *J Vasc Surg* 2007; 46: 204-210.

31 Dias NV, Riva L, Ivancev K et al. Is there a benefit of frequent CT follow-up after EVAR? *Eur J Vasc Endovasc Surg* 2009; 37: 425-430.

15

ENDOVASCULAR TREATMENT OF RUPTURED ABDOMINAL AORTIC ANEURYSMS

NICOLAS LOUIS, FRÉDÉRIC COCHENNEC, JEAN-PIERRE BECQUEMIN

Ruptured abdominal aortic aneurysms (RAAA) are responsible for 2% of all deaths in men over 65 years [1]. In a population-based study from Malmö, Sweden, the incidence increased from 5.6 per 100 000 persons/year in the early 1970s to 10.6 per 100 000 persons/year in the 2000 [2].

Despite advances in intensive care medicine and development of specialized vascular centers, the peri-operative mortality of RAAA has not changed for two decades [3]. In the series from Malmö, the overall mortality reached 85% (95%, CI 80-91). Authors estimated that 66% of patients with RAAA (95% CI 58-73) died before reaching the hospital or before any attempt of aortic repair [4]. For people who survive open repair (OR), recent meta-analysis and population based studies reported incompressible 40% to 50% mortality rates [5,6].

The low peri-operative mortality associated with endovascular aortic repair (EVAR) in the elective setting has been established by three randomized controlled trials [7-9]. Given the poor outcomes after OR for RAAA as well as reduction in peri-operative mortality associated with elective EVAR, an increasing number of centers have established protocols to use EVAR for RAAA (REVAR). Avoidance of laparotomy and aortic clamping, reduction of blood loss and limitation of iatrogenic injury [10] may indeed have a benefit on survival and the overall results.

In this chapter, we will describe the management and the operative technique of EVAR in an emergent setting, present a literature review and summarize the protocols of controlled randomized studies in progress that compare EVAR and OR for RAAA.

Management and operative technique of EVAR for RAAA

Fig.1 shows the current management chart of EVAR for RAAA in our institution.

Prerequisites

Five conditions are necessary to start a program of EVAR for RAAA: 1) a computed tomography (CT)-scan available in the institution; 2) an operating room dedicated to EVAR available day and night; 3) the availability of a large choice of stent-grafts; 4) endovascular expertise of the surgical staff; 5) the presence of two senior vascular surgeons and/or a vascular surgeon and an interventional radiologist.

Pre-operative CT-scan: the pros and cons

As discussed later in this paper, CT-scan should not delay the intervention especially in unstable patients. However, we are convinced that CT-scan is essential for REVAR and it provides more pertinent informations than the intra-operative angiography. Not the least, CT-scan confirms the diagnosis of aneurysm rupture and eliminates other abdominal emergencies such as acute pancreatitis or mesenteric infarction.

Then an accurate sizing can be performed. It is a key point for an endovascular procedure to be successfull. A minimum of four measurements are necessary for a proper planning: 1) the length and diameter of the aortic neck (respectively ≥ 10 mm

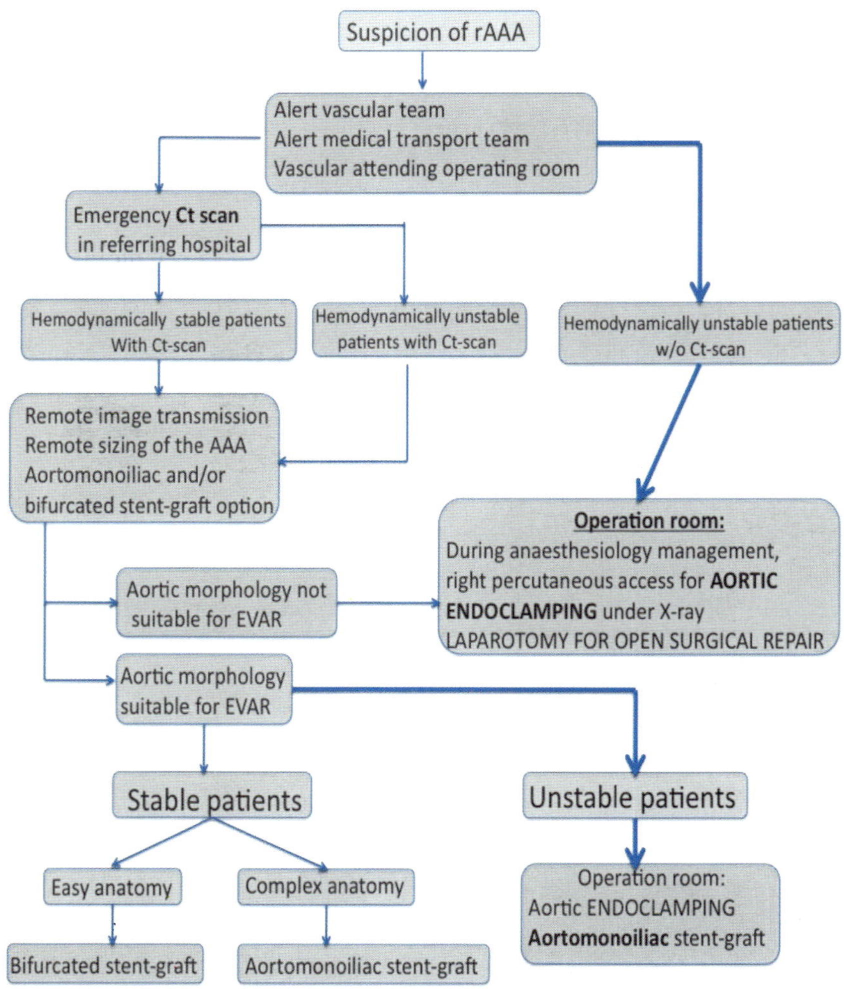

FIG. 1 Chart summarizing the management of ruptured abdominal aortic aneurysms in our institution.

and ≤ 32 mm) to asses EVAR feasibility; 2) the diameters of the common iliac arteries to select the stent-graft.

With these measurements, an aorto-uni-iliac stent-graft with a short main body can be inserted expediently. If too short, an iliac extension is added. Its length is determined on the angiogram with a calibrated catheter.

Resuscitations measures

"Hypotensive hemostasis" is a key point to minimize blood loss. It is achieved by limiting the volume of fluid perfusion and the use of vaso-active drugs. The systolic blood pressure should be maintained around 80/90 mm of mercury. The operating table set up with open and endovascular instruments, the C-arm and the injector need to be ready when the patient enters the operative room. The patient is prepped and draped in supine position. A urinary catheter with an aspiration port is inserted to monitor the intra-abdominal pressure (IAP) by connecting the aspiration port to a pressure transducer. The surveillance of the IAP is essential to detect abdominal compartment syndrome (ACS).

While one surgeon performs the cut down in the groin, the second surgeon validates the feasibility and the sizing of the stent-graft. The analysis on a dedicated platform with a center line such as Osirix, 3 Mensio, Advantage Windows or Terrarecon is essential when the neck is angulated, since with the axial cuts alone, angulations may be misleading for the evaluation length and diameter of the aortic neck. During the procedure systemic anticoagulation is not mandatory and we prefer not to use it, in order to limit the bleeding and to prevent ACS.

General or local anesthesia

The procedure can be performed or at least started under local anesthesia of the groins. The main advantage is to keep the abdominal wall under tension which tends to limit the intra and retro-peritoneal bleeding until the aortic occlusion balloon is in place. However due to brain hypoxia, abdominal pain, and anxiety, the patient may become confused and agitated. Thus the operation can become very demanding. General anesthesia can also be induced when the bleeding is controlled to perform the femoro-femoral bypass graft when an aorto-uni-iliac graft has been inserted or when an abdominal decompression is required.

Approach: pig tail and sheaths positioning

The femoral arteries are approached through a transverse incision of the groin. A 9 Fr introducer sheath is introduced and the aneurysm neck is catheterized with a 0.035 floppy angled guide wire. Whenever catheterization of the upper neck is difficult (angulated neck, large aneurysm), an angulated catheter is used to orientate the guide wire. A calibrated pig tail is then placed in due position. A first shot is taken to verify the anatomy of the aneurysm, the neck features and the positions of the renal and hypogastric arteries. If EVAR is judged feasible, the pig tail is removed and the 9 French introducer sheath is replaced by a 45 cm-lenght 14 F sheath with radiopaque markers. The distal radiopaque markers of the sheath are placed at the level of the low thoracic aorta or the above the renal arteries.

Endo aortic balloon occlusion

Aortic occlusion balloon in hemodynamically unstable patients is a life saving gesture. It stops the hemorrhage, reduces the retroperitoneal hematoma and may prevent abdominal compartment syndrome. The balloon can be inserted via a brachial as well as a femoral approach. We feel that the femoral approach remains the best option. The femoral route is also used for the aortic stent-graft, saving one access. Arterial and venous accesses of both upper limbs are left to the anesthesiologists. Currently available occlusion balloons require 10 to 14 F introducer sheaths, which would need an extra cut down if inserted via the brachial artery (Table I). Getting into the descending aorta from above is sometimes tricky and may waste precious time. To allow rapid management of the patient, we use in our center, a pre-prepared emergency endoclamping kit. There are two different kits. One kit is dedicated to open surgery (Table II) with a 10 Fr sheath which can be inserted percutaneously under local anesthesia of the groin while the anesthesiologists prepare the patient. The second kit is dedicated to endovascular surgery (Figs. 2,3, Table III): it includes the endovascular tools needed for the endoclamping as well as for the placement of an aorto-uni-iliac or a bifurcated stent-graft.

The main difference between the two kits is the size of the sheaths, 10 F versus 14 F. For REVAR we use a 14 Fr introducer sheath. Through the hemostatic valve of the introducer, a compliant occlusion balloon (40 mm in diameter) is pushed up-

Table I PROPERTIES OF COMPLIANT AORTIC OCCLUSIVE BALLOONS

Balloon occlusion	*Sheath size (F)*	*Catheter length (cm)*	*Maximum balloon diameter (mm)*
Coda (Cook, Bloomington, IN)	10	100-120	32-40
Reliant (Medtronic, Santa Rosa, CA)	12	100	46
Equalizer (Boston Scientific, Natick, MA)	14-16	65-110	20-27-33-40

Table II LIST OF INSTRUMENTS WHICH CONSTITUTE THE ENDOCLAMPING KIT FOR OPEN SURGERY

ENDOCLAMPING KIT FOR OPEN SURGERY

- Needle puncture: 1
- 0.035 angle guidewire 180 cm length: 1 (Glidewire®, Terumo)
- 9 F sheath 10 cm length: 1 (Pinnacle®, Terumo)
- Vertebral catheter 5 F, 100 cm length: 1 (Angiographic catheter, vertebral, Terumo)
- 0.035 Extra-stiff wire guide 260 cm length: 1 (LunderquistTM, Cook Medical)
- 10 F sheath 40 cm length: 1 (Check-Flo® introducers with radiopaque tip, Cook)
- 0.035 balloon occlusion 40 mm diameter: 1 (Coda® Balloon Catheter, Cook)

Table III LIST OF INSTRUMENTS WHICH CONSTITUTE THE ENDOCLAMPING KIT FOR eEVAR

KIT FOR eEVAR

- Needle puncture: 1
- 0.035 angle guidewire 180 cm length: 1 (Glidewire®, Terumo)
- 9 F sheath 10 cm length: 1 (Pinnacle®, Terumo)
- Vertebral catheter 5 F, 100 cm length: 1 (Angiographic catheter, vertebral, Terumo)
- 0.035 Extra-stiff wire guide 260 cm length: 1 (LunderquistTM, Cook Medical)
- 14 F sheath 40 cm length: 1 (Check-Flo® introducers with radiopaque tip, Cook)
- 10 F sheath 40 cm length: 1 (Check-Flo® introducers with radiopaque tip, Cook)
- 0.035 balloon occlusion 40 mm diameter: 1 (Coda® Balloon Catheter, Cook)
- Pigteal 5 F, 110 cm length: 1 (Angiographic catheter, PIG, Cordis)
- Headhunter 5 F, 100 cm length: 1 (Angiographic catheter, femoral cerebral headhunter, Terumo)

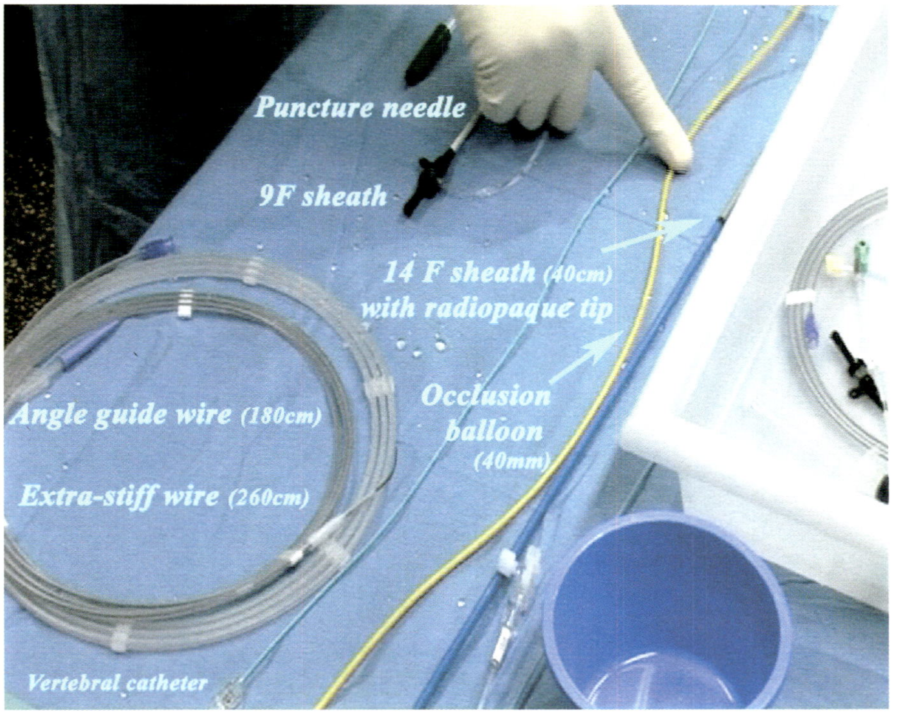

FIG. 2 Kit for endoclamping.

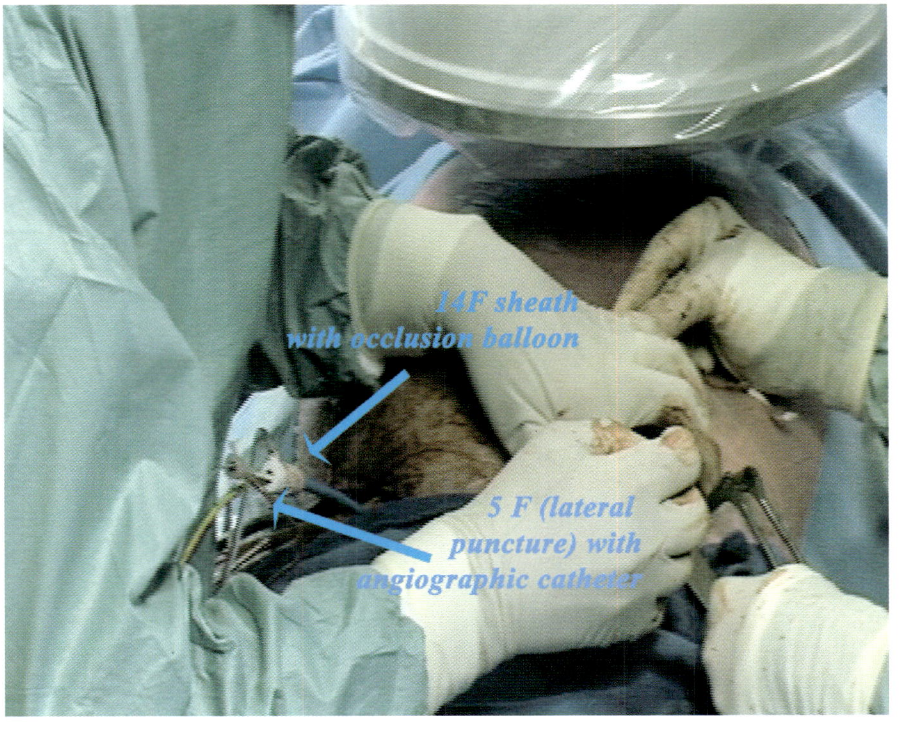

FIG. 3 Lateral puncture of the 14 F sheath to allow the placement of the pig-tail angiographic catheter.

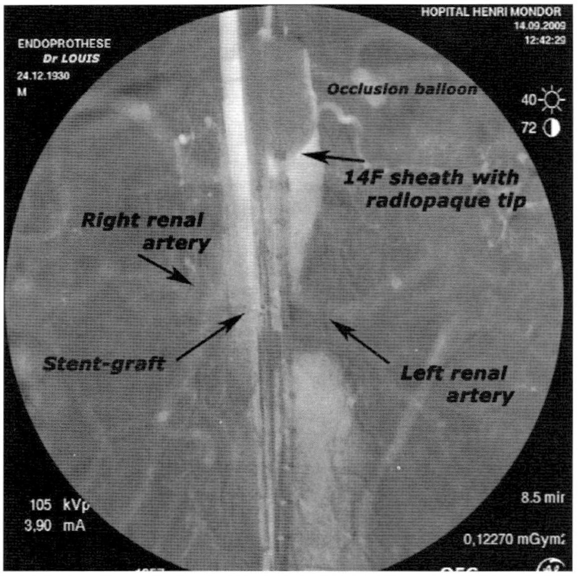

FIG. 4 Intra-operative X-ray imaging of a stent-graft deployed with the endoclamping system.

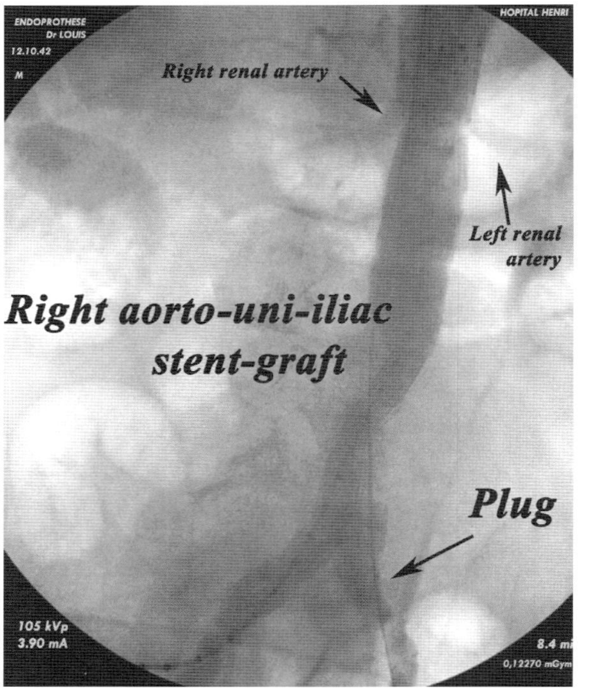

FIG. 5 Intra-operative X-ray imaging of an aorto-uni-iliac stent-graft for RAAA.

ward on a stiff wire, then via a lateral puncture of the valve with a 5 F sheath, the pig tail is replaced into the aorta (Fig. 3). The contralateral femoral artery is then available and can be used for insertion of the aorto-uni-iliac or the main body of the bifurcated graft stent-graft. This trick avoids repeated exchanges of wires and catheters and is less time consuming.

Finally the balloon is inflated into the aorta close to the markers. The sheath blocks the balloon and prevents its drifting into the aneurysm sac (Fig. 4).

STENT-GRAFT CONFIGURATION: CHOICE AND PLACEMENT

Bifurcated versus aorto-uni-iliac stent-grafts

According to patient's condition and aneurysm anatomy, a bifurcated or an aorto-uni-iliac stent-graft can be used. Bifurcated grafts are chosen in relatively stable patients with very favorable anatomy. Otherwise aorto-uni-iliac stent-graft is a better option (Fig. 5). The latter allows stopping the hemorrhage quicker and is more appropriate when the iliac arteries are tortuous or diseased. Bifurcated stent-graft exposes to persistent bleeding during the catheterization of the contralateral limb which can take some time in tortuous anatomy (Fig. 6). When a bifurcated graft has been chosen, catheterization can be performed more quietly following the placement of the occlusion balloon inside the main body of the stent-graft from the opposite groin (Fig. 7).

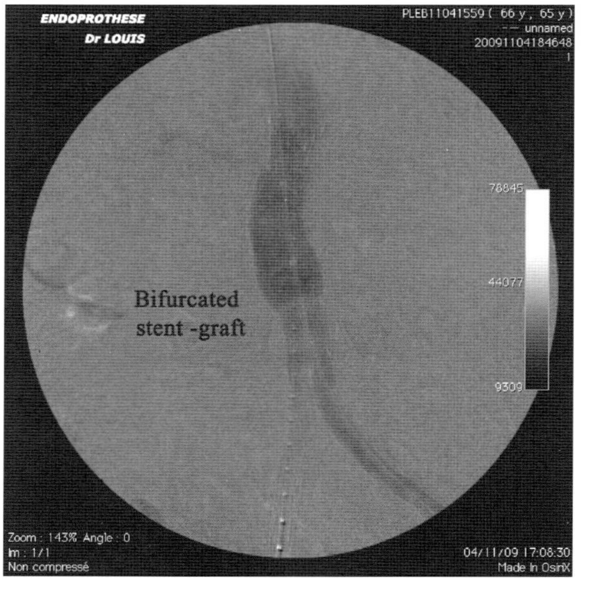

FIG. 6 Intra-operative X-ray imaging of a bifurcated stent graft for RAAA.

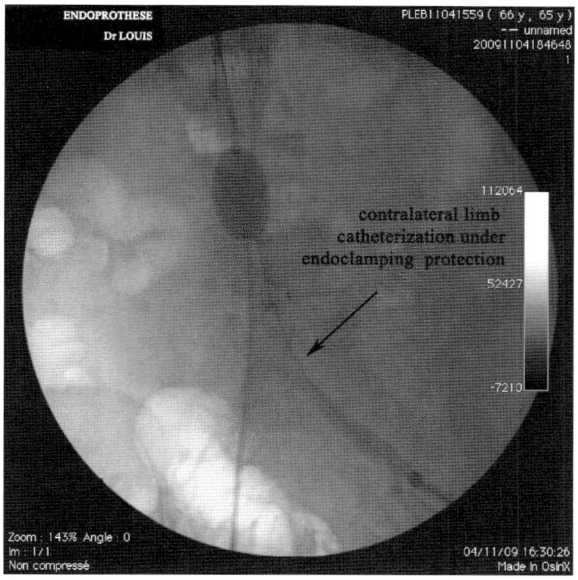

FIG. 7 Intra-operative X-ray imaging of a short limb catheterization while the endoclamping is used.

Balloon occlusion and stent-graft placement management

A 9 F sheath is introduced via the available femoral artery. A hydrophilic guide wire is pushed with a catheter laterally to the occlusion balloon and then exchanged for an extra-stiff guide wire. The stent-graft is then inserted into the aorta. An aortography is performed via the pig tail catheter, and the stent-graft is positioned at the renal arteries' level. They are two options for the deployment of the stent-graft: 1) prior to the deployment of the main body, the aortic occlusion balloon is deflated and pulled downward into the aneurysm sac. Then the graft is quickly deployed. Deflation of the occlusion balloon can lead to severe drop of the blood pressure. If hypotension persists, the occlusion balloon can be replaced through the main body of the stent-graft and inflated into the main body of the graft. 2) The balloon is maintained inflated and the distal tip of the sheath with the stent-graft is carefully passed into the aorta lateral to the inflated balloon. The sheath supporting the balloon must remain above the stent-graft to allow withdrawal of the balloon into the sheath after the stent-graft has been opened. This option is chosen when the patient is hemodynamically unstable.

Aorto-uni-iliac stent-graft

After deployment of an aorto-uni-iliac stent-graft, an angiogram is performed. It focuses on the iliac artery bifurcation (C-arm with 30° left anterior oblique view for the right bifurcation, and right anterior oblique view for the left bifurcation). Complementary graft limbs can then be inserted whenever necessary but great care should be taken to preserve the hypogastric artery. The subsequent step is modeling with the occlusion balloon of the main body's proximal range of stent, the overlap between graft components, and the iliac extension distal rim. Following, the balloon is exchanged for the pig tail catheter and a final angiogram is performed. If the sealing is obtained, an occluder plug is inserted into the contra-lateral common iliac artery. If there is a proximal leak, the contra-lateral access must be available since it may be used for complementary maneuvers. A cross over femoral femoral bypass is then performed with end-to side anastomoses.

Bifurcated stent-graft

Catheterization of the contra-lateral limb can be difficult especially in case of iliac and aneurysm angulations and large aneurysms. When it fails, a cross-over technique with a snare is used. In very rare cases a brachial approach can be the ultimate option. When the limb cannot be cannulated, particularly in unstable patients, the bifurcated stent graft should be converted to an aorto-uni-iliac configuration by using devices such as the Renu device (Cook, Inc., Bloomington, IN).

Abdominal compartment syndrome

The abdominal compartment syndrome is due to the increase of the intra-abdominal pressure (IAP) (Fig. 8). The cause of IAP after EVAR for RAAA is multifactorial: large retroperitoneal hematoma which acts as a space-occupying process; persistent back bleeding from the lumbar and inferior mesenteric arteries, coagulopathy; alteration of flow in the micro vessels of the intestines with subsequent interstitial edema. At a later stage ischemia and intestinal necrosis may occur as well as respiratory and renal failure. The incidence and severity of ACS varies from series to series, largely depending upon the hemodynamic status of the patient.

The normal IAP pressure ranges between 0 and 5 mmHg. Between 10 and 15 mmHg, the cardiac index is usually maintained, respiratory and renal symptoms are unlikely to occur. At this point, intravascular volume optimization is sufficient to correct the alterations. When intra-abdominal pressure is between 15 and 25 mmHg the syndrome can oc-

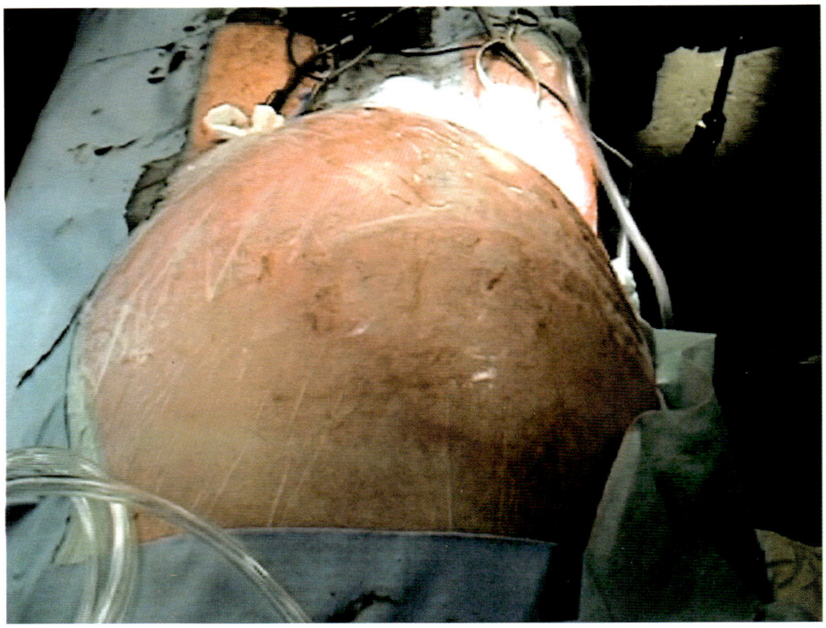

FIG. 8 Picture of a patient with an abdominal compartment syndrome after RAAA treated by EVAR.

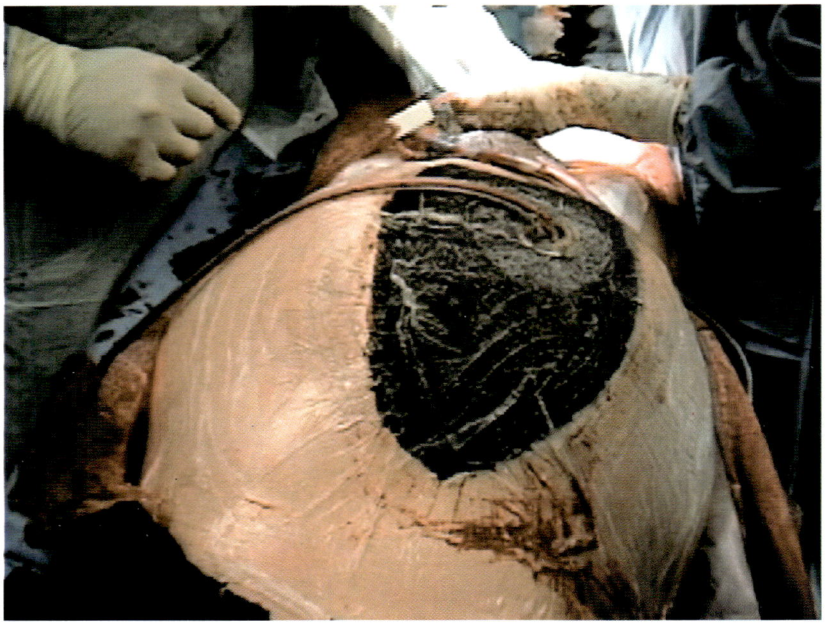

FIG. 9 Picture of a VAC placed on the abdominal wound whch was left open to treat a severe compartment syndrome.

cur, however, it usually responds to aggressive fluid resuscitation and surgical decompression. Above 25 mmHg, urgent surgical decompression, fluid resuscitation and vasoconstrictive agents are mandatory and seem to improve the prognosis.

The abdomen must left open until the edema is cleared. A vacuum-assisted closure (VAC) system placed on the abdominal wound seems to be a promising tool (Fig. 9). After several days the abdomen wall can be closed.

Literature review

To date, four systematic reviews or REVAR have been published [11-14]. The pooled mortality and morbidity rates varied from 18% to 24% and from 28% to 44%, respectively. Results of these studies are summarized in Table IV. Two of them compared results of REVAR and OR. Harkin et al. found a pooled mortality rate of 18% after REVAR as compared with 34% after OR [12]. However, 95% CI were not reported and the calculation of the overall mortality after OR was mainly based on historical control groups. In the Visser et al. study [13] the pooled 30-day mortality rates were 22% (95% CI: 16-29) after REVAR and 38% (95% CI: 32-45) after OR. The pooled rates for total systemic complications were 28% (95% CI: 17-48) for REVAR and 56% (95% CI: 37-85) for OR. A world experience collected from 49 centers by F Veith has shown a total 30-day mortality of 21 % in 1 037 patients.

OPPONENTS OF REVAR UNDERLINE SEVERAL DRAWBACKS

1) Delay in treatment: EVAR, ideally, requires preoperative anatomical assessment by a CT-scan, which can theoretically delay the intervention. In order to limit any delay, some authors have proposed to use intra-operative calibrated angiography [15] rather than CT-scan. However, due to the inability to visualize the luminal thrombus, this approach can be responsible for underestimation of aortic diameter at the level of the proximal sealing zone and subsequent Type I endoleak. Recent studies have shown that delays induced by CT-scan assessment were acceptable [16,17]. In our daily practice, only a small subset of patients with ruptured aneurysm present with hemorrhagic shock that is instable enough to require emergent surgical exploration and the vast majority of patients with RAAA are pre-operatively assessed with a CT scan.
2) Uncontrolled type II endoleak: patients with RAAA treated by EVAR may develop type II endoleak leading to persistent blood loss, retroperitoneal hematoma increase and compartment syndrome. However, this adverse event has been rarely reported [18,19]. It may be that the clots and pressure due the surrounding retroperitoneal hematoma, compress and block the back bleeding, assuring hemostasis.
3) Uncertainty with regard to the sealing zones: contrary to strict anatomical inclusion criteria for elective EVAR, in an emergent setting, experienced interventionalists including ourselves are often more liberal with regard to the length of the proximal neck and iliac tortuosity [20]. Retrospective studies reported significant variations in the anatomical inclusion and exclusion criteria employed, with anatomical suitability rates ranging from 34% to 100% [12]. The consequences are a greater risk of type I endoleak or unintentional renal arteries blockages.
4) Uncertainty with long term benefit: since no long term follow-up data are available after REVAR and additional studies are indeed necessary to assess if REVAR is a durable treatment.
5) Cost effectiveness: EVAR has substantial cost implications in terms of hospital resources consumption such as medical and nurses' staff and equipment. However, given the reduction of blood transfusion and ICU stay, the in-hospital and one-year costs of treating RAAA by EVAR are lower than those following OR [13].

Table IV LITERATURE REVIEW OF EVAR FOR RAAA

First author (ref.)	*Number of studies included*	*Number of patients included*	*Pooled mortality rates, % (95% CI)*
Rayt [11]	31	982	24 (20-28)
Harkin [12]	34	891	18 (ND*)
Visser [13]	10	148	22 (16-29)
Mastracci [14]	18	436	21 (13-29)

6) Improved outcomes uncertainties: there is growing evidence that REVAR may improve the outcome of RAAA. However, no level one evidence is available. Apart from a single controlled randomized trial [21] and a prospective non randomized study [22], all series comparing EVAR with OR were case-control studies or cohort studies. Some groups have not been able to confirm the advantage of REVAR over OR [21,23,24]. In the NEW ERA study [22], a prospective non-randomized international multi-center study that included 100 patients, 30-day mortality rates were 35% after EVAR and 39% after OR (p = NS). The mortality associated with EVAR was indeed higher than previously reported in retrospective studies. The presence of a selection bias in such cohort studies might be an explanation. It has been suggested that the anatomic and hemodynamic eligibility criteria for EVAR (good anatomy in stable patients) select the patients with better prognosis and biases the results. To date, one single randomized control trial comparing REVAR and OR has been published [21]. This study showed no significant difference in terms of mortality (EVAR: 53% versus OR: 53%) and post-operative complications rates (EVAR: 77% versus OR: 80%) between the two groups. However, this result should be interpreted with caution. Although 103 consecutive patients were admit-

Table V DESIGNS OF THE THREE CURRENTLY ONGOING RANDOMIZED TRAILS

	ECAR	*IMPROVE*	*AJAX*
Primary outcome measures:	30-day mortality	30-day mortality	Mortality and severe measured at 30 days, 3 months, and 6 months.
Estimated enrollment:	160	600	120
Randomization:	Week for each center, one week of endovascular treatment in alternation with one week of treatment by conventional repair	Randomization by telephone. Randomization is stratified by trial centre.	
Inclusion criteria:	Age > 18 years, Ruptured aorta-iliac aneurysms diagnosed by CT-scan, infrarenal AAA, stable hemodynamic condition, anatomic criteria, technical constraints.	All non-moribund patients with a clinical diagnosis of ruptured AAA made in hospital, including patients transferred from other hospitals with a diagnostic CT-scan.	Ruptured AAA diagnosed by CT-scan, anatomic criteria, age>18 years
Exclusion criteria:	Unstable hemodynamic condition, anatomic criteria of non-inclusion, non-ruptured symptomatic, supra-renal, mycotic and post-traumatic AAA, infectious false aneurysms, impossibility to obtain a CT-scan with injection	Connective tissue disorders, previous AAA repair, unconscious or moribund patients.	Juxtarenal AAA, anatomical unsuitability, patient unfit for open procedure, extreme instability making CT-scan impossible

ted with RAAA, only 32 were randomized to either open or EVAR. This low rate of patient's randomization (31%) may be in part explained by the broad exclusion criteria applied, including: patient unfit for open repair; death before randomization; inability to give consent; age; refusal of operation; no team available; surgeon preference.

Then, although REVAR provides encouraging results, other appropriate randomized controlled studies are needed to determine the best treatment option.

Randomized controlled studies in progress

Two trials of endovascular versus open repair for ruptured AAA are currently underway: the AJAX trial in Amsterdam, supported by the Dutch Heart Foundation and the ECAR trial in France supported by the delegation Recherche Clinique. In the ECAR trial, patients who are hemodynamically stable undergo CT-scan and if they are anatomically suitable for endovascular repair, are offered randomization. Both trials are small sized: AJAX originally planned to randomize 80 patients but more recently recruitment has been extended to 120 patients and ECAR proposes to recruit 160 patients.

The Immediate Management of the Patient with Rupture: Open Versus Endovascular repair (IMPROVE) trial, has a different design. A total of 600 patients are to be randomized. The point of randomization is the clinical diagnosis of ruptured aneurysm, made in participating hospitals. The patients will be randomized to undergo either immediate CT-scan with endovascular repair whenever possible or open repair, in which case a CT-scan is optional. Patient entry will be unselected and include those who are hemodynamically unstable. The trial is powered to show a difference of 30-day mortality of 14% between the randomized groups: 44% for open surgery versus 30% for intention for endovascular.

The designs of these prospective randomized studies are summarized in Table V.

In summary REVAR is a promising new way of treating patients with ruptured aneurysm. However, level one evidence is required to prove the benefit of this approach. Surgeons, institutions and health care providers should integrate the requirements quoted above to be able to offer this new modality to treat this dreadful life threatening event.

REFERENCES

1 Mayer D, Pfammatter T, Rancic Z et al. 10 years of emergency endovascular aneurysm repair for ruptured abdominal aortoiliac aneurysms: lessons learned. *Ann Surg* 2009; 249: 510-515.

2 Acosta S, Ogren M, Bengtsson H et al. Increasing incidence of ruptured abdominal aortic aneurysm: a population-based study. *J Vasc Surg* 2006; 44: 237-243.

3 Heller JA, Weinberg A, Arons R et al. Two decades of abdominal aortic aneurysm repair: have we made any progress? *J Vasc Surg* 2000; 32: 1091-1100.

4 Bengtsson H, Bergqvist D. Ruptured abdominal aortic aneurysm: a population-based study. *J Vasc Surg* 1993; 18: 74-80.

5 Bown MJ, Sutton AJ, Bell PR et al. A meta-analysis of 50 years of ruptured abdominal aortic aneurysm repair. *Br J Surg* 2002; 89: 714-730.

6 Visser P, Akkersdijk GJ, Blankensteijn JD. In-hospital operative mortality of ruptured abdominal aortic aneurysm: a population-based analysis of 5593 patients in The Netherlands over a 10-year period. *Eur J Vasc Endovasc Surg* 2005; 30: 359-364.

7 Anonymous. EVAR trial participants. Endovascular aneurysm repair versus open repair in patients with abdominal aortic aneurysm (EVAR trial 1): randomised controlled trial. *Lancet*; 365: 2179-2186.

8 Blankensteijn JD, de Jong SE, Prinssen M et al. Two-year outcomes after conventional or endovascular repair of abdominal aortic aneurysms. *N Engl J Med* 2005; 352: 2398-2405.

9 Lederle FA, Freischlag JA, Kyriakides TC et al; Open Versus Endovascular Repair (OVER) Veterans Affairs Cooperative Study Group. Outcomes following endovascular vs open repair of abdominal aortic aneurysm: a randomized trial. *JAMA* 2009; 302: 1535-1542.

10 Alonso-Pérez M, Segura RJ, Sánchez J et al. Factors increasing the mortality rate for patients with ruptured abdominal aortic aneurysms. *Ann Vasc Surg* 2001; 15: 601-607.

11 Rayt HS, Sutton AJ, London NJ et al. A systematic review and meta-analysis of endovascular repair (EVAR) for ruptured abdominal aortic aneurysm. *Eur J Vasc Endovasc Surg* 2008; 36: 536-544.

12 Harkin DW, Dillon M, Blair PH et al. Endovascular ruptured abdominal aortic aneurysm repair (EVRAR): a systematic review. *Eur J Vasc Endovasc Surg* 2007; 34: 673-681.

13 Visser JJ, van Sambeek MR, Hamza TH et al. Ruptured abdominal aortic aneurysms: endovascular repair versus open surgery–systematic review. *Radiology* 2007; 245: 122-129.

14 Mastracci TM, Garrido-Olivares L, Cinà CS et al. Endovascular repair of ruptured abdominal aortic aneurysms: a systematic review and meta-analysis. *J Vasc Surg* 2008; 47: 214-221.

15 Veith FJ, Ohki T, Lipsitz EC et al. Endovascular grafts and other catheter-directed techniques in the management of ruptured abdominal aortic aneurysms. *Semin Vasc Surg* 2003; 16: 326-331.

16 Lloyd GM, Bown MJ, Norwood MG et al. Feasibility of preoperative computer tomography in patients with ruptured abdomi-

nal aortic aneurysm: a time-to-death study in patients without operation. *J Vasc Surg* 2004; 39: 788-791.

17 Boyle JR, Gibbs PJ, Kruger A et al. Existing delays following the presentation of ruptured abdominal aortic aneurysm allow sufficient time to assess patients for endovascular repair. *Eur J Vasc Endovasc Surg* 2005; 29: 505-509.

18 Hartung O, Vidal V, Marani I et al. Treatment of an early type II endoleak causing hemorrhage after endovascular aneurysm repair for ruptured abdominal aortic aneurysm. *J Vasc Surg* 2007; 45: 1062-1065.

19 Hinchliffe RJ, Singh-Ranger R, Davidson IR et al. Rupture of an abdominal aortic aneurysm secondary to type II endoleak. *Eur J Vasc Endovasc Surg* 2001; 22: 563-565.

20 Rose DF, Davidson IR, Hinchliffe RJ et al. Anatomical suitability of ruptured abdominal aortic aneurysms for endovascular repair. *J Endovasc Ther* 2003; 10: 453-457.

21 Hinchliffe RJ, Bruijstens L, MacSweeney ST et al. A randomised trial of endovascular and open surgery for ruptured abdominal aortic aneurysm - results of a pilot study and lessons learned for future studies. *Eur J Vasc Endovasc Surg* 2006; 32: 506-515.

22 Peppelenbosch N, Geelkerken RH, Soong C et al. Endograft treatment of ruptured abdominal aortic aneurysms using the Talent aortouniiliac system: an international multicenter study. *J Vasc Surg* 2006; 43: 1111-1123.

23 Ockert S, Schumacher H, Böckler D et al. Early and midterm results after open and endovascular repair of ruptured abdominal aortic aneurysms in a comparative analysis. *J Endovasc Ther* 2007; 14: 324-332.

24 Visser JJ, Bosch JL, Hunink MG et al. Endovascular repair versus open surgery in patients with ruptured abdominal aortic aneurysms: clinical outcomes with 1-year follow-up. *J Vasc Surg* 2006; 44: 1148-1155.

16

CURRENT PRACTICE AND GUIDELINES FOR AAA TREATMENT

WISSAM AL-JUNDI, JONATHAN BEARD

The management of infra-renal abdominal aortic aneurysm (AAA) has undergone huge changes over the last two decades. Advances include endovascular aneurysm repair (EVAR), better knowledge of the timing of intervention and the introduction of screening programs. These advances have led to a reduction of operative mortality for elective repair of AAA. However, the fate of patients with ruptured AAA (rAAA) may have changed little over the past decade. This chapter presents a brief review of the current evidence underpinning current practice and guidelines for AAA treatment. The specifics of the individual treatments are discussed in the preceding chapters.

Population screening for AAA

Several characteristics of AAA make it an ideal disease for screening:

1) it is a common condition, affecting about 5% of men aged 65 to 74 years;
2) B-mode ultrasound scanning using portable equipment has been shown to be an accurate, fast, inexpensive and acceptable method of screening with an estimated sensitivity and specificity of 98 and 99%, respectively;
3) the majority of AAAs are asymptomatic, with a long latent period between initial development and rupture;
4) elective repair of asymptomatic AAA has a operative mortality < 6% compared to an mortality of 85% for rAAA (30%-50% operative mortality).

Evidence for screening

The benefits of screening to reduce AAA related mortality has become clear following several trials of screening and a recent Cochrane Review [1].

The UK Multicenter Aneurysm Screening Study (MASS) trial [2] has provided convincing evidence that the prevalence of aneurysm-related death is reduced significantly in a screened male population aged 65-74 years, with a 53% reduction in those who attended for screening. Other added benefits included a reduction in the emergency workload for ruptured aneurysms, and cardiovascular risk assessment with appropriate lifestyle advice and pharmacological therapy. Because other causes of death overshadow those due to rAAA, it has not been possible to demonstrate a statistically significant overall survival advantage for the screened population. Nevertheless, the case for population-based screening for AAA is convincing. The MASS trial data showed that over 4 years the mean incremental cost-effectiveness ratio for screening was £ 28 400 per life-year gained, equivalent to approximately £ 36 000 per quality-adjusted life-year. It was estimated that this would fall to approximately £ 8 000 per life-year gained at 10 years. The long-term costs of AAA screening therefore compare favorably with breast and cervical cancer screening programs in terms of cost-effectiveness. The recent Cochrane Review [1] has identified three other randomized controlled trials (RCTs), from Chichester in the UK, Western Australia, and Viborg in Denmark, which assessed screening for AAAs. Results from the review showed a significant decrease in aneurysm-related mortality in men but not in women. In addition, there was a decreased incidence of ruptured aneurysms in men together with a manageable increase in elective surgery. Despite these impressive findings, the cost-effectiveness was questioned and further assessment recommended. A meta-analysis of the mid- and long-term effects of screening for aneurysms[3] has confirmed these findings. National screening programs for AAA in men are now being introduced in many countries in Europe and North America.

Medical management of asymptomatic AAA

Medical management of patients with AAA is important for several reasons:

1) these patients have an increased risk of cardiovascular death and therapy to reduce cardiovascular events is essential;
2) some of these therapies might slow aneurysm growth;
3) medical therapy for those undergoing AAA repair may reduce peri-operative risk.

Treatment is in line with the medical management of coronary, cerebral and peripheral artery disease and includes blood pressure control, cholesterol reduction, antiplatelet therapy and smoking cessation [4]. There have been no randomized trials of cardiovascular risk reduction in patients with AAA, and so current recommendations mostly derive from risk reduction trials in patients with other cardiovascular disease and observational studies (often retrospective) of patients with AAA. The most important modifiable risk factor in those with small AAA is cigarette smoking as this is associated with more rapid expansion rates. Dyslipidemia and hypertension are less powerful risk factors for AAA. The use of statins has been associated with an improved survival after AAA repair, with a more than three-fold reduction in risk of cardiovascular death associated with statin usage, HR 0.3 (95%CI 0.2-0.6) $p < 0.001$ in a retrospective single center series and a similar risk reduction in the EUROSTAR registry [4]. The results of the Heart Protection study suggest that all AAA patients should receive statin therapy, irrespective of serum cholesterol concentration [5]. The preferred first line drug for the treatment of hypertension in most of these older patients is an angiotensin converting enzyme (ACE) inhibitor [6]. Despite an absence of prospective studies investigating the likely benefit of anti-platelet therapy on AAA progression, it should be an important aspect of general cardiovascular risk reduction in the patient with AAA. The use of beta-blockers to improve peri-operative cardiac morbidity and mortality remains controversial [7]. Similarly, the role of antibiotics in treating secondary chlamydial infection to slow progression of aneurysm expansion remains unclear. Large scale randomized trials are necessary to evaluate the effectiveness of these pharmacotherapuetic agents in the medical management of AAA.

Surgical management of asymptomatic AAA

In the absence of symptoms, the principal determinant for intervention in the management of asymptomatic AAA remains the aneurysm diameter, although other parameters such as aneurysm volume have been suggested. Currently, the threshold for repair is accepted as ≥ 5.5 cm in diameter for men and ≥ 5 cm for women. For men, this diameter is based on the results of the UK small aneurysm trial (UKSAT) [8] and the US Aneurysm Detection and Management (ADAM) trial [9]. These studies did not have a sufficient number of women to precisely identify the size threshold for repair. The threshold of 5 cm for women is based on a higher rate of rupture of aneurysms < 5.5 cm in women. For small AAAs (4.0-5.5 cm diameter), there has been considerable debate as to the most beneficial course of treatment, i.e. immediate

Table I CHARACTERISTICS OF UKSAT AND ADAM TRIALS

		UKSAT	*ADAM*
Participants	Country	United Kingdom	United States
	N	1 090	1 136
	Age	60-76 years	50-79 years
	Sex	M (n = 902) F (n = 188)	M (n=1126) F (n=10)
Interventions	Open AAA repair	n = 563	n = 569
	Surveillance	n = 527	n = 567

surgery versus surveillance and selective repair of AAAs that subsequently enlarge. This "grey area" of care led to the design of the UK Small Aneurysm Trial (UKSAT) and the ADAM trials.

SMALL ANEURYSMS TRIALS

Two trials, the UKSAT [8] and ADAM [9] trials, were designed to provide guidelines as to when to offer elective surgery on the basis of aneurysm size (Table I). Both trials addressed the difficult dilemma of how to manage patients in whom the risks of surgery and rupture are similar. Therefore, they enrolled patients with small (4.0 to 5.5 cm) non-tender, asymptomatic AAAs who were considered to be fit for immediate surgery. In both trials, the 30-day operative mortality in the immediate surgery group (5.5% UKSAT and 2.1% ADAM) led to an early disadvantage in terms of survival in this study group. The lower 30-day operative mortality rate observed in the ADAM trial was expected due to restricting inclusion criteria to fit patients with better lung and renal function. On the other hand, there was no statistically significant difference in long-term survival between the immediate surgery and surveillance groups. In the UKSAT study, the long-term mortality rate (range 8 to 12 years, mean 10 years) was 63.9% in the immediate surgery group and 67.3% in the surveillance group (adjusted hazard ratio [HR] 0.88, 95% CI 0.75 to 1.02) (Fig. 1). At the end of the study follow up (range 3.5 to 8.0 years, mean 4.9 years), the observed mortalities for the ADAM trial in the immediate repair and the selective surveillance groups were 25.1% and 21.5%, respectively. A recent Cochrane Review [10] of these two trials performed a meta-analysis of mortality at six years and revealed no overall advantage to early surgery for small AAA (4.0 to 5.5 cm). However, it provided no additional guidelines for "best care" management of subgroups of patients (for example, by age or aneurysm size) due to lack of power in each of the trials for such analyses. Brown et al. [11] demonstrated no evidence to suggest any benefit in operating early in a review of a cohort of the fittest patients from UKSAT trial. The results of the individual patient data (IPD) re-analysis of the UKSAT and ADAM studies are awaited. Future research regarding the management of AAA should focus on non-Caucasians and women, as data regarding these populations are lacking.

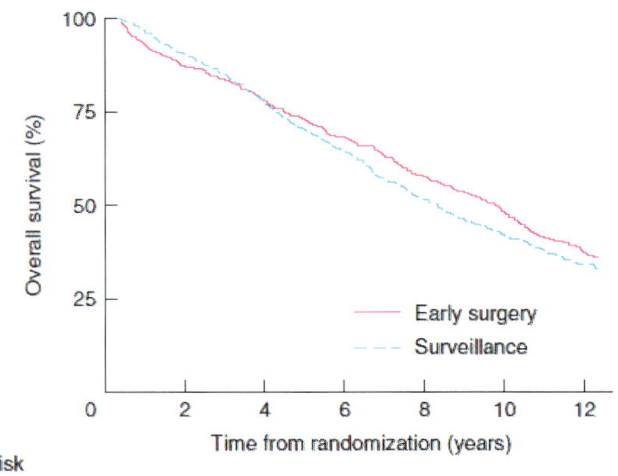

No. at risk							
Surgery	563	488	428	375	318	255	118
Surveillance	527	466	393	329	261	215	69

FIG. 1 Kaplan-Meier estimates of overall survival from UKSAT.

The lower peri-operative mortality associated with EVAR has reopened the debate about intervention for small AAAs. Two trials are currently comparing EVAR with surveillance: the PIVOTAL trial that began in 2005 and the CAESAR trial that began in 2004 [12]. When complete, the results of these trials should provide objective evidence to guide the use of EVAR for small AAAs.

Surveillance of patients with small aneurysms

There is no evidence from the randomized trials about the best surveillance program for small AAAs. Patients with AAAs of < 5.5 cm diameter should be managed conservatively with best medical therapy and regular surveillance by interval ultrasound scanning. The timing of such scans remains controversial, requiring a balance between cost, inconvenience and patient safety. It has recently been shown that an aorta with a diameter of < 3 cm in a male aged 65 years of age or over is associated with minimal risk of eventual rupture, hence there is probably no justification for continued surveillance. For larger aneurysms, there is no robust evidence-base upon which to base a surveillance programme. However, it is generally accepted that screening intervals of one year for aneurysms of 3.5-4.4 cm and 6 months for those of 4.5-5.4 cm would appear to be appropriate. From a meta-analysis of 13 studies, Law et al. [13] have quantified the annual AAA rupture risk in relation to size risk for differing initial size (Table II).

Table II Annual AAA Rupture Risk in relation to size (adapted from Law et al. [13])

AAA size (cm)	*Risk of rupture per year (%)*
< 3.0	0
3-3.9	0.4
4-4.9	1.1
5-5.9	3.3
6-6.9	9.4
7-7.9	24

Elective AAA repair

The therapeutic strategy for a patient with an asymptomatic AAA must be determined on an individual basis, as the risks of treatment must be balanced against the risk of death from rupture of aneurysm. When considering intervention, three key elements need to be considered:

1) Is intervention justified (aneurysm diameter > 5.5 cm)?
2) Is the patient fit enough for intervention?
3) Is the morphology of the AAA suitable for EVAR?

Contrary to open AAA repair (OR), EVAR suitability largely depends upon aneurysm morphology. The number of patients with aneurysms who are suitable for endovascular repair is steadily increasing with increasing operator experience, relaxation of morphological contra-indications and advances in graft technology.

Evidence for EVAR

Since the launch of endovascular repair, there has been a steady accumulation of evidence regarding its safety and efficacy. Most of the published evidence originates from large national and international registries and prospective RCTs. The project of European collaborators on stent-graft technique for AAA repair (EUROSTAR) [14] registry was established in February 1996 with the purpose of collating and investigating an extensive multicenter experience on endovascular repair AAA repair. The Registry for Endovascular Treatment of Aneurysms (RETA) [15] was established to collect data on EVAR from UK Centers since 1996. With one thousand cases submitted to the registry by 2000, it informed the design of the UK randomized trials (EVAR 1 and 2). The EVAR 1 trial recruited 1 082 UK patients aged 60 years or older with AAA of at least 5.5 cm [16]. Patient considered fit for OR and morphologically suitable for EVAR were randomized to EVAR or OR. The EVAR 2 trial assigned 338 patients who were deemed unfit for open repair to receive either EVAR or no intervention [17]. Both trials measured the following outcomes: mortality, postoperative complications, hospitals costs and quality of life. In the Dutch Randomized Endovascular Aneurysm Management (DREAM) trial [18], 345 patients with AAA ≥ 5 cm were randomly assigned to undergo open repair or EVAR. Primary end-points included mortality and complications. In addition to registry data and RCTs, large cohort series and meta-analyses have contributed to the weight of evidence for EVAR.

SHORT-TERM OUTCOMES

The UK EVAR 1 trial reported a 30-day mortality of 1.7% for EVAR versus 4.7% for OR. Similar outcomes were reported for the DREAM trial (30-day mortalities for endovascular repair and open repair of 1.2% and 4.6%, respectively). A slightly higher 30-day mortality following EVAR has been reported in non-randomized trials and case series. The short-term survival advantage of EVAR over open repair is more durable among older patients as shown by a propensity analysis of Medicare population (2.1% difference for those 67 to 69 years old vs. 8.5% for those 85 years and older, $p < 0.001$) [19].

Other procedure-related outcomes from the randomized trials show the differences that one might expect from a minimally invasive procedure, with a shorter stay in hospital, a reduced use of critical care facilities and a lower mean blood loss [1]. The DREAM trial showed EVAR patients had a mean duration of stay in intensive care of 16 hours compared with 72 hours required by open-repair patients ($p < 0.001$) and a total hospital stay of 6 days rather than 13 days ($p < 0.001$). EVAR 1 showed a similarly reduced mean hospital stay of 7 days rather than 12 days ($p < 0.001$). It has become clear now that unless patients have severe co-morbidity, a routine stay on the intensive care unit is unnecessary. The DREAM trial also showed that EVAR is associated with significantly less blood loss (394 mL versus 1 654 mL) and decreased transfusion requirements (6% of patients versus 72%). The development of low-profile endograft delivery systems has enabled wholly percutanous procedures without the need for femoral cut-downs. This can lower blood loss during the procedure and enable earlier ambulation and discharge from hospital. EVAR was associated with specific complications that were not seen following open repair, with technical failure or persistent endoleaks being recorded in 0.2% of patients at 30 days, early rupture within 30 days in 0.3% and primary conversion to open repair in 1.7%.

LONG-TERM OUTCOMES

Although there is little controversy about the short-term benefit of endovascular aortic aneurysm repair compared with open repair, there is concern that the long-term outcomes of endovascular aortic aneurysm repair may be less favourable. There are few large-scale evaluations of the comparative long-term outcomes of EVAR versus open repair. At 4-year follow-up; the EVAR 1 trial revealed maintenance of the early advantage for endovascular repair over open repair with respect to aneurysm-related deaths (4% in the EVAR group versus 7% in the open-surgery group), however the all-cause mortality was similar in both groups at around 28% (Fig. 2). Similarly, the aneurysm-related deaths in

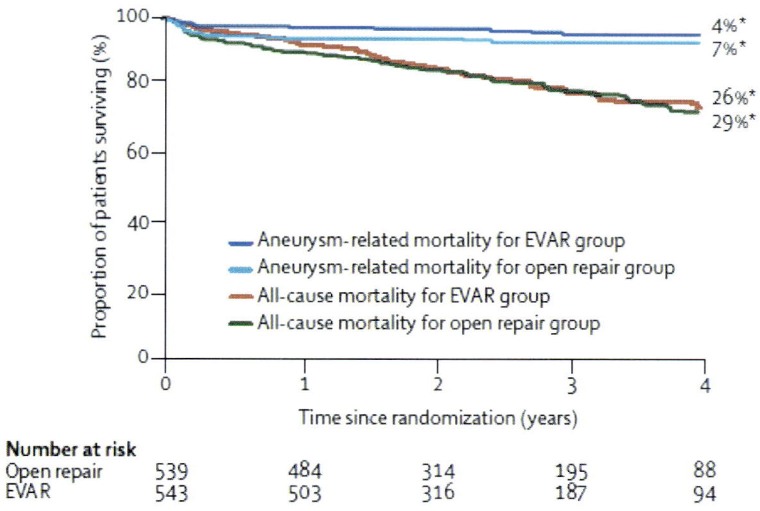

FIG. 2 Kaplan-Meier estimates of survival and survival free from aneurysm-related death (EVAR 1 Trial)
*Mortality 4-year point estimates

the DREAM trial were lower at 2 years in the EVAR group (2.1% versus 5.7%, p = 0.05) and survival of both groups was equivalent at 89.6% and 89.7% for the open repair and endovascular-repair groups, respectively.

The EVAR 1 and DREAM trials showed a significant improvement in the quality of life of EVAR patients during the first 3 months following their procedure. This is hardly surprising given the major trauma, post-operative pain, reduced ambulation and longer hospital stay following open repair. However, it is interesting that this 3-month dip in the quality of life of the OR group disappears thereafter when both groups enjoy a similar quality of life. Moreover, the quality of life of the EVAR group might suffer more on the long term due to the increased surveillance programme and re-intervention, where necessary.

The propensity analysis of Medicare beneficiaries undergoing open and endovascular repair compared 22 830 matched patients in each cohort [19]. Despite expected lower peri-operative mortality after endovascular repair compared to open repair (1.2% vs. 4.8%, p < 0.001), late survival was similar in the two cohorts, although the survival curves did not converge until after 3 years. By 4 years, rupture was more likely in the endovascular-repair cohort than in the open-repair cohort (1.8% vs. 0.5%, p < 0.001), as was intervention related to AAA (9.0% vs. 1.7%, p < 0.001), although most reinterventions were minor. In contrast, by 4 years, surgery for laparotomy-related complications was more likely among patients who had undergone open repair (9.7%, vs. 4.1% among those who had undergone endovascular repair; p < 0.001), as was hospitalization without surgery for bowel obstruction or abdominal-wall hernia (14.2% vs. 8.1%, p < 0.001). Thus, late interventions related to AAA repair are more common after endovascular repair but are balanced by an increase in laparotomy-related reinterventions and hospitalizations after open surgery.

With regard to cost-effectiveness, EVAR 1 reported an increased mean cost of EVAR (£ 13 257) compared with open repair (£ 9 946) at 4 years. This was mainly due to the initial cost of the graft and the cost of graft surveillance and re-intervention, which outweighed the savings in intensive care and hospital stay (Fig. 3). However, most patients with type II endoleaks are now managed conservatively unless there is evidence of aneurysm sac enlargement. This, and advances in graft technology, has significantly reduced re-intervention rates since the trial and graft surveillance is also becoming less expensive (see below).

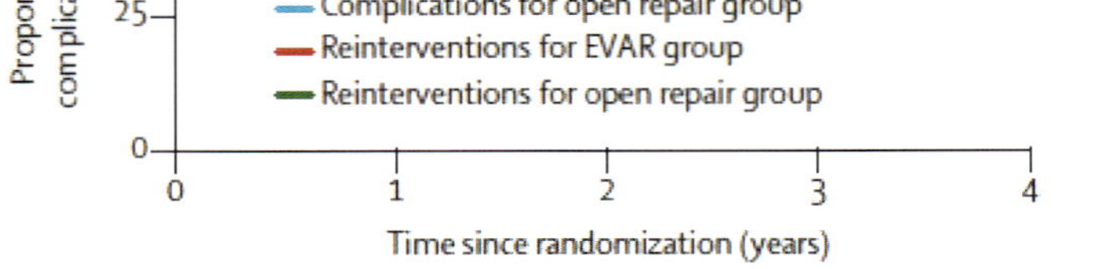

Number at risk for complications					
Open repair	539	466	301	182	82
EVAR	543	386	235	134	67
Number at risk for reinterventions					
No intervention	539	468	304	189	88
EVAR	543	450	278	168	80

FIG. 3 Kaplan-Meier estimates of post-operative complications and re-interventions (EVAR 1 Trial)
*4-year point estimates for patients with complications or re-interventions

Unfit patients

The EVAR 2 trial aimed to identify whether EVAR improves survival compared with no intervention in patients unfit for open repair of aortic aneurysm [17]. It randomized 338 patients who were deemed unfit for open repair to receive either EVAR or no intervention. The trial showed a much higher 30 day mortality rate from EVAR in unfit patients (9%) compared to EVAR in fit patients in the EVAR trial 1 (1.7%). The conclusion was that EVAR is not a safe procedure in such patients, although several non-randomized cohort studies have since reported acceptable mortality rates for high-risk patients (who were perhaps not quite so unfit). There was also a greater difference in hospital costs between EVAR and no intervention (£ 13 632 vs. £ 4 983, respectively), because in the EVAR trial 2, the alternative to EVAR was no surgical intervention which is inexpensive. The main cost in the no intervention arm was from patients who subsequently crossed over and received an EVAR (see later). The all-cause mortality rates were comparable among unfit patients who received EVAR or had no intervention in the EVAR 2 trial (66% vs. 62%, p = 0.25), however, the curves for aneurysm related mortality did cross at about 2 years, raising the possibility of a late benefit for the EVAR group (Figs. 4, 5). Extended follow-up

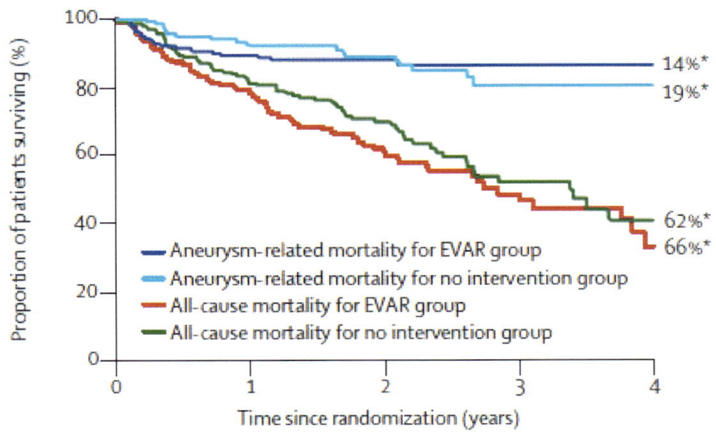

Number at risk

No intervention	172	139	71	29	9
EVAR	166	129	58	23	6

FIG. 4 Kaplan-Meier estimates of survival and survival free from aneurysm-related death (EVAR 2 Trial)
*Mortality 4-year point estimates

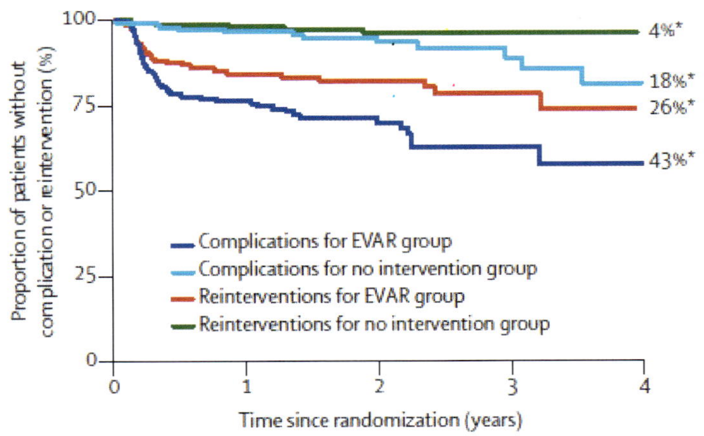

Number at risk for complications

No intervention	172	137	69	26	7
EVAR	166	105	47	14	5

Number at risk for reinterventions

No intervention	172	137	70	29	9
EVAR	166	115	55	20	7

FIG. 5 Kaplan-Meier estimates of post-operative complications and re-interventions (EVAR 2 Trial)
*4-year point estimates for patients with complications or re-interventions

is needed to clarify any association, but given that only one third of these unfit patients are expected to live beyond 4 years, a clear difference is unlikely to emerge. There was no consistent difference in the quality of life between the two randomized groups in the EVAR trial 2. The EVAR trial 2 had several limitations. Firstly, it enrolled a sample size calculated to yield 90% power to detect 10% difference in all cause mortality between the two groups (25% in the no intervention group vs. 15% in the EVAR group). However, the mortality in the no intervention group was lower than that expected while it was higher than predicted in the EVAR group. Thus, another trial with a larger sample size and longer follow-up is needed to demonstrate the presence or absence of difference between the two groups. Secondly, more than a quarter of patients assigned to no intervention for their aneurysm underwent aneurysm repair. Finally, there was sometimes lengthy interval between randomization and surgery in the EVAR group which resulted in ruptures and deaths prior to surgery in the EVAR group. Despite its limitations, the EVAR trial 2 demonstrated that in patients who are unfit for open repair, EVAR is costly and has little benefit. The focus in these patients should be on improving fitness rather than early EVAR. If fitness can be improved, then EVAR may then become justified.

Surveillance after EVAR

Lifelong surveillance is essential for the safe treatment of patients with endoluminal devices to monitor the integrity of the endograft, absence of endoleaks, and shrinkage of the aneurysm sac. Such requirement is often quoted as a disadvantage of EVAR. The standard surveillance protocol requires computed tomography angiography (CTA) before discharge or at 4-6 weeks, and further CTAs at 3 months, 12 months, and at annual intervals thereafter; similar to the follow-up protocol used in the EVAR 1 trial. This surveillance program subjects the patient to a high radiation exposure and is expensive. Duplex ultrasound is not as sensitive in the detection of type II endoleaks compared with CT, but B-mode ultrasound can accurately measure aneurysm sac diameter. Since type II endoleaks without increasing sac diameter are not associated with a significant risk of adverse clinical events, this may be regarded as an acceptable limitation. Plain abdominal radiographs in the anteroposterior and lateral projections can assess graft migration, stent fractures and modular disconnections. It is comparatively inexpensive and usefully complements ultrasound scanning. Used in combination these two methods represent a potentially acceptable, less expensive and less hazardous alternative to CT for surveillance.

Management of acutely symptomatic or rAAA

The overall mortality of ruptured aneurysms (rAAA) exceeds 85%. Many of these patients die in the community. Of those who reach hospital, half or more die before reaching the operating theater. Only about 50% of patients who reach operating theater for open repair will leave hospital alive. These stark figures have changed little over the last 50 years. The question is whether emergency EVAR (eEVAR) can improve the depressing mortality associated with open repair for rAAA. Evidence from several studies has shown that the aneurysm morphology is significantly more challenging compared with those undergoing elective EVAR. In particular many centers accept inferior proximal neck anatomy, which would normally preclude patients from elective EVAR.

eEVAR can be associated with higher survival rate following rAAA and has the potential to reduce the costly in-hospital care of these patients. The lower mortality rate of eEVAR may be due to several reasons, including the avoidance of laparatomy and lesser requirements for anesthetic agents and transfusion. Despite these obvious potential advantages, several recent reports have failed to demonstrate a survival benefit for EVAR over open repair when an attempt has been made to compare the two procedures in a randomized fashion.

Evidence of EVAR for rAAA

There have been four RCTs that compared eEVAR with OR for rAAA. Of these, only one small pilot RCT from Nottingham has published its results [20]. Out of 103 patients with suspected rAAA considered for the trial, it recruited only 32 patients. All patients were suitable for open repair and randomized into EVAR or open repair at time of diagnosis. Those who were to receive EVAR had CT scan to confirm suitability for EVAR. The low rate of patient randomization (31%) could be explained by the broad exclusion criteria applied, including: patient unfit for open repair; death before randomization; inability to give informed consent; age; refusal of operation; no team available; surgeon preference. On an intention to treat analysis, the study revealed a 30-day mortality rate of 53% in both the EVAR group and open repair group. If patients who died after randomization but before intervention are excluded, mortality for EVAR would be 54%, including 2 EVAR failures requiring open conversions (1 survivor; 1 non-survivor), compared to 43% mortality for the open group. Moderate or severe operative complications occurred in 77% in the EVAR group and in 80% in the open repair group. Severe renal complications were significantly more common in the EVAR group compared to open repair (55% vs. 7%, $p < 0.02$). Median total hospital in the EVAR group was 10 days (6-28) and 12 days (4-52) in the open repair group. Median time between diagnosis and operation was 75 minutes (64-126) in the EVAR group and 100 minutes (48-138) in the open repair group. The above study not only lacked sufficient power to generalize the results, but also suffered from selection bias. Despite these limitations, the study showed that it is possible to perform an ethical randomized study of EVAR compared with open repair for rAAA. In addition, it challenged the concerns that CT scanning prior to surgery causes detriment to the patient, as the time interval between arrival and operation was similar in the two groups. However, it highlighted the significant logistical problems in having a fully trained, equipped, and committed endovascular team available at all times.

Three other RCTs have started to evaluate EVAR for rAAA, one in Amsterdam (the AJAX trial), one in France (the ECAR trial) and one in the UK (the IMPROVE trial). The AJAX and ECAR recruit patients who are hemodynamically stable to undergo CT scan and if they are anatomically suitable for endovascular repair, are offered randomization to either EVAR or open repair. The AJAX trial originally planned to randomise 80 patients, but more recently recruitment has been extended to 120 patients because of a better than expected mortality after OR. The ECAR trial proposes to recruit 160 patients. The IMPROVE [21] trial has adopted randomization at the time of clinical diagnosis of ruptured AAA. Starting in 2009, this trial proposes to randomize 600 patients and will also record the outcomes of excluded patients.

The publication of the results of these trials will hopefully provide Level 1 evidence for the efficacy and safety of eEVAR for rAAA. In the absence of these results, the best evidence on the topic comes from systematic reviews. There have been at least three separate systematic reviews, all finding a lower operative mortality for endovascular repair (ranging from 18% to 22%), but all reviews comment on biases in patient selection and publication [22]. A recent appraisal by the UK National Institute for Health and Clinical Excellence (NICE) has concluded that eEVAR is not recommended for patients with rAAA, except in the context of research [21]. It has also been suggested that the expense required to support the infrastructure for eEVAR would be better spent on an AAA screening program.

REFERENCES

1 Cosford PA, Leng GC. Screening for abdominal aortic aneurysm. *Cochrane Database Syst Rev* 2007; 2: CD002945.

2 Thompson SG, Ashton HA et al. Multicentre Aneurysm Screening Study Group. Screening men for abdominal aortic aneurysm: 10 year mortality and cost effectiveness results from the randomised Multicentre Aneurysm Screening Study. *BMJ* 2009; 338: b2307.

3 Lindholt JS, Norman P. Screening for abdominal aortic aneurysm reduces the overall mortality in men. A meta-analysis of the mid and long term effects of screening for abdominal aortic aneurysms. *Eur J Vasc Endovasc Surg* 2008; 36: 167-171.

4 Golledge J, Powell JT. Medical management of abdominal aortic aneurysm. *Eur J Vasc Endovasc Surg* 2007; 34: 267-273.

5 Anonymous. Heart Protection Study Collaborative Group. MRC/BHF Heart Protection Study of cholesterol lowering with simvastatin in 20,536 high-risk individuals: a randomized placebo-controlled trial. *Lancet* 2002;360:7-22.

6 Sever P. New hypertension guidelines from the national institute for health and clinical excellence and the British Hypertension Society. J *Renin Angiotensin Aldosterone Syst* 2006; 7: 61-63.

7 Howell SJ, Vohra RS. Perioperative management of patients undergoing non-cardiac vascular surgery. *Eur J Vasc Endovasc Surg* 2007; 34: 625-631.

8 Powell JT, Brown LC, Forbes JF et al. Final 12-year follow-up of surgery versus surveillance in the UK Small Aneurysm Trial. *Br J Surg* 2008; 94: 702-708.

9 Lederle FA, Wilson SE, Johnson GR et al. Immediate repair compared with surveillance of small abdominal aortic aneurysms. *N Engl J Med* 2002; 346: 1437-1444.

10 Ballard DJ, Filardo G, Fowkes G et al. Surgery for small asymptomatic abdominal aortic aneurysms. *Cochrane Database Syst Rev* 2008; 4: CD001835.

11 Brown LC, Thompson SG, Greenhalgh RM et al. Fit patients with small abdominal aortic aneurysms (AAAs) do not benefit from early intervention. *J Vasc Surg* 2008; 48: 1375-1381.

12 Cao P. CAESAR trial collaborators. Comparison of surveillance *vs* Aortic Endografting for Small Aneurysm Repair (CAESAR) Trial: Study Design and Progress. *Eur J Vasc Endovasc Surg* 2005; 30: 245-251.

13 Law MR, Morris J, Wald NJ. Screening for abdominal aortic aneurysms. *J Med Screen* 1994; 1: 110-115.

14 Harris PL, Buth J, Mialhe C et al. The need for clinical trials of endovascular abdominal aortic aneurysm stent-graft repair: The EUROSTAR Project. EUROpean collaborators on Stent-graft Techniques for abdominal aortic Aneurysm Repair. *J Endovasc Surg* 1997; 4: 72-77.

15 Thomas SM, Beard JD, Ireland M et al. Results from the prospective registry of endovascular treatment of abdominal aortic aneurysms (RETA): mid term results to five years. *Eur J Vasc Endovasc Surg* 2005; 29: 563-570.

16 Greenhalgh RM, Brown LC, Kwong GP et al. EVAR trial participants. Endovascular aneurysm repair versus open repair in patients with abdominal aortic aneurysm (EVAR trial 1): randomised controlled trial. *Lancet* 2005; 365: 2179-2186.

17 Anonymous. EVAR trial participants. Endovascular aneurysm repair and outcome in patients unfit for open repair of abdominal aortic aneurysm (EVAR trial 2): randomised controlled trial. *Lancet* 2005; 365: 2187-2192.

18 Prinssen M, Verhoeven EL, Buth J et al. Dutch Randomized Endovascular Aneurysm Management (DREAM)Trial Group. A randomized trial comparing conventional and endovascular repair of abdominal aortic aneurysms. *N Engl J Med* 2004; 351: 1607-1618.

19 Schermerhorn ML, O'Malley AJ, Jhaveri A et al. Endovascular vs. open repair of abdominal aortic aneurysms in the Medicare population. *N Engl J Med* 2008; 358: 464-474.

20 Hinchliffe RJ, Bruijstens L, MacSweeney ST et al. A randomised trial of endovascular and open surgery for ruptured abdominal aortic aneurysm - results of a pilot study and lessons learned for future studies. *Eur J Vasc Endovasc Surg* 2006; 32: 506-513.

21 Powell JT. Time to IMPROVE the management of ruptured abdominal aortic aneurysm: IMPROVE trialists. *Eur J Vasc Endovasc Surg* 2009; 38: 237-238.

22 Rayt HS, Sutton AJ, London NJ et al. A systematic review and meta-analysis of endovascular repair (EVAR) for ruptured abdominal aortic aneurysm. Eur J Vasc Endovasc Surg 2008; 36: 536-544.

17

THE IDEAL EDUCATIONAL CURRICULUM OF THE VASCULAR SPECIALIST

THOMAS KOEPPEL, MICHAEL JACOBS

In most European countries, the profile of the classical "vascular surgeon" has evolved towards that of a "vascular specialist" within the last decade. Not only do vascular surgeons perform open vascular procedures, but nowadays they also routinely perform endovascular techniques. Consequently, national training programs for vascular fellows have to be adapted to this "new qualification profile" to provide a basis for these trainees to acquire state-of-the-art technical skills and a profound theoretical background in vascular medicine. Because of a lack of medical doctors in European Union (EU) countries, it is moreover challenging to create attractive boundary conditions for training in vascular surgery so as to engage the interest of students and graduates to embrace this field. Therefore, an ideal educational curriculum consists of a modular training program that bolsters the trainee's experience level in both vascular as well as endovascular procedures. In addition, this training program may also provide a basis for an academic vascular surgery fellowship that combines both basic laboratory research and comprehensive clinical training. Even though the Union of Medical Specialists in Europe (UEMS) has proposed guidelines for coordinating the training in vascular surgery, there are still enormous deviations in the various curricula in Europe that reflect national priorities and boundary conditions. To counter these discrepancies, it is important to introduce uniform and binding educational aims and curricula in vascular surgery/medicine in order to facilitate excellent yet equal standards of open and endovascular procedures in Europe.

Background

Cardiovascular disease (CVD) is the main cause of death in Europe and accounts for 49% of all deaths and 30% of all premature deaths before the age of 65. Even though age-specific mortality rates from CVD have decreased by half in western Europe in the last 20 years, the prevalence of CVD is actually increasing due to an ageing population [1]. In the future, the demand for medical care, especially in cardiovascular medicine, will increase. Thus, it is not surprising that in some European countries the number of vascular departments has continuously grown in recent years, in parallel with an increasing demand for specialized and qualified vascular surgeons [2].

In the near future, these developments will lead to further problems, because already now, highly qualified doctors are lacking in the job market [3]. There are many reasons for this. First of all, since there is a general lack of doctors in European countries, there is already enormous competition among the various disciplines and industry to attract the best graduates. Moreover, fewer medical graduates are deciding to enter a surgical discipline, thereby aggravating the situation [4,5]. In order to effectively counter this negative development, attractive boundary conditions have to be created to entice medical graduates to train in vascular surgery. Besides favorable working conditions and an attractive salary in the field of vascular surgery, the actual quality of the education determines their career perspectives [6]. This, in itself, is a criterium for students to decide vascular surgery as their vocation.

Traditionally, vascular surgery has been incorporated as a subspecialty of general surgery. In recent years, however, vascular surgery has developed as an independent discipline with a high degree of specialization in most European countries [7]. This development has been accompanied by a change in the qualification profile of the so-called "modern" vascular surgeon. Besides classical open vascular reconstruction techniques, endovascular interventions are increasingly becoming a priority in this discipline. Thus, vascular surgeons are evolving to "vascular specialists" [8]. These changes demand that the training curriculum be fitted to accommodate these new requirements. In this regard, there have been many national initiatives to improve the curriculum in vascular surgery. These initiatives, however, often vary with respect to length of training, accreditation requirements, operative volume and type of procedures learned [7].

Up to now, each individual country of the EU has defined the specific vascular surgery curriculum as well as the accreditation of the training programs nationally [7]. Consequently, the training programs of the various countries often strongly deviate from one another. To ensure uniform standards in vascular surgical training throughout Europe, the European Board of Vascular Surgery (EBVS), which is a part of the Union of Medical Specialists in Europe (UEMS), has created a logbook that recommends open vascular and endovascular procedures that should be taught during vascular surgery training [9]. Furthermore, the EBVS gives the opportunity to acquire a European qualification, whereby candidates have to pass a theoretical and practical examination. Nonetheless, this particular specialist qualification does not replace an accreditation by the national medical board.

Because of this lack of uniform standards in vascular surgical training, it is utmost important from an European point of view, to create an "ideal educational curriculum" that facilitates uniform training programs and standardizes accreditation procedures in the individual European countries. Nevertheless, not only should the ideal curriculum meet the requirements of the state-of-the-art surgical and endovascular techniques, but it should also stay flexible by taking into account national boundary conditions. Thus, this "ideal educational curriculum" should be a guideline rather than a strict regulation. Therefore, it is important to prioritize specific educational aims in order to attain the desired qualification level. Ultimately, it is essential to clearly define the qualification profile of the "vascular specialist" in collaboration with all national European vascular societies. Even though the training of the vascular specialist takes place on a national platform, it has to be ensured that the targets of the curriculum have been attained. Furthermore, to guarantee better comparability among the various national vascular surgery programs, the final national board examinations each must meet uniform criteria for assessing the candidate's practical skills and knowledge in vascular surgery/medicine.

The ideal educational curriculum: principles and modular concept

The Logbook of the European Section and Board of Vascular Surgery already provides an excellent basis for a uniform European educational curriculum [9]. The "ideal educational curriculum" should provide a structured, modular training program (from "basic" to "advanced" procedures) in vascular and endovascular surgery. Moreover, candidates should acquire a profound theoretical background in vascular medicine. A continuous standardized assessment of the training success should be performed and documented. In addition to the technical skills, so-called "soft skills", i.e. interpersonal communication skills should also be evaluated and coached [10]. In addition, it would be useful to outline an academic curriculum for vascular surgery that includes basic laboratory research in conjunction with comprehensive clinical training to facilitate an academic career pathway.

Profile of the vascular specialist

Before one can establish the specific curriculum, it is important to first of all formulate what a vascular specialist should be able to do. Specifically speaking, what exact surgical and non-surgical procedures constitute expertise in vascular surgery/medicine? The aim for the candidate is to gain medical competence and personal confidence to effectively treat a broad spectrum of vascular patients. With respect to very specific and rather rare vascular diseases such as complex suprarenal, thoracic and thoraco-abdominal aortic aneurysms, it is not necessary to incorporate the teaching of how to treat such complex vascular pathologies in a standard educational curriculum. For these patients it has been documented, however, that the success of the treatment depends on the expertise of the surgeon and also on the volume of patients treated in a particular vascular center [11]. Consequently, it would be useful to train "high-end procedures" only in highly specialized vascular centers within a clearly defined framework of continuing education towards becoming a "vascular expert".

Thus, within the scope of an "ideal educational curriculum" in vascular surgery/medicine the following didactic aims should be considered:

- Open vascular procedures:
  - arterial reconstructions for aneurysms and occlusive disease;
  - venous surgical procedures (e.g. varicose veins, venous leg ulcerations);
  - major and minor limb amputation;
  - surgical management of chronic wounds;
  - treatment of vascular compression syndromes;
- Endovascular procedures:
  - percutaneous transluminal balloon and stent angioplasty;
  - intra-operative endovascular (hybrid) repair of iliac and femoro-popliteo-crural vessels;
  - endovascular aneurysm repair of thoracic (TEVAR) and abdominal aortic aneurysms (EVAR);
  - endovenous obliteration of varicose veins;
  - catheter-directed lysis of arterial and venous occlusion.
- Diagnostic procedures:
  - ankle brachial pressure index (ABPI) assessment;
  - measurement of walking distance and speed in patients with peripheral arterial disease;
  - B-mode sonography and color-coded Duplex sonography, plethysmography;
  - evaluation of magnetic resonance (MR)-angiographies (MRA), computed tomography (CT)-angiographies (CTA), digital subtraction angiography (DSA) and phlebographies;
  - assessment of cardiovascular risk factors, evaluation of diagnostic procedures (e.g. ECG, exercise ECG)
- Non-invasive procedures, adjuvant medical therapy:
  - management of thrombophilia, deep venous thrombosis and other venous pathologies (e.g. postthrombotic syndrome), inflammatory vascular disease;
  - intravenous treatment with vasodilatative drugs;
  - anticoagulant therapy;
  - comprehensive (non-surgical) wound management;
  - adjuvant medical therapy (e.g. treatment of hypertension, hyperlipidemia).

Structure of the educational curriculum

The duration of the training may vary and depends on the national speciality status (vascular surgery is either independent or subspeciality) and training requirements. However, it appears reasonable that the first two years of an integrated vascular training program should be devoted to a core surgical training, followed by at least four years of specific training in vascular and endovascular surgery (e.g. 2+4 program).

Core surgical training

In the first section (e.g. 2 years) of the training, the trainee should take core surgical training in general surgery but also in intensive care. During that time, trainees have to acquire general surgical and professional competencies which will enable the evaluation of a trainee's suitability for a career in vascular surgery. Furthermore, the core surgical training should deliver speciality-specific competencies that allow progress to higher surgical training.

Basic, intermediate and advanced training level

The special training in vascular surgery takes 4 years (in a 2+4 program) and can be based on the logbook of the European Section and Board of Vascular Surgery (Table). This training comprises all aspects of in-patient and out-patient care as well as postoperative care. In all, the surgical training may consist of different modules. In the basic training modules, the trainee learns to access various vascular regions as well as to master basic vascular reconstruction and suture techniques (e.g. embolectomy/thrombectomy, patch plasty). The endovascular basic training (e.g. percutaneous transluminal angioplasty with or without stent placement in the iliofemoral vascular axis) is likewise a fundamental component of the basic curriculum as well as the education in diagnostic techniques (Duplex sonography, angiography). To complement clinical training on actual patients, it is recommendable that the candidates take part in particular courses using simulators [12]. The basic training in vascular procedures is followed by an intermediate training level which involves more complex reconstructive procedures, such as anatomic/extra-anatomic bypasses, open and/or remote endarterectomies and various patching procedures in patients with stenotic or aneurysmal vascular disease. Moreover, candidates should be trained in vascular access surgery. The final training year should focus on advanced vascular and endovascular procedures for all types of vascular pathology. These procedures include the open and endovascular repair of abdominal and thoracic aortic aneurysms, treatment of visceral and renal artery stenotic/occlusive disease, management of supra-aortic vessel pathology and reconstruction/endovascular repair of very distal (e.g. crural/pedal) arteries. Furthermore, trainees should be able to diagnose and manage peri- and postprocedural complications, such as graft infections.

Assessment of skills

Quality control: The success of the candidate should be continuously checked by a mentor who evaluates the overall skills of a candidate from many perspectives (so-called "360°-evaluation"). Assessed here are: 1) surgical operative capabilities (such as preparation-operation planning, dexterity, theoretical knowledge, operation catalogue/logbook); 2) communicative and organizing skills (such as interaction with doctors, patients and nursing staff, time and patient management).

The curriculum leading to an academic career

In some countries (e.g. United Kingdom, United States of America), programs promoting young people in academia have long been established [13,14]. There, the career planning begins already at the end of university study or upon beginning professional life: students can decide whether they wish to pursue an academic career and can be directed towards teaching, or either clinical or basic research [15]. The analysis of individual educational programs has shown that basic research as a solid part of the clinical training significantly influences the scientific output, generation of third-party funding, and career perspectives (such as attaining professorships and chairs) [16,17]. Consequently, an "ideal educational curriculum" should encompass a structured academic education for novice vascular surgeons trained in academic institutions, such as university hospitals. Another objective of an "academic curriculum" is to provide the candidate with enough time and freedom to address a specific research theme in vascular medicine besides acquiring clinical and theoretical knowledge (Fig.).

Theoretical education

In the first part of training, interdisciplinary courses are offered for the trainees in the core surgical training program in collaboration with other surgical departments. The essential subjects of the curriculum encompass: 1) the introduction in the fundamentals of health economics; 2) the teaching of basic knowledge in scientific methods and statistics; 3) guidelines for critical appraisal of papers and scientific writing; and 4) courses in tutoring and oral presentation skills; furthermore,

Table THE LOGBOOK OF THE EUROPEAN SECTION AND BOARD OF VASCULAR SURGERY

OPEN VASCULAR PROCEDURES

I. Basic

- Embolectomy/thrombectomy with or without patch closure (excl. mesenteric and renal)
- Elements of arterial procedures: i.e. one anastomosis or arterial exposure without further reconstruction
- Miscellaneous:
  - Ligation (e.g. of traumatic bleed)
  - Suture closure (e.g. false aneurysm)

II. Intermediate

- All arterial procedures not specified as class I or III, including: bypass (anatomic or extra-anatomic), endarterectomy (open or remote), patching, interposition, or other reconstruction of stenotic, occlusive, or aneurysmal disease at the following levels: iliac, femoral, or popliteal and any sequential combination of these levels
- Access surgery (e.g. cimino, gracz, or loop arterio-venous fistula) (excl. catheters)

III. Advanced

- Bypass (anatomic or extra-anatomic), endarterectomy, patching, interposition, or other reconstruction of stenotic, occlusive, or aneurysmal disease of supra-aortic, arm, hand, thoracic aortic, juxta/suprarenal abdominal aortic, infrarenal aortic, tibial, or pedal arteries and any sequential combination of these levels
- Carotid endarterectomy or other carotid artery surgery (glomus tumors)
- Mesenteric or renal artery procedures (incl. embolectomy/thrombectomy)
- Venous reconstructions (except all superficial venous and perforator incompetence procedures)
- Vascular reconstructions for graft infection
- Microvascular repair of small blood vessels
- Porta-systemic shunts
- Renal, liver, or pancreas transplantation

ENDOVASCULAR PROCEDURES

I. Basic

- Diagnostic (percutaneous) arteriography (excl. intra-operative bypass flush angiograms)
- PTA with or without stent placement of stenotic (not occlusive) lesions at the following levels: infrarenal aortic, iliac, femoral, popliteal, tibial, or pedal (or transition zones)
- Miscellaneous:
- Vena cava filter placement

II. Intermediate

- PTA with or without stent placement of stenotic lesions at all other levels as specified in Class I (excl. carotid artery stent placement)
- PTA with or without stent placement of any occlusive lesion except tibial or pedal arteries
- PTA with or without stent placement of access surgery
- Fluoro-assisted thrombectomy (open or percutaneous)
- Thrombolysis
- Miscellaneous:
  - Coil-embolization / detachable balloons, etc
  - Vena cava filter retrieval

III. Advanced

- PTA with or without stent placement of occlusive lesions of tibial or pedal arteries
- Carotid artery stent placement
- Any kind of stent graft anywhere (EVAR, TEVAR, covered stent for SFA occlusion, etc)
- Miscellaneous:
  - TIPPS
  - Neurointerventions

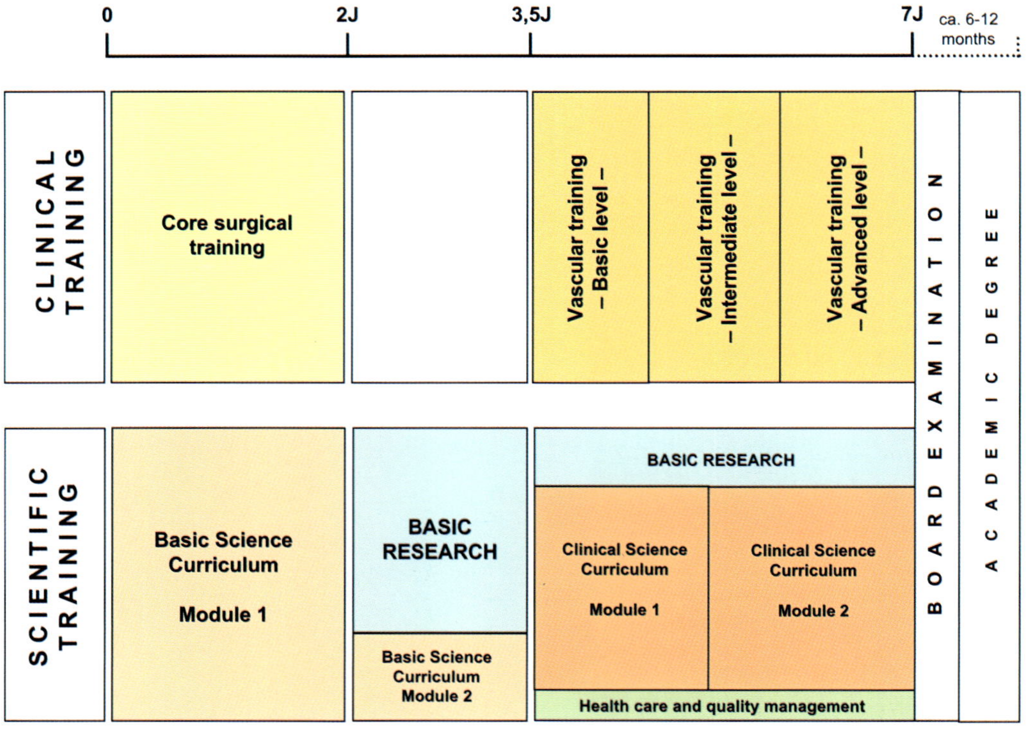

FIG. The proposed academic route — 2+2+4 program.

5) the trainees are expected to gain competence in pathophysiological fundamentals in vascular medicine by learning independently and together with other colleagues and students (also with the help of an e-learning platform). Hereby the contents of the "*Basic Science Curriculum*" *of* "*Association of Program Directors in Vascular Surgery (APDVS)*" of the United States of America could serve as a basis (http://apdvs.vascularweb.org) and be easily adapted towards European requirements and boundary conditions.

During the first two years of training to become a vascular specialist, the post-doctoral fellows should be acquainted with local research structures and should decide for a scientific focus in their respective specialty. The continuation of the theoretical education should take place according to a "*Clinical Science Curriculum*", such as also provided by the *APDVS* (http://apdvs.vascularweb.org). For this continuing education, seminars, journal clubs and an e-learning platform should be offered. As an option, candidates may also participate in introductory courses in health care and quality management.

Scientific training

An essential component of an "academic curriculum" is a research fellowship (e.g. 18 months) in a multidisciplinary research project in vascular medicine in the candidates' respective faculties. During this time, the candidates will be completely released from their clinical duties in order to focus on their particular research project in close collaboration with the scientific mentor. This mentor professionally helps each candidate in project planning and routine laboratory work. Furthermore, the candidates are supported in coordinating funding proposals with their research directors and collaboration partners. Thus, this ensures the successful continuation of existing research projects when the fellows have returned to clinical work and training.

Completion of the academic training

As research activities are a basic component of the "academic curriculum", completion of the training program in vascular surgery/medicine within six years will not be realizable. By presuming that the research fellowship takes 18 months and that continuation of the research projects requires 20% of the working time, the total length of the academic training program should comprise eight years (e.g. 2+"2"+4 program). As soon as the candidates have met the specific clinical requirements for a national board certification (in accordance with the EVBS guidelines), an internal examination should take place (meeting the *Clinical Science Curriculum* guidelines) and should precede the actual national medical board. Upon passing the national board examination, the candidates have completed the "academic curriculum". Ideally, candidates should also fulfill the requirements of the local medical faculty (publications in peer-reviewed journals, successful fund-raising, teaching activities) to receive an academic degree (e.g. Ph.D.) at this time.

Prerequisites regarding personnel, infrastructure and funding

A candidate may only be freed of his/her clinical duties provided that enough staff is present to assume these responsibilities. Thus, it is important, especially for small vascular departments, to optimize their work procedures to allow the candidate freedom to do research. Moreover, it is advantageous that the university entertains good networks with other departments of the medical faculty working in vascular science. In addition, a cross-linking between medicine and engineering as well as the natural sciences is conducive for innovation and technology transfer. These collaborations allow the postdoctoral fellow an ideal opportunity to broaden his/her expertise. Ideally, research fellowships are supported by the medical faculty by seed funds or, alternatively, by third-party funding.

Conclusion

In recent years, vascular surgery has evolved from open surgery to less invasive endovascular surgery. To successfully accommodate these advances in medicine, it is very important to train young vascular specialists accordingly. Even though the Union of Medical Specialists in Europe has proposed guidelines for coordinating the training in vascular surgery, there are still enormous deviations in the various curricula in Europe that reflect national priorities and boundary conditions. To counter these discrepancies, it is important to introduce uniform and binding educational aims and curricula in vascular surgery/medicine to facilitate excellent yet equal standards of open and endovascular procedures in Europe. Integration of an optional, basic-research training program that encourages trainees to pursue an academic pathway in vascular surgery will complement the "ideal educational curriculum" for the vascular specialist.

The future responsibility of national vascular societies is to promote and complete the restructuring within the next decade. This uniformity will strengthen the role of vascular surgery as an independent and highly specialized medical discipline that ensures comprehensive treatment of vascular disease. Within Europe, this stronger collaboration will help vascular specialists to advance their interests in policy-making regarding health care issues in the European Union. Moreover, this better position will enable European vascular specialists to promote their expertise on an international platform.

REFERENCES

1 Rayner M, Petersen S. European cardiovascular disease statistics. British Heart Foundation: London, 2008 [Internet]. Available from: *http://www.heartstats.org/homepage.asp* [cited 2009, Dec 3].

2 Eckstein HH, Knipfer E. Current status of vascular surgery: in vascular medicine and general surgery. *Chirurg* 2007; 78: 583-592.

3 Anonymous. "Health Worker Migration in the European Region: Country Case Studies and Policy Implications"; Report by WHO Europe about the migration of healthcare workers in Europe [Internet] Available from: *http://www.euro.who.int/document/e88366.pdf* [cited 2009, Dec 3].

4 Currie S, Coughlin PA, Bhasker S et al. Vascular surgery is an unattractive career option for current basic surgical trainees: a regional perspective. *Ann R Coll Surg Engl* 2007; 89: 792-795.

5 Calligaro KD, Dougherty MJ, Sidawy AN et al. Choice of vascular surgery as a specialty: survey of vascular surgery residents, general surgery chief residents, and medical students at hospitals with vascular surgery training programs. *J Vasc Surg* 2004; 40: 978-984.

6 Berman L, Rosenthal MS, Curry LA et al. Attracting surgical clerks to surgical careers: role models, mentoring, and engagement in the operating room. *J Am Coll Surg* 2008; 207: 793-800.

7 Cronenwett JL, Liapis CD. Vascular surgery training and certification: an international perspective. *J Vasc Surg* 2007; 46: 621-629.

8 Avgerinos ED, Dalainas I, Liapis C. The transformation of vascular surgeons to vascular specialists: policy or necessity? *Vasc Endovascular Surg* 2009; 43: 233-237.

9 van Bockel JH, Bergqvist D, Cairols M et al. Education in vascular surgery: critical issues around the globe-training and qualification in vascular surgery in Europe. *J Vasc Surg* 2008; 48 (Suppl 6): 69S-75S.

10 Joshi R, Ling FW, Jaeger J. Assessment of a 360-degree instrument to evaluate residents' competency in interpersonal and communication skills. *Acad Med* 2004; 79: 458-463.

11 Cowan JA Jr, Dimick JB, Henke PK et al. Surgical treatment of intact thoracoabdominal aortic aneurysms in the United States: hospital and surgeon volume-related outcomes. *J Vasc Surg* 2003; 37: 1169-1174.

12 Neequaye SK, Aggarwal R, Van Herzeele I et al. Endovascular skills training and assessment. *J Vasc Surg* 2007; 46: 1055-1064.

13 Staveley-O'Carroll K, Pan M, Meier A et al. Developing the young academic surgeon. *J Surg Res* 2005; 128: 238-242.

14 Nuttall MC, van der Meulen JH, Browne JP et al. An analysis of the Research Fellowship Scheme of the Royal College of Surgeons of England. *J Am Coll Surg* 2005; 200: 186-190.

15 Gabram SG, Espat NJ, Jacobs LM et al. Academic careers in surgery: the many paths from which to choose. *J Surg Educ* 2007; 64: 27-35.

16 Robertson CM, Klingensmith ME, Coopersmith CM. Long-term outcomes of performing a postdoctoral research fellowship during general surgery residency. *Ann Surg* 2007; 245: 516-523.

17 Henke PK, Kish P, Stanley JC. Relevance of basic laboratory and clinical research activities as part of the vascular surgery fellowship: an assessment by program directors and postfellowship surgeons. *J Vasc Surg* 2002; 36: 1083-1091.

18

SHOULD VASCULAR SURGERY BE CENTRALIZED?

PETER HOLT, MATT THOMPSON

Vascular surgery is an evolving specialty that has developed from the generality of surgery. Along with the traditional delivery of general surgical services, vascular surgery has evolved with a partially devolved model of care. This has meant that vascular services have been available in most hospitals with surgical capabilities, even when this has meant that the workload of individual units and surgeons was small. In tandem with other areas of surgery such as cardiothoracic surgery and hepatopancreatobiliary surgery, there is an increasing body of evidence that these vascular surgical procedures might be best placed within a centralized model of care to attain best outcomes.

The healthcare political landscape is evolving rapidly, with many countries now advocating specialization in surgical practice and regionalization of complex services, which would include arterial surgery. The change in delivery of specialized services has been driven by the increasing complexity of cases undertaken and the advent of new technology, in tandem with a focus on reporting health outcomes [1,2]. With an emphasis being placed on the public reporting of these outcomes, used to inform patient choice, elective mortality may be used as a barometer of quality.

This chapter reviews the current evidence towards centralization of vascular surgical services compiling evidence from a number of healthcare systems. The index procedures of abdominal aortic aneurysm (AAA) repair, carotid endarterectomy (CEA) and lower extremity arterial bypass (LEAB) are discussed.

AAA repair

Elective AAA

Elective AAA repair remains the key indicator procedure for vascular surgical practice. The mainstay of management for patients with large AAA is elective surgical repair, although endovascular procedures have become more common in recent years. Elective aneurysm surgery remains a procedure with significant morbidity and mortality as patients have co-morbid risk factors including significant cardio-respiratory disease and renal dysfunction. AAA repair fulfils many of the requirements for a generalizable model of care for high-risk surgery and any relationship between volume and outcome for AAA repair might be extrapolated to other high-risk procedures.

A large number of studies have been performed in recent years to attempt to quantify this relationship using ever more advanced statistical techniques. Studies published before 2006 were subjected to meta-analysis to try to gain an estimate of the overall effect across a number of healthcare systems. The results were strongly in favour of the centralization of care with an odds ratio of 0.66 (0.65-0.67) at a threshold of 43 AAA repairs per annum arising from 421 229 elective repairs (Fig. 1) [3-21].

Even when highly risk-adjusted data are used these relationships remain robust and highly significant across different healthcare systems. The nature of the relationship needs further determination but at least for modest annual volumes (up to 50 elective AAA repairs per annum) the relationship appears to be linear with each extra case performed being associated with lower mortality rates. It is likely that the improvements seen per additional case at very high annual volumes might be more modest than those at the lower end of the spectrum. This aside, the existence and strength of this relationship is not now disputed.

Surgeon volume

As well as a relationship existing between hospital-volume and outcome, significant relationships have been described between the annual caseload of individual surgeons and mortality. To determine the strength of this relationship the available data were subjected to meta-analysis [22] and after exclusions, 14 articles provided information on the

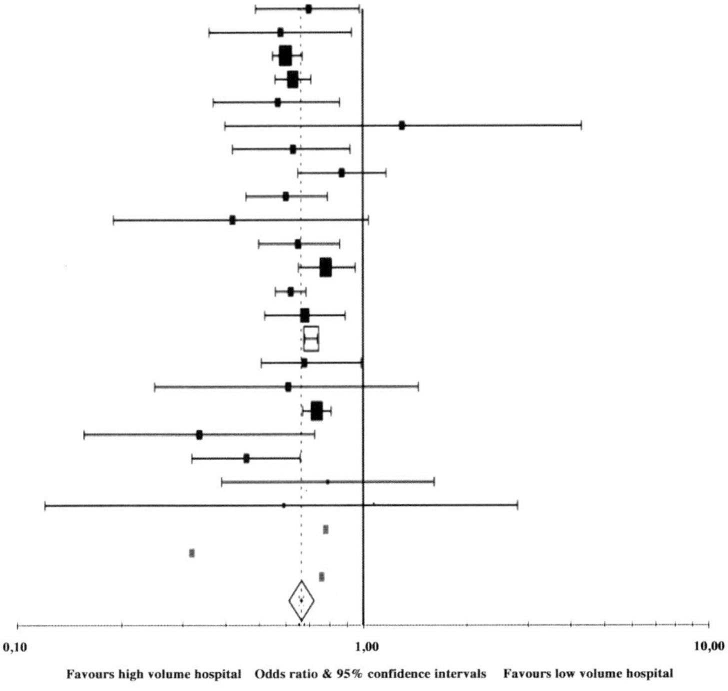

FIG. 1 Forest plot for the relationship between hospital-volume and outcome for elective AAA repair. From Holt et al. Br J Surg 2007; 94: 395-403 [18].

annual surgeon volume of elective AAA repair and mortality [3,4,8,15,20,23-31]. A total of 115 273 elective AAA repairs were considered with a mean mortality rate of 5.56%. It was shown that the observed mortality rate fell as a surgeon's annual operative volume increased.

Overall, from the meta-analysis, the pooled effect estimate for mortality rates of higher as compared to lower-volume surgeons was 0.57 (95% confidence intervals 0.53 to 0.62) at a weighted mean threshold between higher- and lower-volume surgeons of 13 AAA per annum (Fig. 2). This result was robust in terms of heterogeneity and sensitivity analyses.

The relative contributions of surgeon volume and hospital volume on outcome have been usefully debated. It is likely that for higher-risk conditions such as AAA repair the relationships hold roughly equal weight [27]. The reasons behind this are that outcomes are in part reliant on surgeons operating within an appropriate hospital infrastructure, with the provision of expert intensive care units, specialist vascular anesthetists and the effective working of large multidisciplinary teams. In fact, it has been demonstrated that a low-volume surgeon operating in a high-volume hospital can adopt a mortality rate close to that of a high-volume surgeon operating in a high-volume hospital for some procedures.

Surgeon specialty

A number of studies have investigated the relationship between surgeon specialty and outcome [3,25,26] and all found that operations performed by vascular specialist surgeons were associated with significant reductions in mortality, when compared to surgery by general surgeons. This advantage was in addition to the benefits gained through the provision of higher-volume services at the level of both the hospital and the surgeon [3]. Therefore, high-volume specialist vascular surgeons operating in high-volume hospitals achieve the lowest mortality for elective AAA repairs.

Open versus endovascular repair

To achieve low mortality rates, vascular surgeons are likely to employ an increased use of endovascular aneurysm repair (EVR), which has a lower mortality rate than open repair. As experience of these techniques increases, and technology improves, it is likely that an increasing proportion of cases will be within the scope of routine endovascular management in specialist centers. Consequently,

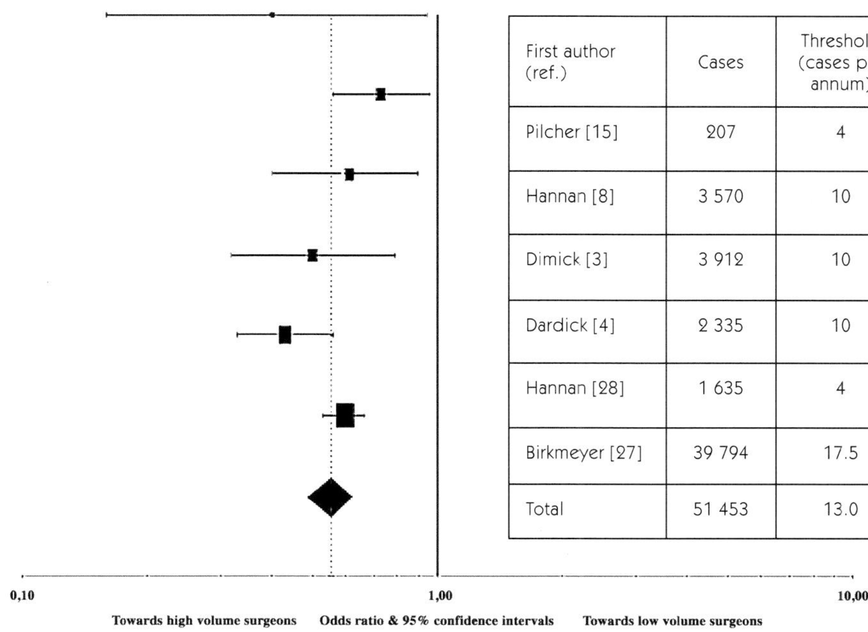

First author (ref.)	Cases	Threshold (cases per annum)	Weight (%)	OR (95% CI)
Pilcher [15]	207	4	6.2	0.40 (0.16-0.94)
Hannan [8]	3 570	10	12.9	0.73 (0.56-0.96)
Dimick [3]	3 912	10	10.7	0.60 (0.40-0.88)
Dardick [4]	2 335	10	11.0	0.50 (0.32-0.79)
Hannan [28]	1 635	4	22.4	(0.33-0.56)
Birkmeyer [27]	39 794	17.5	36.8	0.60 (0.53-0.67)
Total	51 453	13.0	100	0.63 (0.52-0.75)

FIG. 2 Forest plot for the relationship between surgeon volume and outcome for elective AAA repair. From Young et al. J Vasc Surg 2007; 46: 1287-1294 [22].

in England, the National Institute for Health and Clinical Excellence has suggested that EVR should only be performed in specialized centers with appropriate expertise in endovascular aortic surgery. This alone implies the centralisation of aneurysm services.

To date only two studies have investigated the specific volume-outcome relationship for EVR [32,33]. The findings of these large population-based studies were very similar and provide a convincing, although small, evidence base regarding the effective delivery of these procedures. The scale of effect, including the finding of a higher magnitude of effect for EVR than open repair, was consistent between the English [33] and the North American studies [32]. The absolute mortality rates for English practice are given (Fig. 3). Further agreement was found between these two studies in the low uptake of EVR on a national basis in both England and the USA, which may be inappropriate given the proven survival advantage delivered through EVR. Even from population-based studies, which are known to have higher absolute mortality rates than clinical trials, the reductions in mortality with EVR were significant supporting a move for an increased uptake of this technique. In the current climate, and in light of the volume-outcome relationships demonstrated, this will require a move towards centralization.

Ruptured AAA

The preceding literature has focused on the delivery of elective AAA repair with positive volume-outcome relationships being demonstrated for both open and EVR and elective mortality has been used as a barometer of quality [34-36]. It is likely that if centralization occurs for elective cases, then non-elective care is likely to undergo reconfiguration along similar pathways. Although this does not mandate an investigation of the volume-outcome relationship for ruptured AAA, the existence of such relationships would strengthen the case towards centralization. This might be particularly important when considering the delivery of EVR in non-elective situations as both single center case series and larger reports based on administrative datasets have suggested a survival benefit for EVR in non-elective AAA cases.

When considering the configuration of emergency aneurysm services two major questions must be addressed. The first is that the population survival rates of ruptured AAA repair must be es-

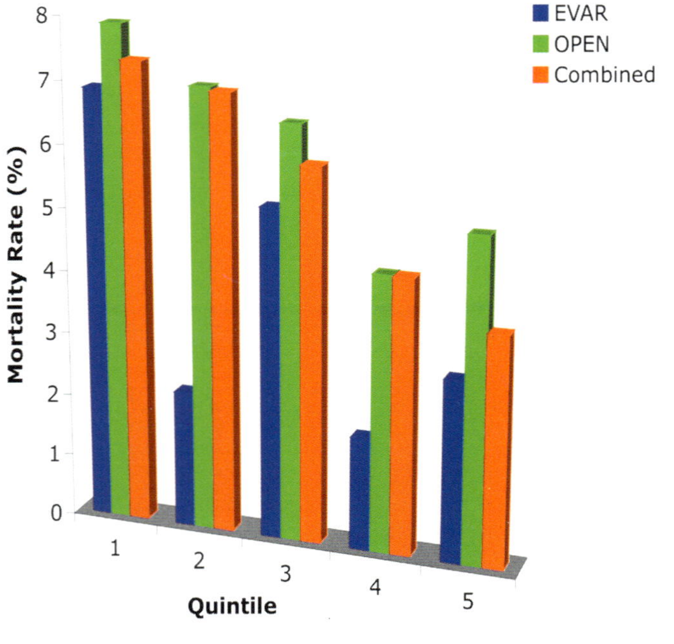

FIG. 3 In-hospital mortality rates for elective open AAA repair (OPEN) and elective endovascular AAA repair (EVAR) and all repairs (Combined) in England by hospital volume. From Holt et al. Circ Cardiovasc Qual Outcomes 2009 [In press] [33].

tablished along with treatment rates at individual centers. Second, the role of EVR in the care pathway for these patients needs quantification.

Recent data from England [37], which were similar to that from the USA [38-40], suggested that EVR was associated with a significant risk-adjusted reduction in in-hospital mortality for ruptured AAA (odds ratio 0.527 [95% CI 0.416 to 0.668]; $p < 0.0001$) and urgent aneurysm repair (odds ratio 0.531 [95% CI 0.415 to 0.680]; $p < 0.0001$). Both ruptured AAA ($p < 0.0001$) and urgent ($p = 0.0146$) repairs were associated with lower mortality rates when performed in hospitals performing a greater number of elective cases. These results equated to a hospital performing 50 elective cases per annum conferring an odds of mortality of 0.61 on any ruptured case ($p < 0.0001$). When a hospital performed a high proportion of EVR electively, patients had lower mortality rates for rAAA that were performed either as open repairs ($p < 0.0001$) or EVR ($p < 0.0001$).

In terms of the proportion of the overall workload, the denominator, hospitals with a high total aneurysm experience (i.e. elective, urgent, emergency and non-operated ruptured aneurysms combined) operated on a greater proportion of rAAA as a percentage of their total workload than lower volume hospitals ($p = 0.0003$).

Higher-volume hospitals for elective cases were also more likely to operate on ruptured aneurysms presenting to the hospital ($p = 0.0332$). This was true both in terms of their total workload and their emergency workload (Fig. 4).

LENGTH OF STAY, DISCHARGE DESTINATION AND READMISSIONS

Although for AAA repair, mortality might be the best surrogate marker of quality of care, a number of other factors have also been considered [41]. It has been found that in addition to lower mortality rates, higher-volume hospitals also have a reduced length of hospital stay. Furthermore, patients are more likely to be discharged home, as opposed to nursing care, from higher-volume hospitals and less likely to be readmitted as an emergency.

AAA SCREENING AND CENTRALIZATION

The elective mortality rate for repair of AAA has assumed a greater importance since the announcement of national screening programmes for AAA, which to be cost effective should be based around a limited number of screening centers, each covering a population of one million [42]. The delivery of surgical repair of screen-detected aneurysms must be performed at the lowest possible mortality rate if it is to be an acceptable treatment for these asymptomatic patients and radical models of service delivery, based on outcomes data, have been suggested [43].

It is likely that the future delivery of aneurysm repair will follow the credentialing of screening centers. With this in mind it is important the preferences of the screened population are determined and account taken of them. One study made an assessment of the preferences of patients attending a regional AAA screening service with the aim of determining their willingness to travel to a service

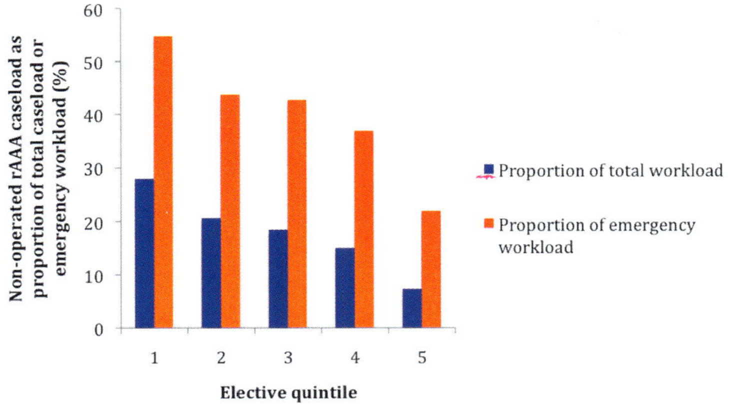

FIG. 4 Palliation rates for ruptured AAA by hospital volume quintile with respect to total workload (blue) and emergency workload (red). From Holt et al. Br J Surg 2009; [In Press] [37].

providing specific attributes [44]. It also provided information on the impact of providing information to patients on their strength of preference.

In this study, 92-95% of respondents demonstrated willingness to travel at least one-hour to access services with a lower post-operative mortality rates ($p < 0.0001$) and stroke rate ($p < 0.0001$) and amputation rates ($p < 0.0001$), a routine availability of minimally invasive surgery ($p < 0.0001$), the demonstration of safety ($p < 0.0001$) and an experienced surgical team ($p < 0.0001$). Factors such as car parking, waiting lists, seeing the same doctor every day and having a shorter length of hospital stay appeared to carry the least importance for respondents when compared with mortality ($p < 0.0001$).

These findings are of critical importance to the argument for centralization for AAA services, as the results do not support a hypothesis that patients are unwilling to travel to access care.

CEA

CEA is undertaken to reduce the risk of stroke in both symptomatic and asymptomatic patients with carotid artery stenosis. CEA has been shown to be superior to medical management in defined subgroups of patients with carotid stenosis [45]. With prompt surgery following a carotid territory event, highly significant absolute risk reductions in subsequent stroke may be attained with low numbers of patients requiring treatment to prevent a neurological event [46].

The absolute risk reduction in stroke depends upon the natural history of the disease and the peri-procedural risk of stroke and death. The lower the peri-operative event rate, the greater the absolute risk reduction. Selected single center series and trial participants have produced very low 30-day stroke rates, but there have been some studies that have questioned whether these results are reproducible in the community [47]. It has been suggested that the number of adverse events related to CEA may be associated with the annual hospital volume undertaken. To investigate this claim the published literature were meta-analyzed.

After exclusions, 25 articles (935 156 cases) provided information on the annual hospital volume and outcome of CEA. The mean death rate was 1.6% (range 0.3% to 5.2%), and the mean disabling stroke rate was 2.7% (0.23% to 6.1%). The results from 885 034 CEA were suitable for meta-analysis and were sub-divided into three groups depending on the focus of the published article. The pooled effects for each group were all in favour of surgery in higher volume hospitals (odds ratio [95% confidence intervals]):

- Stroke rate 0.84 [0.79-0.88]
- Death rate 0.76 [0.74-0.81]
- Combined stroke/death rate 0.73 [0.68-0.78].

Overall, stroke and death attributable to CEA occurred less frequently in higher-volume hospitals 0.78 (0.64-0.92). The critical volume threshold between higher- and lower-volume hospitals was between 70 and 80 CEA per annum, although the values in individual studies varied considerably between different healthcare systems.

One criticism of this study would be that the included studies contained outcomes data from both symptomatic and asymptomatic patients, and consequently the overall stroke and death rates were lower than might have been expected, especially when compared to European data based on performing the majority of procedures on symptomatic patients. Despite this, the results demonstrated that CEA performed at higher-volume hospitals had improved outcome quantified through significantly lower stroke and death rates.

Lower extremity arterial bypass

The evidence for a volume-outcome relationship for LEAB remains limited. This is likely to be due to the complexity of accurately adjusting data for the burden of peripheral vascular disease and any previous endovascular interventions. Whilst it is conceivable that CEA and AAA repair might be centralized with little effect on the majority of most surgeons overall workload, for the majority of surgeons the management of peripheral vascular disease and the diabetic foot remain the mainstay of their work.

Ten studies have addressed the question of a relationship between volume and outcome for LEAB encompassing 539 188 cases. These were subjected to meta-analysis examining both post-operative mortality and subsequent amputation as outcome measures [48]. With respect to post-operative mortality, 385 833 cases were meta-analyzed giving a pooled effect estimate of 0.81 (0.71 to 0.91; $p = 0.0004$) in favour of higher-volume hospitals (Fig. 5) [13,49-51]. In total, five of these studies showed that mortality was significantly lower at HVH compared to LVH [13,19,49-51]. Four studies did not find a significant relationship between hospital volume and rates of mortality [25,52-54]. Fewer ar-

First author [ref.]	HVH Events	HVH Tota	LVH Events	LVH Tota	Weight	Odds ratio M-H Random 95% CI
Birkmeyer [13]	8307	156 553	6371	107 054	42.9%	0.89 [0.86, 0.92]
Dimick [49]	22	995	77	2 085	5.4%	0.59 [0.36, 0.95]
Ebaugh (50)	158	5 649	399	10 773	21.2%	0.75 [0.62, 0.90]
Feinglass [51]	742	19 240	433	8 888	30.4%	0.78 [0.69, 0.88]
Total (95% CI)		182 437		128 800	100.0%	0.81 [0.71, 0.91]
Total events	9229		7280			

Heterogeneity: Tau² = 0.01; Chi² = 8.94, df = 3 (p = 0.03); I² = 66%

Test for overall effect: Z = 3.56 (p = 0.0004)

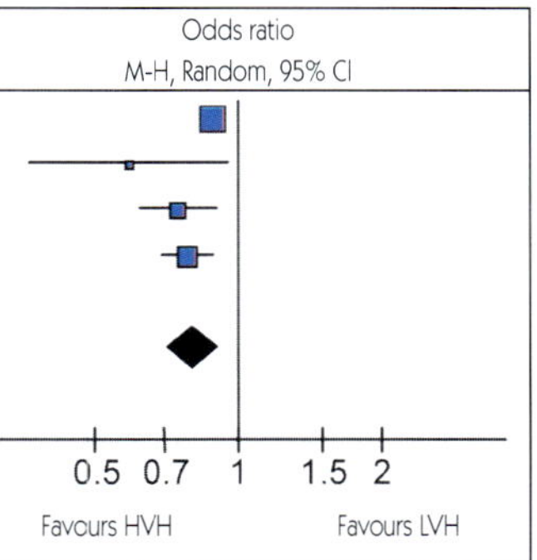

HVH: high volume hospital
LVH: low volume hospital

FIG. 5 Forest plot for the volume-outcome relationship for LEAB. From Awopetu et al. Br J Surg 2009; [In press] [48].

ticles addressed amputation as an outcome. Despite this, 46 311 cases were subjected to meta-analysis and demonstrated a significant result in terms of subsequent limb salvage, with a pooled odds ratio of 0.88 (95% CI 0.79 to 0.98; p = 0.02) [50,51,53].

Can the benefits of centralized model be quantified?

Whilst the previous summary of the published literature has presented a strong case for the centralization of vascular surgery, it has been unclear how this centralization might be best implemented. There are a number of models of care that have been suggested from a collaboration of district hospitals sharing an on-call rota to fully centralized models. It is likely that in many healthcare systems the model most likely to be successful is a hub-and-spoke model whereby major surgery takes place within a central hub unit. Peripheral spoke hospitals are formally attached to the hub, with arrangements for the transfer of elective and emergency patients for surgery. Whether the spoke hospitals are routinely serviced through in-reach or out-reach services is a matter for debate, but it is likely that the two models are much the same.

On this basis, an attempt at quantifying the benefits of a centralized model of care have been made using a theoretical model in England [43]. Based on adherence to minimum annual case volumes and the statistical demonstration of procedural safety, hub hospitals were identified. Hospitals local to the hub were designated as spoke hospitals. The model was quantified in terms of peri-operative deaths and travel times. The proposed model had definable transfer times and suggested that service reconfiguration by centralization may improve outcomes. Highly significant potential reductions in mortality were suggested through the centralization of care, basing English AAA and CEA services around only 48 vascular networks rather than the current 242 vascular services. The majority of patients in England would have to travel for less than one hour to access elective or emergency vascular services.

These results of this model referred particularly to vascular services in England, but they may be extrapolated to inform discussion regarding the provision of specialized surgical services in other healthcare systems. There is substantial evidence supporting the centralization of cancer and major trauma services in England, Europe and North America and where these services have been centralized, the subsequent impact of reconfiguration has generally been positive.

Difficulties of centralization

Centralization of care is not without difficulties, beyond those of local politics. It is important that vascular specialists continue to give appropriate support to all networked hospitals. The prime example of this would be the necessity to provide an in-reach or out-reach service for diabetic patients to ensure that these patients are appropriately managed for the complications of diabetic feet, and unnecessary amputations are avoided. A further example would be patients presenting to peripheral hospitals with a transient ischemic attack must be assessed and provided with a full vascular and neurological work-up in order to provide prompt CEA, avoiding unnecessary strokes and achieving the maximum benefit from these procedures.

Conclusion

Vascular services must be centralized using a hub-and-spoke model. Vascular units should comprise specialist high-volume vascular surgeons and both surgeons and hospitals should achieve a minimum annual volumes. We would suggest an absolute minimum of 50 AAA and 50 CEA per annum. The case for the centralization of LEAB is more limited, but it is probable that more distal revascularisation attempts should be performed in specialist units.

For the best results vascular centers should be on the same site as key support services including an ITU experienced with vascular cases and dialysis facilities. Multidisciplinary assessment should be made prior to surgery for all surgical interventions.

REFERENCES

1 Anonymous. Department of Health. Measuring for Quality Improvement: The approach. London; 2009.

2 Darzi A. High quality care for all: NHS Next Stage Review final report. London; 2008.

3 Dimick JB, Cowan JA Jr, Stanley JC et al. Surgeon specialty and provider volumes are related to outcome of intact abdominal aortic aneurysm repair in the United States. *J Vasc Surg* 2003; 38: 739-744.

4 Dardik A, Lin JW, Gordon TA et al. Results of elective abdominal aortic aneurysm repair in the 1990s: a population-based analysis of 2335 cases. *J Vasc Surg* 1999; 30: 985-995.

5 Goodney PP, Lucas FL, Birkmeyer JD. Should volume standards for cardiovascular surgery focus only on high-risk patients? *Circulation* 2003; 107: 384-387.

6 Dimick JB, Pronovost PJ, Cowan JA Jr et al. Should older patients be selectively referred to high-volume centers for abdominal aortic surgery? *Vascular* 2004; 12: 51-56.

7 Wen SW, Simunovic M, Williams JI et al. Hospital volume, calendar age, and short term outcomes in patients undergoing repair of abdominal aortic aneurysms: the Ontario experience, 1988-92. *J Epidemiol Community Health* 1996; 50: 207-213.

8 Hannan EL, Kilburn H Jr, O'Donnell JF et al. A longitudinal analysis of the relationship between in-hospital mortality in New York State and the volume of abdominal aortic aneurysm surgeries performed. *Health Serv Res* 1992; 27: 517-542.

9 Amundsen S, Skjaerven R, Trippestad A et al. Abdominal aortic aneurysms. Is there an association between surgical volume, surgical experience, hospital type and operative mortality? Members of the Norwegian Abdominal Aortic Aneurysm Trial. *Acta chir Scand* 1990; 156: 323-328.

10 Sollano JA, Gelijns AC, Moskowitz AJ et al. Volume-outcome relationships in cardiovascular operations: New York State, 1990-1995. *J Thorac Cardiovasc Surg* 1999; 117: 419-430.

11 Urbach DR, Bell CM, Austin PC. Differences in operative mortality between high- and low-volume hospitals in Ontario for 5 major surgical procedures: estimating the number of lives potentially saved through regionalization. *CMAJ* 2003; 168: 1409-1414.

12 Katz DJ, Stanley JC, Zelenock GB. Operative mortality rates for intact and ruptured abdominal aortic aneurysms in Michigan: an eleven-year statewide experience. *J Vasc Surg* 1994; 19: 804-817.

13 Birkmeyer JD, Siewers AE, Finlayson EV et al. Hospital volume and surgical mortality in the United States. *N Engl J Med* 2002; 346: 1128-1137.

14 Urbach DR, Baxter NN. Does it matter what a hospital is "high volume" for? Specificity of hospital volume-outcome associations for surgical procedures: analysis of administrative data. *Qual Saf Health Care* 2004; 13: 379-383.

15 Pilcher DB, Davis JH, Ashikaga T et al. Treatment of abdominal aortic aneurysm in an entire state over 7 1/2 years. *Am J Surg* 1980; 139: 487-494.

16 Birkmeyer JD, Dimick JB. Potential benefits of the new Leapfrog standards: effect of process and outcomes measures. *Surgery* 2004; 135: 569-575.

17 Kazmers A, Jacobs L, Perkins A et al. Abdominal aortic aneurysm repair in Veterans Affairs medical centers. *J Vasc Surg* 1996; 23: 191-200.

18 Holt PJ, Poloniecki JD, Gerrard D et al. Meta-analysis and systematic review of the relationship between volume and outcome in abdominal aortic aneurysm surgery. *Br J Surg* 2007; 94: 395-403.

19 Manheim LM, Sohn MW, Feinglass J et al. Hospital vascular surgery volume and procedure mortality rates in California, 1982-1994. *J Vasc Surg* 1998; 28: 45-58.

20 Veith FJ, Goldsmith J, Leather RP et al. The need for quality assurance in vascular surgery. *J Vasc Surg* 1991; 13: 523-526.

21 Khuri SF, Daley J, Henderson W et al. Relation of surgical volume to outcome in eight common operations: results from the VA National Surgical Quality Improvement Program. *Ann Surg* 1999; 230: 414-432.

22 Young EL, Holt PJ, Poloniecki JD et al. Meta-analysis and systematic review of the relationship between surgeon annual caseload and mortality for elective open abdominal aortic aneurysm repairs. *J Vasc Surg* 2007; 46: 1287-1294.

23 Dueck AD, Kucey DS, Johnston KW et al. Long-term survival and temporal trends in patient and surgeon factors after elective and ruptured abdominal aortic aneurysm surgery. *J Vasc Surg* 2004; 39: 1261-1267.

24 Kantonen I, Lepantalo M, Salenius JP et al. Mortality in abdominal aortic aneurysm surgery–the effect of hospital volume, patient mix and surgeon's case load. *Eur J Vasc Endovasc Surg* 1997; 14: 375-379.

25 Pearce WH, Parker MA, Feinglass J et al. The importance of surgeon volume and training in outcomes for vascular surgical procedures. *J Vasc Surg* 1999; 29: 768-778.

26 Tu JV, Austin PC, Johnston KW. The influence of surgical specialty training on the outcomes of elective abdominal aortic aneurysm surgery. *J Vasc Surg* 2001; 33: 447-452.

27 Birkmeyer JD, Stukel TA, Siewers AE et al. Surgeon volume and operative mortality in the United States. *N Engl J Med* 2003; 349: 2117-2127.

28 Hannan EL, O'Donnell JF, Kilburn H Jr et al. Investigation of the relationship between volume and mortality for surgical procedures performed in New York State hospitals. *JAMA* 1989; 262: 503-510.

29 Huber TS, Seeger JM. Dartmouth Atlas of Vascular Health Care review: impact of hospital volume, surgeon volume, and training on outcome. *J Vasc Surg* 2001; 34: 751-756.

30 Kelly JV, Hellinger FJ. Physician and hospital factors associated with mortality of surgical patients. *Med care* 1986; 24: 785-800.

31 AbuRahma AF, Robinson PA, Boland JP et al. Elective resection of 332 abdominal aortic aneurysms in a southern West Virginia community during a recent five-year period. *Surgery* 1991; 109: 244-251.

32 Birkmeyer JD, Dimick JB. Understanding and Reducing Variation in Surgical Mortality. *Annu Rev Med* 2009; 60: 405-415.

33 Holt PJE, Poloniecki JD, Khalid U et al. Effect of endovascular aneurysm repair on the volume-outcome relationship in aneurysm repair. *Circ Cardiovasc Qual Outcomes* 2009:10.1161/CIRCOUTCOMES.109.848465.

34 Dimick JB, Upchurch GR Jr. Endovascular technology, hospital volume, and mortality with abdominal aortic aneurysm surgery. *J Vasc Surg* 2008; 47: 1150-1154.

35 Holt PJ, Poloniecki JD, Loftus IM et al. Epidemiological study of the relationship between volume and outcome after abdominal aortic aneurysm surgery in the UK from 2000 to 2005. *Br J Surg* 2007; 94: 441-448.

36 Holt PJ, Poloniecki JD, Loftus IM et al. Demonstrating safety through in-hospital mortality analysis following elective abdominal aortic aneurysm repair in England. *Br J Surg* 2008; 95: 64-71.

37 Holt PJE, Karthikesalingam A, Poloniecki JD et al. Ruptured aneurysms in England: A propensity scored analysis of outcomes. *Br J Surg* 2009; [In press].

38 Giles KA, Hamdan AD, Pomposelli FB et al. Population-based outcomes following endovascular and open repair of ruptured abdominal aortic aneurysms. *J Endovasc Ther* 2009; 16: 554-564.

39 Giles KA, Pomposelli FB, Hamdan AD et al. Comparison of open and endovascular repair of ruptured abdominal aortic aneurysms from the ACS-NSQIP 2005-07. *J Endovasc Ther* 2009; 16: 365-372.

40 Egorova N, Giacovelli J, Greco G et al. National outcomes for the treatment of ruptured abdominal aortic aneurysm: comparison of open versus endovascular repairs. *J Vasc Surg* 2008; 48: 1092-1100.

41 Holt PJ, Poloniecki JD, Hofman D et al. Re-interventions, readmissions and discharge destination: modern metrics for the assessment of the quality of care. *Eur J Vasc Endovasc Surg* 2009; [Epub ahead of print].

42 Ashton HA, Buxton MJ, Day NE et al. The Multicentre Aneurysm Screening Study (MASS) into the effect of abdominal aortic aneurysm screening on mortality in men: a randomised controlled trial. *Lancet* 2002; 360: 1531-1539.

43 Holt PJ, Poloniecki JD, Hinchliffe RJ et al. Model for the reconfiguration of specialized vascular services. *Br J Surg* 2008; 95: 1469-1474.

44 Holt PJE, Gogalniceanu P, Murray S et al. Screened patients' preferences in the delivery of abdominal aortic aneurysm repair: A rating scale analysis. *Br J Surg* 2009; [In press].

45 Rothwell PM, Eliasziw M, Gutnikov SA et al. Endarterectomy for symptomatic carotid stenosis in relation to clinical subgroups and timing of surgery. *Lancet* 2004; 363: 915-924.

46 Rothwell PM, Eliasziw M, Gutnikov SA et al. Analysis of pooled data from the randomised controlled trials of endarterectomy for symptomatic carotid stenosis. *Lancet* 2003; 361: 107-116.

47 Wennberg DE, Lucas FL, Birkmeyer JD et al. Variation in carotid endarterectomy mortality in the Medicare population: trial hospitals, volume, and patient characteristics. *JAMA* 1998; 279: 1278-1281.

48 Awopetu AI, Moxey P, Hinchliffe RJ et al. Meta-analysis and systematic review of the relationship between hospital volume and outcomes for lower limb vascular surgery; *Br J Surgery 2009* [In press].

49 Dimick JB, Cowan JA Jr, Henke PK et al. Hospital volume-related differences in aorto-bifemoral bypass operative mortality in the United States. *J Vasc Surg* 2003; 37: 970-975.

50 Ebaugh JL, Feinglass J, Pearce WH. The effect of hospital vascular operation capability on outcomes of lower extremity arterial bypass graft procedures. *Surgery* 2001; 130: 561-569.

51 Feinglass J, Sohn MW, Rodriguez H et al. Perioperative outcomes and amputation-free survival after lower extremity bypass surgery in California hospitals, 1996-1999, with follow-up through 2004. *J Vasc Surg* 2009; 50: 776-783.

52 Bates EW, Berki SE, Homan RK et al. The challenge of benchmarking: surgical volume and operative mortality in Veterans Administration Medical Centers. *Best Pract Benchmarking Healthc* 1996; 1: 34-42.

53 Kantonen I, Lepantalo M, Luther M et al. Factors affecting the results of surgery for chronic critical leg ischemia–a nationwide survey. Finnvasc Study Group. *J Vasc Surg* 1998; 27: 940-947.

54 Troeng T, Bergqvist D, Janson L. Incidence and causes of adverse outcomes of operation for chronic ischaemia of the leg. *Eur J surg* 1994; 160: 17-25.

19

COST-EFFECTIVENESS OF VASCULAR PROCEDURES

FRANK VERMASSEN

The affordability of the costs related to health care is a rising issue in almost every country. In a constrained health care budget choices have to be made by health insurers and policy makers on what the money can best be spent. This choice not only has to be made between two treatments for the same pathology but also between treatments for different pathologies, between treatments that offer a small benefit for a large group of patients and treatments that offer a large benefit for a small group of patients and even between preventive care, therapeutic care or care for the elderly. As the budget that is available is limited, in order to make the right decisions, objective criteria are necessary to compare the utility of these expenses. In the absence of such criteria it is inevitable that health care resources will be inefficiently allocated, resulting in reduced or sub-optimal health benefits for the total population. Cost-effectiveness studies try to evaluate objectively the benefit of a certain treatment in relation to its costs. When the same outcome unit is used in these studies they enable us to compare different, at first sight incomparable, treatments and allow us to make the right decisions. Therefore, in an era of budget limitation, cost-effectiveness studies gain growing interest and importance and surgeons should have some knowledge and understanding of the methods used in these analyses to be able to examine these studies critically [1].

Methods and definitions

Several methods have been used in order to relate the cost of an intervention to its benefit. At large all these different methods are referred to as cost-effectiveness evaluations but the method and outcome unit that is used is different.

- In a cost-minimization study a comparison is made between the costs of different health-care strategies that are assumed to have similar effectiveness.
- In a cost-benefit analysis monetary units (€, $) are used to compare the costs of health interventions to its health benefits. It converts all benefits to a cost equivalent so that the same unit is used

for cost and benefit. This is a basic technique in the world of finance but has limited success in health care because of the difficulty to assign a monetary value to a health scenario or to a life. In a cost-effectiveness analysis the effectiveness is expressed as an objective figure. Examples are: the number of cancers detected in a screening program (e.g.: the cost per cancer detected with the 1st, 2nd, 3rd guaic stool test), the reduction in length of stay in number of days, the number of life-years saved in cancer treatment. This method is useful when the time horizon is short and an accompanying reduction or improvement in quality of life is unlikely. It does not allow direct comparison between two interventions with different endpoints.

- In a cost-utility analysis the method is comparable but the unit used to measure effectiveness also takes subjective criteria such as quality of life into account and explicitly incorporates patient preferences. The most commonly used measure of effectiveness is quality adjusted life years (QALY). For instance, when evaluating screening programs for BRCA positive women, the benefit in life years gained is adjusted by the reduction in quality of life due to mastectomy and oöphorectomy. It also enables us to compare treatments that only improve the quality of life (and not life expectancy) and as such is the preferred method, certainly in the evaluation of vascular procedures [2,3].

The principle behind the calculation of QALY is that one year with a substantial morbidity or impairment of physical or mental functions values less than one year in full health. Each health state gets a preference weight on a scale of 0 (death) to 1 (full health). This figure is referred to as the "utility" own to a certain health state. The number of QALY is the number of life years multiplied by the utility score. For example: 5 years with a full stroke (utility score: 0.4) will be considered as 2 QALY. This example clearly illustrates the importance of the utility score that is given to a certain condition in the calculation of QALY.

Different methods can be used to assign utilities. The three most used techniques are:

- Standard gamble: the patient with a certain condition is offered the choice to gamble so that he can gain a perfect health when he wins, but dies when he loses. The greater the risk the patient takes, the lower the utility (e.g.: 1 chance out of 2 to win: utility: 0.5)
- Time trade off: how many years of his life a patient wants to give in for perfect health (e.g.: when he considers 3 year in perfect equivalent to 5 year in its present condition: utility: 0.6)
- Visual Analogue Scale: the patient is asked to evaluate its present health state on a scale of 0 (dead) to 100 (full health). When he puts a mark at 80 the utility score is 0.8.

In studies that include quality of life measurement in their protocol using quality of life scales like SF-36 or EQ 5D validated conversion tables can be used to evaluate the utility score in each patient and in each group. In most analyses these data are not available and therefore we have to refer to tables that assign utility scores to different health conditions (Table I) [4]. The question remains by whom these utility scores should be determined: by healthcare professionals, patients or the general population. Arguments exist for each of these alternatives. In general health professionals tend to assign lower ratings than the general public.

In a cost-utility study the total cost of the procedure or intervention, including direct costs, indirect costs and costs of complications is compared to the effectiveness including prevented costs and life-years gained adjusted for their quality. The cost-effectiveness ratio (CE-ratio) is the total net cost/QALY gained.

Table I EXAMPLES OF PUBLISHED UTILITY VALUES

Health conditions	*Utility scores*
Full health	1.00
Mild angina	0.90
Minor stroke	0.80
Moderate claudication	0.80
Moderate angina	0.70
Severe claudication	0.60
Severe angina	0.50
Moderate to severe stroke	0.39
Rest pain	0.30
Death	0.00

Table II MARKOV MODEL

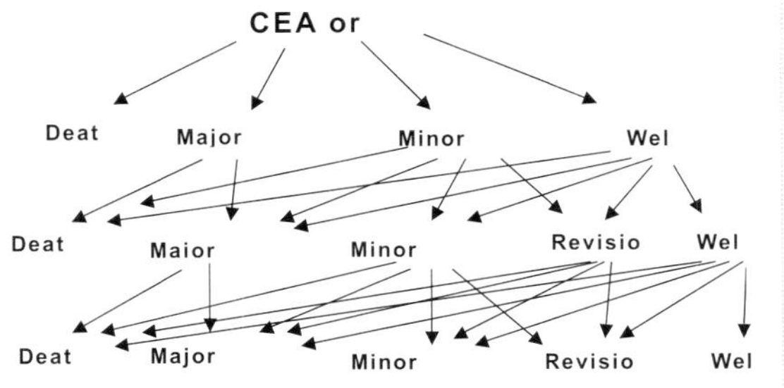

- For each health state a utility is defined
- For each time interval the frequency of transition from one health state to another is defined

Table III DECISION ANALYSIS

	Benefit A > B	*Benefit B > A*
Cost B > A	A dominant	CE-ratio?
Cost A > B	CE-ratio?	B dominant

In order to get a precise and complete image one also has to take into account the changes that can occur over time and their influence on costs or health state. The disease adjusted death-rate shall have to be taken into consideration as well as the chance to incur considerable changes in health state (e.g.: the chance to get a stroke or a myocardial infarction (MI) in a patient with carotid stenosis) especially when this chance is different in two groups that are compared. When starting with a specific cohort each year a number of patients will make a transition to a different health state. All this can be included in a Markov-model (Table II). In such a model for each time interval the probability that the patient is going to make a transition in health state is defined. Each health state has its own utility and cost. In that way the total cost and QALY over a certain time frame can be calculated and compared. Thereby we have to take into account that costs and benefits that will be obtained in the future should be discounted to present value (e.g. at 3-5%/y) [3].

When comparing two different procedures, each with his cost and benefit (QALY gained) there are 4 possible outcomes (Table III). When procedure A is both cheaper and yields more benefit then procedure B this procedure is called "dominant" in the decision analysis and has to be preferred. When procedure A is more costly but is also beneficial the incremental CE-ratio can be calculated which is the incremental cost over the difference in QALY (Table IV). The decision to prefer A over B then depends on how much we or the society wants to spend for one QALY. This will be differ-

Table IV COST-EFFECTIVENESS ANALYSIS

	COST	*Marginal cost*	*Effectivity*	*Marginal effectivity*	*CE-ratio*
SCENARIO I					
Nothing	0	0	0	0	
Treatment A	$ 50 000	$ 50 000	5.5 years	5.5 years	$ 9 091/yr
SCENARIO II					
Nothing	0	0	0	0	
Treatment B	$ 5 000	$ 5 000	5 years	5 years	$ 1 000/yr
Treatment A	$ 50 000	$ 45 000	5.5 years	0.5 years	$ 90 000/yr

Cost-effectiveness analysis
In scenario I treatment A is cost-effective with a CE-ratio of 10 000 €/QALY.
In scenario II a new treatment has become available was is more cost-effective. Although treatment A was cost-effective compared to no treatment and although the results are better, it is no longer cost-effective when compared to treatment B.

ent from one society to another but in general it can be said that in Western Europe a cost below 30 000 €/QALY is considered as good value for money and consequently as cost-effective. This, however, does not mean that CE-ratio is the only criterion that can be used to decide on reimbursement as the goal of the treatment will also play a role in the willingness of the society to pay for it. It can easily be shown that Viagra increases QALY at a price well below 20 000 €/QALY, while hospital hemodialysis costs around 50.000€/QALY (Table V). Nevertheless most societies do not provide reimbursement for the former but do so for the latter. In general, the more severe the disease the more willingness exists in the society to pay for it.

Cost-effectiveness studies also have their limitations. From the previous paragraphs it is clear that when performing a cost-utility analysis one has to try to use as specific and correct data as possible. This is not always easy. On the cost side there is often a difference between what is paid by the health insurer (important for the government or insurance companies), the real cost of the procedure (important for the health care provider) and the total cost for the patient (important for the society). Some indirect costs are also difficult to quantify. On the benefit side the assignment of utilities to health conditions remains a matter of discussion. Although each of the assessments methods is internally consistent, they can provide different utility scores for the same health state. So utilities obtained through rating scale estimates are consistently lower than those obtained via the standard gamble or time trade-off methods.

In a Markov-model for each transition a frequency has to be determined. In most studies this is based on existing literature but in many cases different figures can be used. Often a lot of assumptions have to be made, not the least with regard to the utility scores that are being used when no direct QOL-measurement was performed. Therefore it is always useful to complete a cost-utility analysis with a sensitivity analysis to allow for the uncertainty in the estimates of costs and consequences. In a sensitivity analysis it is calculated what would be the effect on the outcome when one of the data that were used would change (e.g.: in an analysis of the cost-effectiveness of carotid endarterectomy: to use a stroke rate of 4% instead of 3%). In Table VI a practical guide is given of how to proceed when one wants to perform a cost-utility analysis.

Table V EXAMPLES OF PUBLISHED CE-RATIO'S (BASED ON 1990 VALUES)

Treatment	*CE-ratio*
Total hip replacement	$ 4 600
CABG for LM-disease	$ 7 000
Screening for colon CA	$ 14 000
Elective surgery for AAA	$ 17 400
Taxol for advaced ovarian CA	$ 20 000
Clopidrogel vs. aspirin in sec stroke prevention	$ 26 500
Heart transplant	$ 33 000
CABG vs. medical treatment for SV disease	$ 40 500
Yearly screening for cervical CA vs. every 3 yrs	$ 51 000
Hemodialysis for ESRD	$ 53 000
Ondansetran vs. metoclopramide in chemoR/	$ 150 000

Table VI PRACTICAL GUIDE TO PERFORM A COST-UTILITY ANALYSIS

Problem definition
- Define study population
- Reference case
- Study population from randomized trial
- Define strategies-interventions to be studied
- Define time-horizon

Build model
- Define health states used in the model
- Build tree structure
- Assign costs (all) to each intervention and state
- Assign utility to each health state
- Assign probability of transition between states in each time interval

Analysis
- Calculate cost and benefit in QALY
- Calculate ICER = Cost/QALY
- Sensitivity analysis

Cost-effectiveness of vascular procedures

During the last years several new techniques and materials have been developed for the treatment of patients with vascular disease. In general these techniques had the goal to improve the results, or to minimize the invasiveness of the procedures. Most of these new developments also have in common that they are more expensive.

Also, many vascular procedures, especially in lower extremity arterial disease will have no influence on patient survival and are only performed to improve quality of life (e.g.: in claudicants). Without hard end-points it is sometimes difficult to persuade decision makers that these interventions are valuable. Consequently there is growing interest in the use of cost-utility analyses to compare the relative value of different therapies for the same condition as well as to value some procedures. In the next paragraphs we will give some examples of cost-effectiveness analyses that have been performed with regard tio the treatment of carotid stenosis and abdominal aortic aneurysms.

Carotids

Based on the Nascet and ACAS study data several studies in the 1990s have shown carotid endarterectomy (CEA) to be cost-effective in the treatment of symptomatic carotid stenosis [5-7]. For asymptomatic patients, equivocal results have been reported [6,8]. When analyzed separately also carotid stenting shows to be cost-effective in symptomatic patients. The real question after the introduction of carotid artery stenting (CAS) was, however, whether this new treatment would be cost-effective over CEA. Several studies were published on this subject, most with many methodological shortcomings and equivocal results [9,10].

We therefore performed a cost-effectiveness analysis based on cost calculations in our own department and on the results of recently published randomized trials. The hospital costs of all patients treated with CAS or CEA in 2007 were analyzed. In this analysis the cost of CAS was € 1 440 higher than the cost of CEA (€ 5 567 vs. € 4 127). Some assumptions were made with regard to the cost of complications and the utility of the different health states based on literature (Table VII). The results

Table VII Cost utility analysis CAS vs CEA Assumptions

Costs	*QALY*	
Procedure	Utilities	
CEA: € 4 127	Death:	0
CAS: € 5 567	Major stroke:	0.4
Cost of disabling stroke	Minor stroke	
Stroke: € 16 000	1st year:	0.75
Yearly: € 33 000	Following	0.85
Cost of minor stroke	Myocardial infarction	
Stroke: € 5 800	1st year:	0.85
Yearly: € 5 600	Following	0.95
Cost of AMI	Cranial nerve injury	
AMI: € 17 000	1st year:	0.85
Yearly: € 1 180	Following	0.95
Cost of cranial nerve injury comparable to minor stroke	Operation	
	CEA: - 0.02 Qaly (1 week)	
	CAS: - 0.01 Qaly (3 days)	
Cost of reoperation: € 6 000	Mortality: 6%/year; 12% after stroke	

CEA: carotid endarterectomy; CAS: carotid artery stenting; AMI: acute myocardial infarction of Sapphire, Space and Eva-3S trial were put in a model. Not unexpectedly CAS proved to be dominant over CEA when the results of the Sapphire trial were used and CEA dominant over CAS with the results of EVA-3S. When the results of SAPCE were put in the model the CE-ratio of CAS over CEA was a prohibitively high € 193 000 at one year and CEA became dominant (both cheaper and more effective) in the longer run. When CAS would have the same results as CEA with regard to death, stroke and reintervention rate the CE-ratio would be 37 500 €/QALY gained, taking into account the higher cost on one side and the faster recovery, lesser cranial nerve injuries and lower myocardial infarction rate on the other side. In a sensitivity analysis CAS would then obtain a 20 000 €/QALY gained threshold if the supplementary cost could be kept below € 800 per procedure or results could be improved so that the major stroke-rate is 0.5% better than with CEA (Figure). Similar results were obtained in a recent analysis made by Janssen et al. [11]. The conclusion from this study was that procedural costs of CAS were higher than of CEA by € 1 488 mainly due to the higher material cost which was not offset by the shorter hospitalisation time. Similar conclusions were reached in 3 more studies since [12-14]. Consequently CAS can only be cost-effective when the clinical results are superior. As long as this is not the case CAS should be advised against in routine clinical practice and should be restricted to controlled settings.

Aneurysms

Open elective repair of aneurysms > 5.5 cm has proven its cost-effectiveness consistently at a CE-ratio below 20 000 €/QALY gained. For this indication too, more than a decade ago a new technique, endovascular aneurysm repair (EVAR), became available that was less invasive and had a lower operative mortality and morbidity but was probably more expensive as the higher cost for the material is not completely offset by the shorter hospital stay.

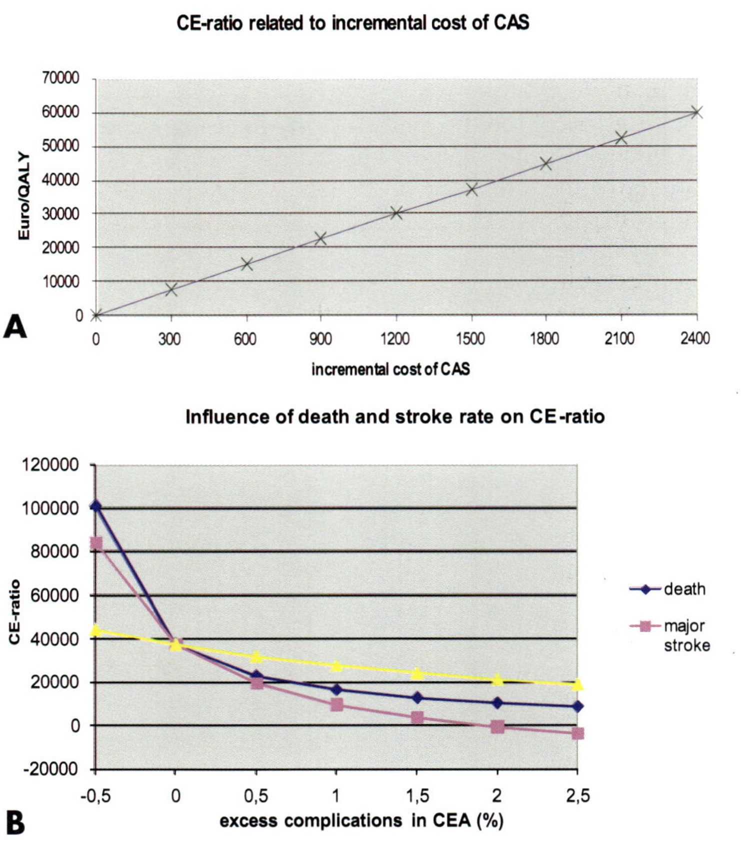

FIG. A - Sensitivity analyses

As such this is an ideal problem to be solved by a cost-effectiveness analysis. Up to 2003, 14 studies were published with regard to this subject mostly limited to a cost-comparison between both techniques [3]. In 2002 Bosch et al. [15] published a cost-effectiveness analysis based on a Markov-model between both techniques showing an incremental CE-ratio of 9 905 $ /QALY for EVAR, meaning that EVAR was more expensive but also yielded an advantage in QALY. In sensitivity analyses this result was insensitive to immediate conversion rate and procedure mortality rate but sensitive to systemic-remote complications, long-term failures and rupture rate. The result suggested that EVAR is a cost-effective alternative compared with open surgery for the elective repair of AAA.

A bit surprisingly a cost-effectiveness analysis based on the results of the DREAM trial [16] came to the conclusion that open treatment was dominant over EVAR during the first year. In this study the presumed advantage with regard to quality of life in the EVAR group was only present during the first months and thereafter the patients in the open surgical group evaluated their QOL based on the EQ-5D questionnaire higher than did the patients in the EVAR group, and for some domains even higher than pre-operatively. One can only speculate about the reason for this difference but it illustrates the difficulty in quantifying subjective feelings such as QOL and maybe the difference in perception between health care professionals and patients. As EVAR was also 4 293 € more expensive, open repair (OR) was more cost-effective.

Similar results were obtained in the EVAR-1 trial [17]. Here too, the advantage in QOL observed in the EVAR group at 0-3 months had disappeared in the 3-12 and 12-24 month evaluation where no significant difference was observed. The cost difference for the primary hospitalization was 10 819 vs. 9 204 UK£, difference that grew during the 4-year follow-up due to the higher number of follow-up examinations and secondary procedures to 13 258 vs. 9 945 UK£.

The situation seems different when treating high surgical risk patients. In patients unfit for surgery Michaels et al. [18] showed through economic modelling and probability sensitivity testing that EVAR was cost-effective over conservative management at a CE-ratio of 8 579 UK£/QALY. In a study based on 192 patients at high risk of surgical complications in Canada Tarride et al. [19] showed that, with a time horizon of one year, EVAR dominated open repair, however, with a substantial degree of uncertainty in a sensitivity analysis.

In an extensive survey by the Health Technology Assessment programme, part of the National Institute for Health Research (NIHR, UK) it was concluded that open repair is more likely to be cost-effective then EVAR on average in patients considered fit for open surgery [20]. EVAR is likely to be more cost-effective than open repair for a subgroup of patients at higher risk of operative mortality. These results are based on extrapolation of mid-term results of clinical trials.

These results with regard to the best treatment option for AAA illustrate the fact that cost-effectiveness analyses depend largely on the correctness of the data and assumptions that are used in the model. The growing number of patients, also fit for surgery, that are treated with EVAR in most European countries illustrates the fact that, despite cost-effectiveness analyses, other factors and arguments play an important role in the preference of patients and physicians and in the adoption of a new technique.

Conclusion

By focusing the attention on the tradeoffs between cost and benefit, cost-effectiveness analysis offers a systematic way of assessing the relative value of competing interventions. Given the increased awareness of the importance of cost-effectiveness and cost control in health care the importance of these analyses will only grow in the future. As these analyses can be very sensitive to changes in the model they should be performed with methodological rigor and use as correct data as possible. The measurement and evaluation of quality of life remains a difficult issue.

New technologies are especially apt to be evaluated by cost-effectiveness analyses. In two examples it is shown that the higher cost of a new procedure is not easily offset by the supposed improvement in quality of life. It also shows that the adoption of a new technology by the medical community is not always based on objective arguments especially with regard to its socio-economic cost. As policy makers increasingly use these analyses when deciding on the implementation and reimbursement of new technologies it is important for health practitioners to become familiar with the methodology and terminology of these studies.

REFERENCES

1 Finlayson SRG, Birkmayer JD. Cost-effectiveness analysis in surgery. *Surgery* 1998; 123: 151-161.

2 Singer ME, Applegate KE. Cost-effectiveness analysis in radiology. *Radiology* 2001; 219: 611-620.

3 Zierler BK, Gray DT. The principles of cost-effectiveness analysis and their application. *J Vasc Surg* 2003; 37: 226-234.

4 Tengs TO, Wailace A. One thousand health-related quality-of-life estimates. *Medical Care* 2000; 38: 583-637.

5 Nussbaum ES, Heros RC, Erickson DL. Cost-effectiveness of carotid endarterctomy. *Neurosurgery* 1996; 38: 237-244.

6 Kuntz KM, Kent KC. Is carotid endarterectomy cost effective? An analysis of symptomatic and asymptomatic patients. *Circulation* 1996; 94 (suppl II): 194-198.

7 Patel ST, Haser PB, Korn P et al. Is carotid endarterectomy cost-effective in symptomatic patients with moderate (50-69%) stenosis. *J Vasc Surg* 1999; 30: 1024-1032.

8 Cronenwett JL, Birmeyer JD, Nuckman GB et al. Cost-effectiveness of carotid endarterectomy in asymptomatic patients. *J Vasc Surg* 1997; 25: 298-311.

9 Kilaru S, Korn P, Kasirajan K et al. Is carotid angioplasty and stenting more cost effective than carotid endarterectomy? *J Vasc Surg* 2003; 37: 331-338.

10 Gray WA, White HJ, Barett DM et al. Carotid stenting an endarterectomy – A clinical and cost comparison of revascularisation strategies. *Stroke* 2002; 33: 1063-1070.

11 Janssen MP, de Borst GJ, Mali WP et al. Carotid stenting versus carotid endarterectomy: evidence basis and cost implications. *Eur J Vasc Endovasc Surg* 2008; 36: 258-264.

12 Park B, Mavanur A, Dahn M et al. Clinical outcomes and cost comparison of carotid artery angioplasty with stenting versus endarterectomy. *J Vasc Surg* 2006; 44: 207-276.

13 Pawaskar M, Satiani B, Balkrishan R et al. Economic evaluation of carotid artery stenting versus carotid endarterectomy for the treatment of carotid artery stenosis. *J Am Coll Surg* 2007; 205: 413-419.

14 Wolf O, Heider P, Weiss W et al. Analyisis of cost-effectiveness. Comparison of carotid endarterectomy and carotid stenting in a university hospital. *Gefasschirurgie* 2007; 12: 435-439.

15 Bosch JL, Kaufman JA, Beinfeld MT et al. Abdominal aortic aneurysms: Cost-effectiveness of elective and open surgical repair. *Radiology* 2002; 225: 337-344.

16 Prinsen M, Buskens E, de Jong SE et al. Cost-effectiveness of conventional and endovascular repair of abdominal aortic aneurysms: Results of a randomized trial. *J Vasc Surg* 2007; 46: 883-890.

17 Greenhalgh RM, Brown LC, Epstein D et al. Endovascular aneurysm repair versus open repair in patients with abdominal aortic aneurysm (EVAR trial 1): randomized controlled clinical trial. *Lancet* 2005; 365: 2179-2186.

18 Michaels JA, Drury D, Thomas SM. Cost-effectiveness of endovascular abdominal aortic aneurysm repair. *Br J Surg* 2005; 92: 960-967.

19 Tarride JE, Blackhouse G, De Rose G et al. Cost-effectiveness analysis of elective endovascular repair compared with open surgical repair of abdominal aortic aneurysms for patients at a high surgical risk: A 1-year patient-level analysis conducted in Ontario, Canada. *J Vasc Surg* 2008; 48: 779-787.

20 Chambers D, Epstein D, Walker S et al. Endovascular stents for abdominal aortic aneurysms: a systematicreview and eceonomic model. *Health Technol asses* 2009; 13: 1-189, 215-318, iii.

20

HYBRID OPERATING ROOM: THE NEW WORKING ENVIRONMENT

RAO VALLABHANENI

Image-guided procedures have emerged as an important and sometimes overwhelming component of cardiovascular therapeutics in the recent years. Clinicians have adapted their existing working environment and available equipment in order to carry out the newer techniques. This occurred as a rapid evolution, during which developments in endovascular techniques and the demands on ideal specification of operating rooms within which they ought to be carried out, outstripped the improvements in operating room infrastructure for most clinicians.

Most clinicians conduct their complex endovascular procedures either in a conventional operating room with a mobile imaging system or in an interventional radiology suite/cathlab. The objective of this chapter is to discuss some of the limitations of either of these options and to highlight the utility of hybrid operating rooms in this context. Additional impetus to acquire a hybrid operating room arises from increasing popularity of hybrid approach to therapeutics, where conventional and image guided techniques are combined into one operation.

Benefits of hybrid approach to techniques

When a patient requires a conventional operation and also an image guided intervention (e.g. a patient requiring femoropopliteal bypass surgery also requiring angioplasty of the iliac system to ensure adequate inflow), it is acceptable to undertake them in consecutive stages (percutaneous angioplasty of the iliac system in the interventional radiology suite in the first instance and separately undertake femoropopliteal bypass in the conventional operating room). The trend, however, is towards conducting both procedures at the same time within a hybrid operating room. Expeditious completion of treatment, shorter cumulative hospital stay, lower cumulative complication rates and lower healthcare costs are some of the potential benefits envisaged.

There are some operations, however, where staging is not possible and the very paradigm of the operation is based on concomitant open surgical and transluminal intervention; e.g. carotid to subclavian bypass in combination with endovascular repair of thoracic aortic aneurysm with seal zone extending over the left subclavian ostium.

Minimally invasive aortic valve replacement is a rapidly expanding procedure, although currently confined to patients at high risk or even unfit for conventional surgery. Transapical aortic valve replacement is associated with a lower risk of stroke compared to transfemoral route and requires to be performed in an operating room for the mini-thoracotomy. Even transfemoral aortic valve replacement is best performed in a fully equipped cardiac operating room so that an occasional serious complication requiring the back up with extracorporeal circulation could be dealt with safely. Treatment of complicated acute type B aortic dissections is a challenging area where endoluminal and hybrid options have found a rapidly expanded role.

There are quality-related advantages to utilizing image guidance for operations traditionally been performed without intra-operative imaging, e.g. peripheral arterial embolectomy. Intra-operative imaging and over-the-wire guided embolectomy ensures that the embolus fragments have been removed completely and that no iatrogenic damage has occurred to the vasculature. This represents a significant improvement over the traditional approach where it is a matter of guesswork or judgement to evaluate the effect of embolectomy. Intraoperative angiography identifies technical issues with bypass grafts and has been shown to reduce early failure rates following coronary revascularization. This trend is also catching on in peripheral bypass surgery.

In the treatment of multivessel coronary disease, rather than considering bypass surgery and transluminal angioplasty as mutually exclusive choices, treating each lesion by the most appropriate technique for its anatomical features, a hybrid approach, has advantages. Reports of internal mammary bypass to the left anterior descending artery through a minithoracotomy combined with angioplasty of additional lesions has been reported to decrease morbidity and mortality.

The current trend of integrating imaging, image guided intervention and conventional surgery to achieve the best results has effected every area of cardiovascular intervention. For most centers, the solution is to utilize a mobile C-arm that can be wheeled into the operating room for specific procedures. There are some perceived advantages with mobile systems. They cost only a fraction of that of a fixed system. They can be moved between different operating rooms, supporting the needs of different specialities. Although many endovascular programmes depend upon mobile imaging systems, they have significant limitations, thus creating the need to re-evaluate the working environment.

Limitations of mobile imaging systems

The first limitation of mobile systems to note is the obvious inferiority of the images they generate in terms of quality. Despite improvements, mobile imagers are less powerful at usually less than 25 kW compared to fixed systems that operate at 80-100 kW. Imaging an obese patient, particularly in lateral angle, could therefore produce an unsatisfactory image.

The majority — if not all of the mobile systems — are equipped with image intensifiers and not flat panel detectors despite the latter's ability to produce better contrast resolution and distortion-free images. Another drawback of mobile systems is their propensity to overheat during operation. Dissipation of the heat produced at the anode is a significant limiting factor upon the operating power of the X-ray generator. The anode cooling mechanisms of most mobile systems are generally not effective enough to prevent overheating. While conducting long and complex procedures it is often necessary to take steps to slow down the heating process, thereby causing either deliberate slowing down the pace of the procedure or accepting poorer quality imaging or both. Incidents of automatic and unstoppable shutdown from overheating during a procedure are well known. Therefore conducting complex endovascular procedures using mobile imaging system without backup imaging equipment could be considered unsafe practice.

Mobile equipment need to be stored or parked at a safe place and kept connected to electrical charge when not in use, creating a logistical problem. Moving the equipment between the site of parking and operating room, setting up the equipment and network connections etc. consume time and have the potential to slow down the intervention.

This is not to say that mobile systems do not have a role to play. A proportion of imaging requirements within operating rooms could be done quite satisfactorily with mobile systems, e.g. orthopedic, general surgical support etc., a factor sometimes leading to purchasing committees under budgetary constraints settling for mobile systems. It is the case, however, that mobile systems are not necessarily the best for areas such as endovascular surgery. More and more complex interventions within the cardiovascular system are being undertaken and the degree of complexity of procedures is increasing too. This calls for good quality, reliable and sophisticated intra-operative imaging, something mobile systems fail to deliver. Most hospitals have the best of their imaging systems within the interventional radiology suite. Therefore it may appear that conducting complex endovascular procedures there might resolve some of these issues. Such arrangement, however, would create another set of problems.

Interventional radiology suite

The alternative location to undertake complex endovascular procedures is the interventional suite. A vast array of consumables such as catheters, sheaths and guidewires are required to conduct complex interventions and in majority of the centers, this inventory is stored within or near the interventional radiology suite. This advantage and the better imaging available, however, are outweighed by many disadvantages. Majority of the problems stem from the fact that it is rare for consideration to have been given at the time of designing the suite, to accommodate regularly, complex procedures requiring multidisciplinary input. A number of design considerations to create an ideal environment to carry out such procedures are discussed in the chapter later and it is rare that standard interventional radiology suites satisfy most or even some of them. This realization has lead to pioneering centres develop hybrid operating rooms.

Hybrid operating room

The term hybrid operating room is used to describe an operating room with fixed imaging equipment, specifically designed to carry out both conventional surgery and image guided intervention. The facility would have been built incorporating as many as possible the best features of both standard operating rooms and standard interventional suites, in order to create the best working environment to carry out complex procedures (Fig. 1).

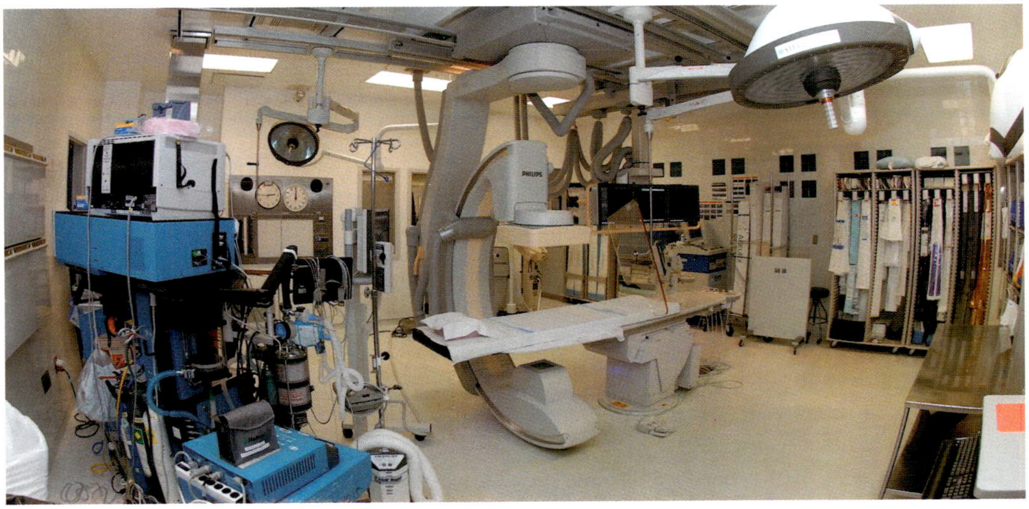

FIG. 1 Hybrid operating room.

Design considerations

Whether a hybrid operating room is being designed from scratch or an existing operating room/interventional suite is being modified, paying attention to detail in designing the facility is crucial for its users to get the best out of it. Rectifying deficiencies later could be difficult, expensive or even impossible.

Deciding the location of an hybrid operating room is important. There should be easy access to and from various other departments within the hospital such as emergency rooms, computed tomography (CT)/magnetic resonance (MR) scanners, intensive care unit, inpatient wards etc. Support facilities such as blood bank, pharmacy, clinical laboratory areas etc. should also be accessible without difficulty even out of hours. Despite the need for easy access, operating rooms, including hybrid facilities ought not be located upon thorough fares within the hospital for infection control reasons.

Another important consideration that is often difficult to satisfy is the space required to accommodate an ideal hybrid operating room. Space is required for the following purposes: 1) area for induction of anesthesia/anesthetic room; 2) scrub room for personnel to wash hands before and after operations; 3) prep area for scrub nurses to set up their trolleys of instruments; 4) control room for locating controls of imaging and archiving system; 5) storage area, considerable space is necessary to store the vast array of consumables needed to be kept handy for complex interventions; 6) equipment such as cardiopulmonary bypass machines, trans-esophangeal echocardiography, intra-operative monitoring equipment etc. occupy considerable space; 7) the operating table, imaging equipment and their displays, anesthetic apparatus, electrodiathermy, intra-operative red cell salvage equipment etc. all occupy space; 8) complex and hybrid procedures often require the presence of a greater number of personnel within the operating room compared to standard procedures. Anesthetists, intensivists, radiologists, cardiologists, surgeons, perfusionists, radiographers, operating department practitioners, surgical assistants, product specialists from companies, observers, proctors and a variety of other personnel are often required to be within the operating room.

Different areas of a hybrid operating room are often compartmentalized for convenience and improved working environment. For example, a central large operating room of approximately 60 sq m surrounded by smaller rooms that serve distinct purpose, with the total floor area of the hybrid facility reaching 100 sq m. The minimum recommended space to install a hybrid operating room is 70 sq m, although examples of 45 sq m facilities exist.

Adequate general lighting and operating lighting is clearly imperative. Operating lights are traditionally ceiling mounted and thus compete for space with other components that too require ceiling mounting. The imaging C-arm itself, image display panels, radiation protection shields, physiological monitoring displays, anesthetic gases etc. may all require ceiling mounts, often via booms.

The operating table is a major component and the ideal table depends upon the nature of procedures being undertaken. Carbon fibre floating tables are popular with cardiovascular surgeons. Sterility of the operating room is of paramount importance. Ideally, hybrid operating room should be served by the traditional double corridor system; a clean corridor for movement of patients, personnel, clean equipment etc. and a separate dirty corridor for the transit of waste and contaminated clinical material. Ventilation should be of positive pressure type with the requisite number of air changes appropriate for the type of operations conducted. Laminar flow systems require special considerations. Ceiling rails carrying the C-arm reduce the efficacy of vertical laminar airflow systems. It is important to realize that a C-arm will always interfere with laminar flow, whether it is floor or ceiling mounted and whether the airflow is vertical or horizontal. Facilities for transmission and reception of a variety of audiovisual signals should be considered at the time of installation of the operating room. Such facilities are imperative for teaching and conference transmission purposes and not easy to install as an afterthought.

Benefits of a fixed imaging system

Complex procedures require more than the basic functions of subtraction angiography. Fixed imaging systems provide better quality images, larger field of vision, greater range of magnification and also a range of advanced functions such as post-processing, calibration and measurement, image referencing functions, etc. Increasing pro-

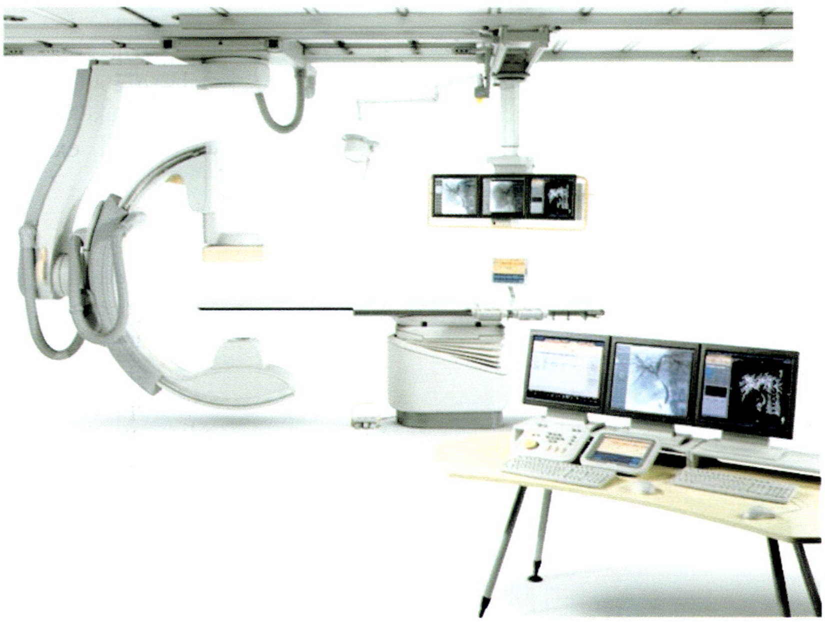

FIG. 2 Philips Allura Xper FD20 system.

portion of fixed systems are being equipped with flat panel detectors, which employ completely digital processing. This allowed the development of some new and exciting possibilities of generating CT like images and rotational angiography, with levels of radiation exposure comparable to that of standard helical multidetector CT (Fig. 2). Excellent quality images allow drastic reduction in the dose of radiographic contrast material, thus attenuating their nephrotoxic effects. It is also possible to glean the necessary information through low frame rates, thus reducing exposure to ionizing radiation. The combination of reliability and better quality imaging with advanced tools leads to significant reduction of operator fatigue, which is an important factor, particularly in relation to procedures that require concentration over extended periods of time, like side-branched endovascular aneurysm repair.

Conclusion

Rapid establishment of image-guided intervention as an important component of therapeutic armamentarium resulted in the logistics of creating appropriate work environment to carry out the complex, long or the hybrid procedures failing to keep pace. The fact that the hybrid operating room is an essential component of the infrastructure of a modern cardiovascular service is being recognized by both the clinicians and the industry providing the equipment. Making the best use of a hybrid operating room is dependant upon robust and careful planning before the suite is being commissioned. Imaging equipment manufacturers also provide technical support and advice regarding all aspects of design and commissioning and ought to be involved from the early stages.

PRINTED BY
EDIZIONI MINERVA MEDICA
FEBRUARY 2010
SALUZZO (ITALY)
CORSO IV NOVEMBRE, 29-31